Advances in Shoulder Surgery

Kazuya Tamai • Eiji Itoi • Kenji Takagishi
Editors

Advances in Shoulder Surgery

Springer

Editors
Kazuya Tamai
Department of Orthopaedic Surgery
Dokkyo Medical University
School of Medicine
Mibu, Tochigi
Japan

Eiji Itoi
Department of Orthopaedic Surgery
Tohoku University School of Medicine
Sendai, Miyagi
Japan

Kenji Takagishi
Department of Orthopaedic Surgery
Gunma University School of Medicine
Maebashi, Gunma
Japan

ISBN 978-4-431-55986-3 ISBN 978-4-431-55988-7 (eBook)
DOI 10.1007/978-4-431-55988-7

Library of Congress Control Number: 2016946969

Printed on acid-free paper

This Springer imprint is published by Springer Nature
The registered company is Springer Japan KK

Foreword

The late 1970s were an exciting time for advancement of surgery of the shoulder. For example, at that time Masaki Watanabe was publishing material in English about clinical applications of shoulder arthroscopy. Shoulder societies had not yet formed except in Japan, and there were few forums to discuss newer ideas or procedures. Luckily, I was able to visit Japan professionally in 1979 and experience the Japan Shoulder Society investigational approach to the science of shoulder surgery. I made a second trip in 1998 and most recently returned for the magnificent International Congress of Shoulder and Elbow Surgery meeting in Nagoya. These on-site experiences gave me greater insight into the Japanese approach to shoulder surgery and made it easy to relate to shoulder surgeons from Japan. Over the years the Society has contributed substantially to the international scene with active participation in the *Journal of Shoulder and Elbow Surgery* and the International Board of Shoulder and Elbow Surgery. It is timely for the Society's publication of a stimulating text in English so that many of us can be made aware of the advances and thinking of a number of Society members.

All physicians with a focus in this anatomic region will find the book enjoyable and educational. There are of course chapters rather typical of textbooks, such as those on the frozen shoulder, nerve injuries, fractures, and reverse arthroplasty, but they are written from the perspective of a Japanese surgeon with useful twists on these subjects. Other chapters have different approaches. The chapter on anatomy is "anatomy for surgeons", not an overview of the subject. The biomechanics chapter pinpoints recent and hot topics in the field. The chapter on instability focuses on the important contemporary issues. New approaches to thinking are covered in other chapters: 3D motion analysis, advanced MRI, and superior capsule reconstruction. Still other chapters have a procedural focus: evolving arthroscopic techniques, mini-open rotator cuff repair with long-term results, and consideration of tissue regeneration instead of repair or reconstruction for massive cuff tears.

Wow! And each chapter is short and to the point, fitting in nicely to our rapid-paced lifestyle. Lucky for us all to have this Society effort available.

Robert H. Cofield, M.D.
Professor of Orthopedics, Mayo Clinic College of Medicine
Past-President, American Shoulder and Elbow Surgeons
Founding Editor, *Journal of Shoulder and Elbow Surgery*
Former Chairman, International Board of Shoulder and Elbow Surgery

Preface

The shoulder joint had been called "the forgotten joint", but the situation has changed dramatically during the past 25 years. This is the case in most parts of the world, including Europe, America, Asia, and Oceania, with a remarkable increase in the number of orthopedic surgeons who have a keen interest in shoulder surgery. The reason is that many more shoulder disorders have become treatable due to the elucidation of the pathologies of the rotator cuff and the glenohumeral joint, the spread and technical progress of arthroscopic surgery, the development of implants for fracture treatment, and the global spread of reverse shoulder arthroplasty. At the same time, new findings, which were clarified by anatomical, biological, and biomechanical studies, have contributed greatly to the establishment of treatment strategies. In addition, progress in diagnostic imaging has enabled us to understand shoulder disorders more precisely than ever before.

When younger and mid-career doctors learn shoulder surgery, they are required to be trained in a mentoring program by experienced instructors at an experienced facility. In their training, it is necessary for them to read detailed monographs and newly published articles in journals, but concise, cultivated reviews are also very useful for studying. We editors aimed to provide the doctors who want to learn shoulder surgery with a book in which high-quality reviews are collected. Fortunately, the Japan Shoulder Society, which in 1974 was the first such society to be established in the world, has made many unique achievements by pioneering surgeons in its more than 40-year history. We owe a great deal of gratitude to the efforts of these individuals. This book was written in the spirit of education and the belief that updated knowledge, combined with the achievements fostered in Japan, will stimulate and encourage all shoulder surgeons both in Japan and abroad.

We included 17 topics in this book: anatomy, biomechanics, kinematics and motion analysis, MR imaging, transosseous-equivalent Bankart repair, management of instability, arthroscopic rotator cuff repair, complications of arthroscopic surgery, mini-open rotator cuff repair, management of massive and irreparable cuff tears, superior capsular reconstruction for irreparable rotator cuff tears, tendon transfer for irreparable rotator cuff tears, frozen shoulder, nerve lesions, proximal humeral fractures, reverse shoulder arthroplasty, and rehabilitation. We sincerely hope that the chapters on these topics will contribute to the progress of knowledge and skills of every shoulder surgeon who yearns to be a true shoulder professional.

Tochigi, Japan Kazuya Tamai
Sendai, Japan Eiji Itoi
Maebashi, Japan Kenji Takagishi

Acknowledgments

We acknowledge the work and efforts of Ms. Saki Kasai and Ms. Makie Kambara at Springer. Their dedication to this book has resulted in a high-quality publication. We would also like to acknowledge and thank the contributing authors for their work and expertise of. This book would not have been possible without their extraordinary efforts.

Tochigi, Japan	Kazuya Tamai
Sendai, Japan	Eiji Itoi
Maebashi, Japan	Kenji Takagishi

Contents

Chapter 1
Anatomy

Akimoto Nimura, Hisayo Nasu, Tomoyuki Mochizuki, and Keiichi Akita

Abstract The supraspinatus inserts into the anteromedial area of the highest impression. The anteriormost region of the infraspinatus almost reaches the anterior margin of the highest impression. The teres minor muscle can be separated into the superior bundle, which inserts to the lowest impression as an oval footprint, and the inferior bundle, which inserts into the distal to the lowest impression as a linear shape. At the border between the infraspinatus and teres minor, the thick attachment of the articular capsule compensates for the lack of tendinous insertion. The coracohumeral ligament could be divided into two parts: one part spreads fibers over the rotator interval to the posterior portion of the greater tuberosity, and the other part extends fibers to envelop the subscapularis muscle. When the inlet of the suprascapular notch is observed from the craniocaudal and mediolateral view, it is recognized to be a triangular space that is bordered by the coracoid process, the subscapularis, and the superior transverse scapular ligament. The axillary nerve divides into the anterior and posterior branch, and is distributed to the deltoid muscle, teres minor muscle, and also the subacromial bursa and the area around the long head of the biceps.

Keywords Rotator cuff muscles • Articular capsule • Coracohumeral ligament • Suprascapular nerve • Axillary nerve

1.1 Introduction

Research in anatomy has been divided approximately into macroscopic and microscopic anatomy. Microscopic anatomy has recently achieved advances by its connections with developmental or molecular biology. In contrast, although

---

A. Nimura (✉) • H. Nasu • K. Akita
Department of Clinical Anatomy, Graduate School of Medical and Dental Sciences, Tokyo Medical and Dental University, 1-5-45 Yushima, Bunkyo-ku, Tokyo 113-8519, Japan
e-mail: nimura.orj@tmd.ac.jp

T. Mochizuki
Department of Joint Reconstruction, Graduate School, Tokyo Medical and Dental University, Tokyo, Japan

K. Tamai et al. (eds.), *Advances in Shoulder Surgery*,
DOI 10.1007/978-4-431-55988-7_1

macroscopic methods have focused on detailed structures, basic knowledge has not increased for a 100 years. The classical knowledge of anatomy could not catch up with the advances in medicine, especially in shoulder surgery. In other words, progress in arthroscopic techniques and the latest imaging methods have made it necessary for us to understand the detailed structures that could not be confirmed with the naked eye. In the age of arthroscopic surgery, anatomy has to cover not only histological characteristics but also the spatial relationships between structures. Based on these concepts, we have recently accumulated anatomic knowledge related to shoulder surgery. In the present chapter, we introduce some anatomic concepts about the rotator cuff muscles, including surrounding structures and representative nerves around the shoulder joint.

1.2 Rotator Cuff Muscles

1.2.1 The Supraspinatus and Infraspinatus Muscles

1.2.1.1 Humeral Insertions

Most anatomy textbooks and the authors of several anatomic studies have stated that the supraspinatus inserts into the highest impression of the greater tuberosity and the infraspinatus inserts into the middle impression of the greater tuberosity. However, Clark and Harryman [1] indicated the difficulty of separating these tendons with their integrated fibers. Minagawa et al. [2] reported overlapping areas of these two tendons on the footprint and claimed the footprint of the supraspinatus to have a wider area than had been previously described.

The supraspinatus muscle originates from the supraspinatus fossa and the superior surface of the spine of the scapula, and it runs laterally. The infraspinatus muscle originates from both the infraspinatus fossa and the inferior surface of the spine of the scapula, and it runs superolaterally (Fig. 1.1). Recently, Mochizuki et al. [3] reported new findings about the humeral insertions of the supraspinatus and infraspinatus. The supraspinatus and infraspinatus appear to mingle into one structure at their insertions on the humerus (Fig. 1.1). However, after removal of the coracohumeral ligament and the loose connective tissues overlying the supraspinatus and infraspinatus, the anterior border of the infraspinatus could be clearly traced and the border between the two muscles became more apparent. The anterior margin of the infraspinatus is slightly protuberant compared with the posterior margin of the supraspinatus. The anterior part of the infraspinatus partially covers the posterolateral part of the supraspinatus (Fig. 1.2).

The upper surface of the greater tuberosity has been generally described as being marked by three impressions: the highest, the middle, and the lowest. However, the humeral insertion of the infraspinatus actually occupies about half of the highest impression and all the middle impression (Fig. 1.3). The anteriormost region of the humeral insertion of the infraspinatus almost reaches the anterior margin of the

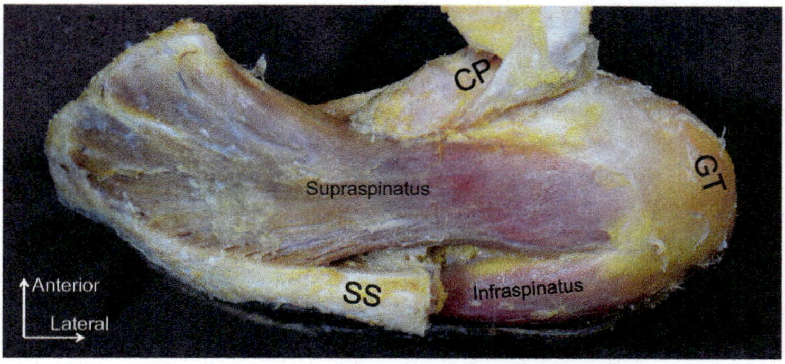

Fig. 1.1 Superior view of the supraspinatus and infraspinatus (right shoulder; acromion has been removed and reflected to anterior). Both tendons appear to mingle into one structure at the greater tuberosity (*GT*). *SS* scapular spine, *CP* coracoid process. (From Nimura et al. [8])

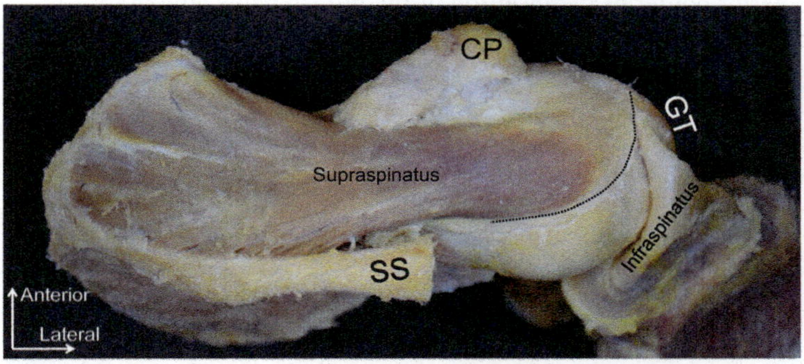

Fig. 1.2 Superior view of border between supraspinatus and infraspinatus (*black dotted line*). The infraspinatus has been detached from the scapula and the articular capsule and reflected to lateral. *SS* scapular spine, *CP* coracoid process. (From Nimura et al. [8])

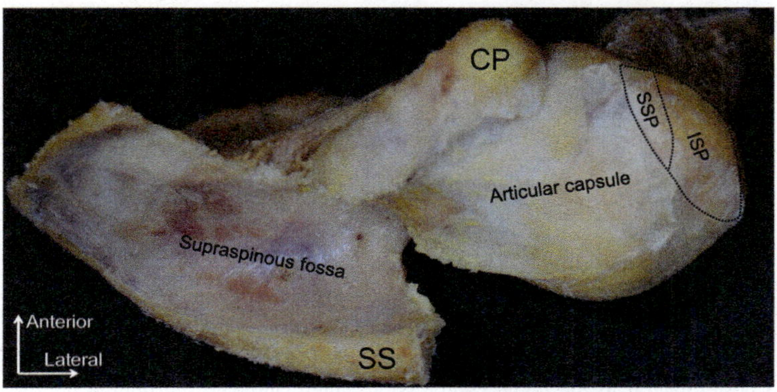

Fig. 1.3 Humeral side insertions of the supraspinatus and infraspinatus. Note articular capsule of the shoulder joint is completely separated from the supraspinatus and infraspinatus and preserved. *SSP* supraspinatus, *ISP* infraspinatus. (From Nimura et al. [8])

highest impression of the greater tuberosity. The supraspinatus inserts into the anteromedial area of the highest impression of the greater tuberosity (Fig. 1.3). The footprint of the supraspinatus is in the shape of a right triangle, with the base lying along the articular surface. In addition to the greater tuberosity, the supraspinatus also inserts in the lesser tuberosity in one fifth of specimens. In these specimens, the anteriormost portion of the supraspinatus tendon covers the superior part of the bicipital groove.

Based on anatomic textbooks, the greater tuberosity is marked by three flat impressions: the highest impression gives insertion to the supraspinatus muscle, and the middle to the infraspinatus. In these descriptions, the shapes of impressions of the greater tuberosity have been simply described as adjacent squares [4]. However, based on the recent study, the "lateral impression," which could be consistently identified, was composed of the border with the highest impression, the border with the middle impression, and the border with the lateral wall of the greater tuberosity (Fig. 1.4). The "lateral impression" was confirmed to correspond to the anterior border of the insertion of the infraspinatus tendon [5].

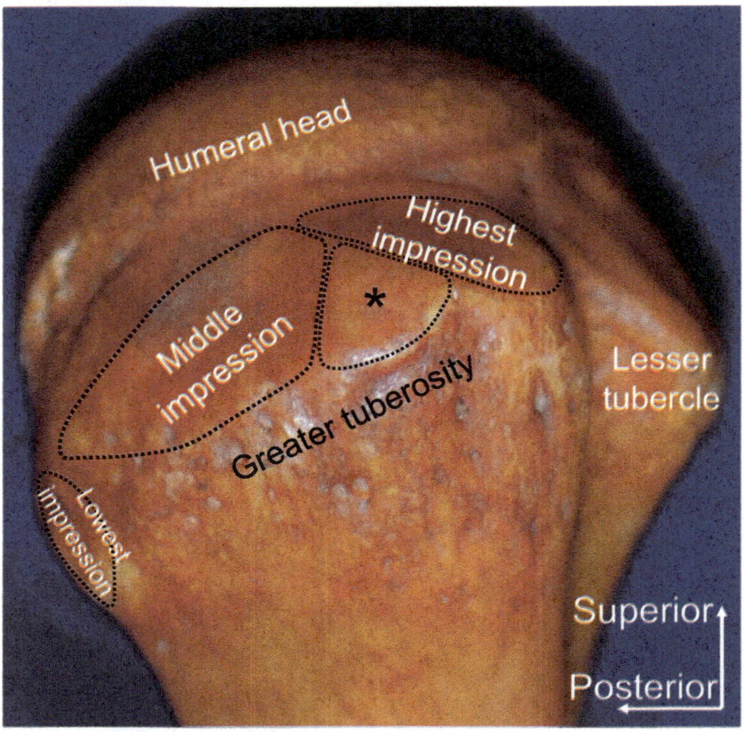

Fig. 1.4 "Lateral impression" of the greater tuberosity. Another impression (*asterisk*) could be observed posterolateral to the highest impression, anterolateral to the middle impression, and medial to the lateral wall of the greater tuberosity

1.2.1.2 Muscular and Tendinous Portions

Most of the muscle fibers of the supraspinatus, especially those of its superficial layer, run anterolaterally toward the anterior tendinous portion, whereas the rest of the fibers from the deep layer run laterally toward the medial margin of the highest impression on the greater tuberosity. The supraspinatus tendon is composed of two portions: the anterior half is long and thick, and the posterior half is short and thin (Fig. 1.5).

The superoanterior two thirds of the infraspinatus is composed of a thick and long tendinous portion. A thin and short tendinous portion that occupied the rest of the infraspinatus muscle joined the thin and short tendinous portion of the teres minor.

1.2.1.3 Oblique and Transverse Part of the Infraspinatus

The infraspinatus is identified to be composed of oblique and transverse parts according to the direction of muscle fibers (Fig. 1.6) [6]. The oblique part is a fan-shaped muscle bundle and originates from the infraspinatus fossa running superolaterally. The transverse part originates from the inferior surface of the spine and runs laterally; it is then attached to the oblique part of the middle portion of the tendinous part. The two parts are connected to each other at the superior area of the muscular portions; however, in the distal tendinous portions they can be clearly separated. Although the oblique part attached to the greater tuberosity, the

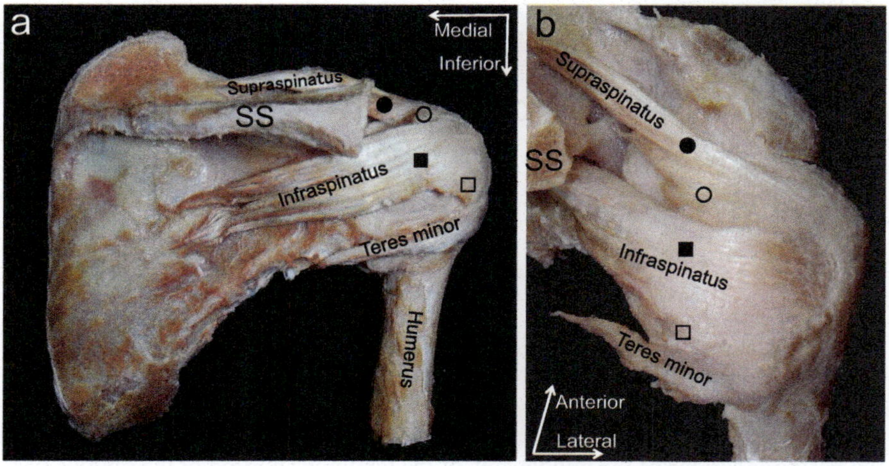

Fig. 1.5 Tendinous geometry of the supraspinatus and infraspinatus. Photographs of right shoulder after removing the acromion, muscular part of the rotator cuffs. (**a**) Posterior aspect. (**b**) Posterolateral aspect. The supraspinatus tendon is composed of two portions: anterior half is long and thick (*black circle*), and posterior half is short and thin (*open circle*). In the same way, the superior half of the infraspinatus tendon is long and thick (*black square*), and the posterior half is short thin (*open square*). *SS* scapular spine

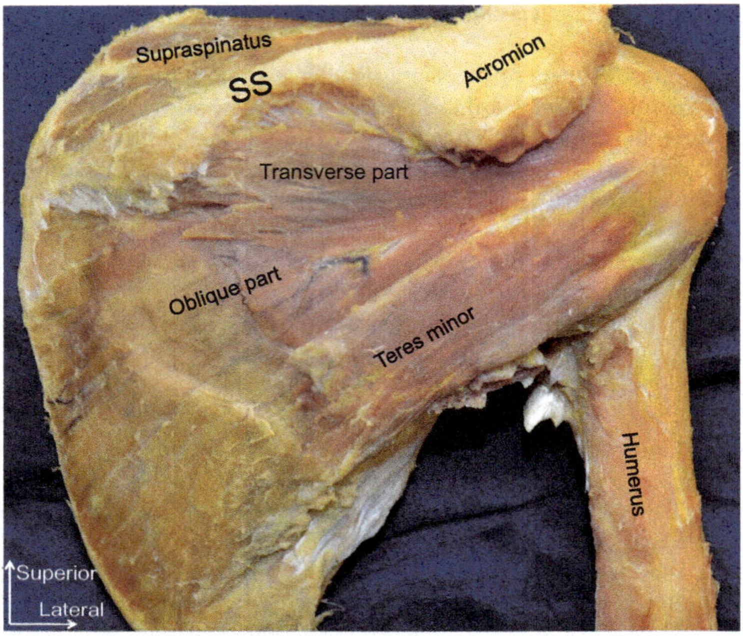

Fig. 1.6 Posterior view of right shoulder. Transverse part of the infraspinatus is shown to attach to the oblique part. (From Nimura et al. [8])

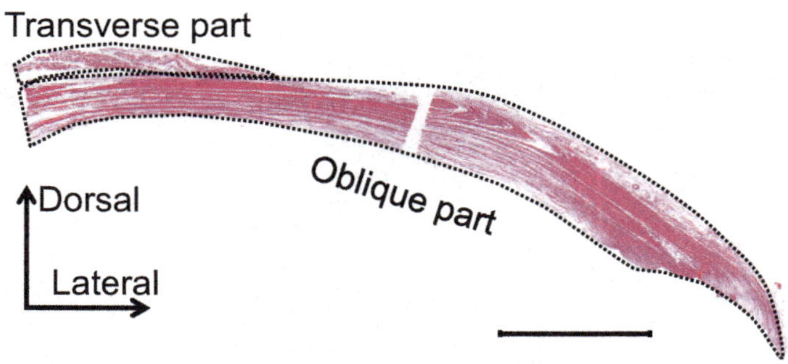

Fig. 1.7 Histological section of distal part of infraspinatus stained by hematoxylin and eosin showing longitudinal section through distal part of infraspinatus. Transverse part shown as *dorsal dotted* area; oblique part shown as *ventral dotted* area. *Bar* 10 mm. (From Kimura et al. [8])

transverse part does not reach the tuberosity (Fig. 1.7). The transverse part adjoins the posterior surface of the middle area of the tendinous portion of the oblique part. It is suggested that significant strength from the oblique part of the infraspinatus can focus more anteriorly and contribute to shoulder abduction; on the other hand, the transverse part may have only a supportive role in the infraspinatus function and stabilize the tendinous portion of the oblique part during the shoulder motion from above.

Origins of the innervating branch of the suprascapular nerve to the transverse part of the infraspinatus are variable. Branches arise from the branch to the supraspinatus muscle, and/or from the main trunk of the suprascapular nerve after branching off the branches to the supraspinatus muscle. No branch is found to pierce the transverse part to innervate the oblique part and vice versa. Although the transverse part is a part of the infraspinatus, according to its innervation, the transverse part might be closely related to the supraspinatus.

1.2.2 The Subscapularis Muscle

The subscapularis muscle insertion is composed of the superior two-thirds tendinous insertion and the inferior one-third insertion where the muscle attaches to the humerus almost directly by way of a thin membranous structure [7]. The superior-most insertion of the subscapularis tendon is wide in the uppermost margin of the lesser tuberosity, whereas the rest of the subscapularis tendon inserts into the anteromedial portion of the lesser tuberosity (Fig. 1.8). Moreover, the superior-

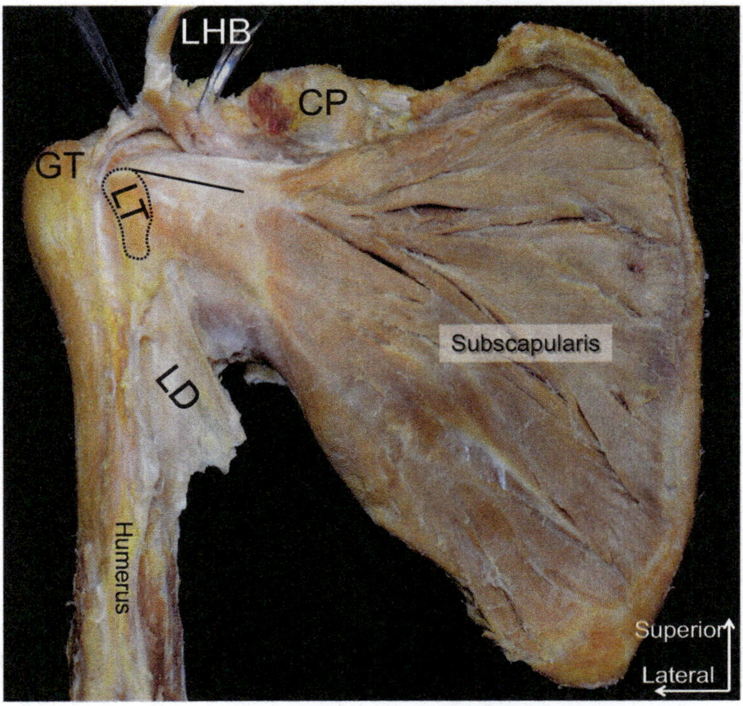

Fig. 1.8 Anterior view of right shoulder. Long head of biceps tendon (*LHB*) is reflected. Coracoid process (*CP*) is partially resected. Cranial part of subscapularis tendon inserts superior to uppermost margin (*black line*) of lesser tuberosity (*LT*, *dotted area*). *GT* greater tuberosity, *LD* latissimus dorsi. (From Kimura et al. [8])

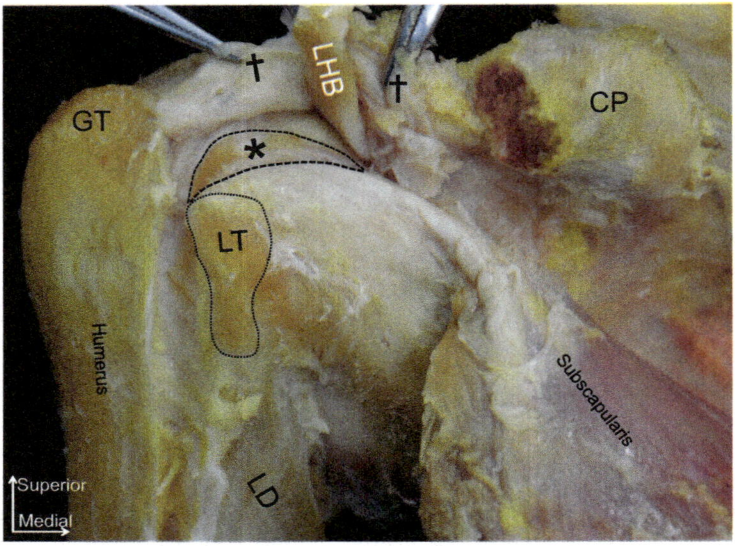

Fig. 1.9 Superior-most insertion of subscapularis tendon. Long head of biceps tendon (*LHB*) is reflected. The coracohumeral ligament is also detached from the subscapularis tendon and reflected with forceps (*cross*). The coracoid process (*CP*) is partially resected. The subscapularis muscle is detached from the scapular origin and reflected to anterior. The superior-most insertion of the subscapularis tendon extends a thin tendinous slip, which attaches to the fovea capitis of the humerus (*dotted area* marked with *asterisk*). (From Kimura et al. [8])

most insertion of the subscapularis tendon extends a thin tendinous slip, which attaches to the fovea capitis of the humerus (Fig. 1.9).

By removing muscular tissues, several intramuscular tendons can be observed. Those tendons aggregate laterally and form a tendinous insertion. The superior-most insertion of the subscapularis tendon is derived from the cranial part of the intramuscular tendons. The superior-most insertion, the lateral portion of the cranial part of the intramuscular tendons, and the tendinous slip comprise a structure that is in direct contact with the inferior side of the corner portion of the long head of the biceps tendon. This structure continues the pathway of the long head of the biceps tendon proximally from the osseous medial wall of the intertubercular groove.

1.2.3 The Teres Minor Muscle

The teres minor muscle locates inferior to the infraspinatus and originates from the lateral edge of the dorsal scapula. The teres minor muscle inserts to the lowest impression of the greater tuberosity of the humerus, and additionally inserts to the posterior side of the surgical neck of the humerus (Fig. 1.10). The border between the infraspinatus and the teres minor is separated by the tendinous fascia, which is sometimes unclear and disappears at their insertion.

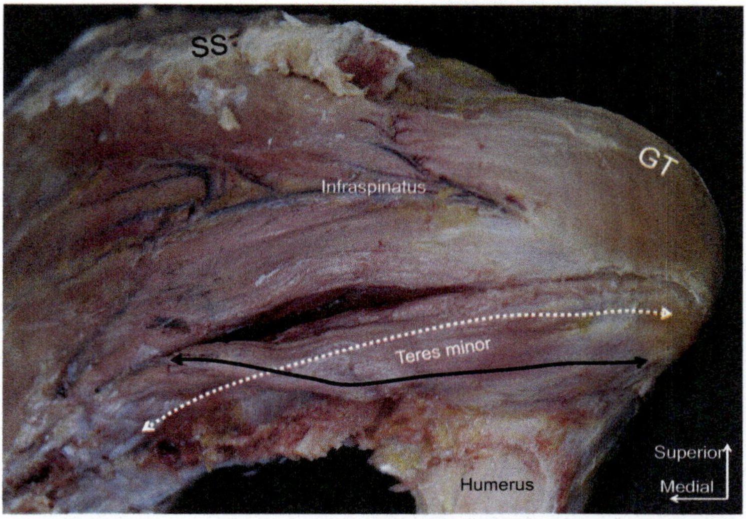

Fig. 1.10 Posterior view of right shoulder. Acromion is resected. The running course of the superior bundle of the teres minor at the insertion is indicated as *white double-headed arrow* with *dotted line*. The running course of the inferior bundle at the insertion is indicated as *black double-headed arrow*. *GT* greater tuberosity, *SS* scapula spine. (From Kimura et al. [8])

At the musculotendinous junction of the teres minor muscle, it can be separated into the superior and inferior bundles. The superior bundle at the insertion originates from the lateral edge of the dorsal scapula and inserts to the lowest impression as a oval footprint (Fig. 1.11) [8]. The inferior bundle at the insertion mainly originates from the tendinous fascia, which forms a septum between the infraspinatus and the teres minor, and partially originates from the lateral edge of the dorsal scapula. The inferior bundle of the teres minor runs dorsal to the superior bundle and inserts into the distal to the lowest impression as a linear shape (Fig. 1.11). At the origin of the teres minor, there is no structure that separates the two bundles. Both bundles are innervated by the branch of the axillary nerve that supplies from the dorsal or inferior side of the teres minor muscle, not from its ventral side.

1.3 Surrounding Structures of the Rotator Cuff

1.3.1 The Superior Capsule of the Shoulder Joint

In the shoulder joint, the deepest layer of the rotator cuff is a thin continuous sheet of interwoven collagen fibrils, which is the capsule that extends from the glenoid labrum medially to the humerus laterally [1]. Although the structure of the articular

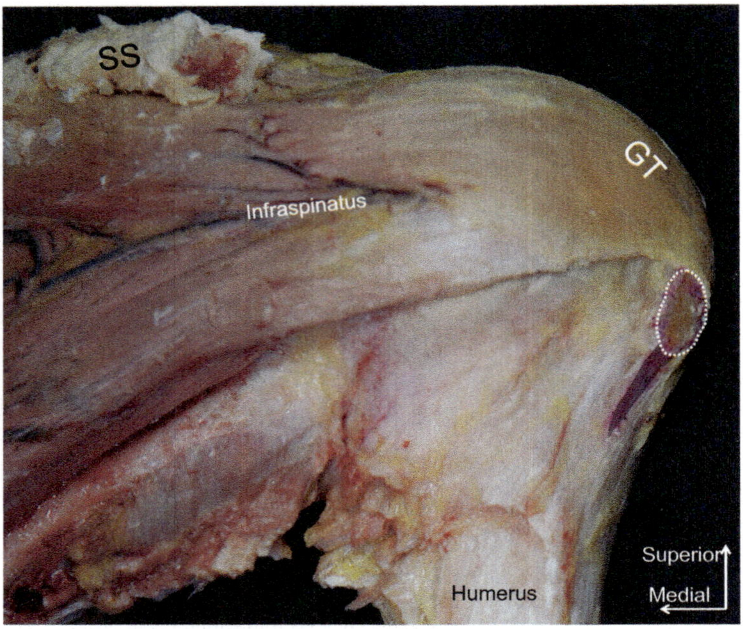

Fig. 1.11 Insertion of teres minor muscle. The teres minor muscle is detached from the humeral insertion. The insertion of the superior bundle of the teres minor is shown as a *white dotted area*. The insertion of the inferior bundle of the teres minor is shown as a *black area* with *arrowhead* shape. *GT* greater tuberosity, *SS* scapula spine. (From Kimura et al. [8])

capsule of the shoulder joint is very sturdy and it is assumed to have functional significance, studies that precisely refer to the function of the articular capsule are rare.

When the supraspinatus, infraspinatus, and teres minor are removed from the humerus, and in addition, the articular capsule is reflected posteriorly, the attachment of the articular capsule on the greater tuberosity is exposed. The attachment of the articular capsule occupies a substantial area of the greater tuberosity (Fig. 1.12) [9]. Near the anterior edge of the supraspinatus and the posterior edge of the infraspinatus, the articular capsule has a relatively thick footprint. In particular, at the border between the infraspinatus and teres minor, the very thick attachment of the articular capsule compensates for the lack of tendinous insertion (approximately 9 mm).

The thinnest point of the capsule attachment is located approximately 11 mm posterior to the anterior margin of the greater tuberosity along the articular cartilage border. At this point, the posterior edge of the supraspinatus insertion is very close and the infraspinatus inserts with a relatively thick attachment. The region in which degenerative rotator cuff tears are most commonly observed [10] is near the thinnest point of the articular capsule. If the thinnest point of the articular capsule attachment is hypothesized as mechanically being the most fragile area, it follows that it may be related to the initiation of degenerative rotator cuff tears.

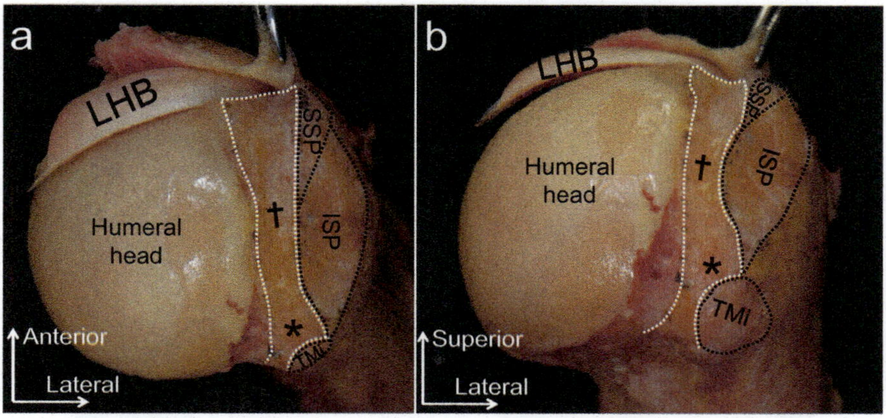

Fig. 1.12 Attachment of superior capsule of shoulder joint. Rotator cuffs and articular capsule are removed from humerus. Attachment area of articular capsule is shown as *white dotted area*. Thinnest point of the articular capsule indicated with a *cross*; thickest point indicated with *asterisk*. (**a**) Superior view of right humerus. (**b**) Posterior view. *ISP* infraspinatus, *LHB* long head of biceps, *SSP* supraspinatus, *TMi* teres minor

On the other hand, at the inferior margin of the infraspinatus where no muscular components are attached, the articular capsule has the thickest attachment (Fig. 1.12b, *asterisk*). Given that, the articular capsule might functionally complement the insertion of the rotator and facilitate maintenance for the endurance of the rotator cuff footprint.

1.3.2 The Coracohumeral and the Superior Glenohumeral Ligaments

The coracohumeral ligament (CHL) was classically described to originate in the outer margin of the horizontal limb of the coracoid process, insert into the greater and lesser tuberosities, and cover the rotator interval, which is the space between the supraspinatus and subscapularis muscles. The CHL was considered to have a key role in the function of the rotator interval. The posterior extension of the CHL from the rotator interval has become well known since the anatomic study of Clark and Harryman [1]. Their study showed that both the superficial and deep branches of the CHL envelop the anterior part of the supraspinatus tendon; the superficial branch fans out laterally and posteriorly over the supraspinatus tendon, extending as far as the infraspinatus, and merges with the periosteum of the greater tuberosity. This envelope-like structure of the CHL should act as a stabilizer of the posterosuperior side of the glenohumeral joint.

However, to date, the anterior extension of the CHL has not been well known. The recent study showed that the CHL could be divided into two parts: one part

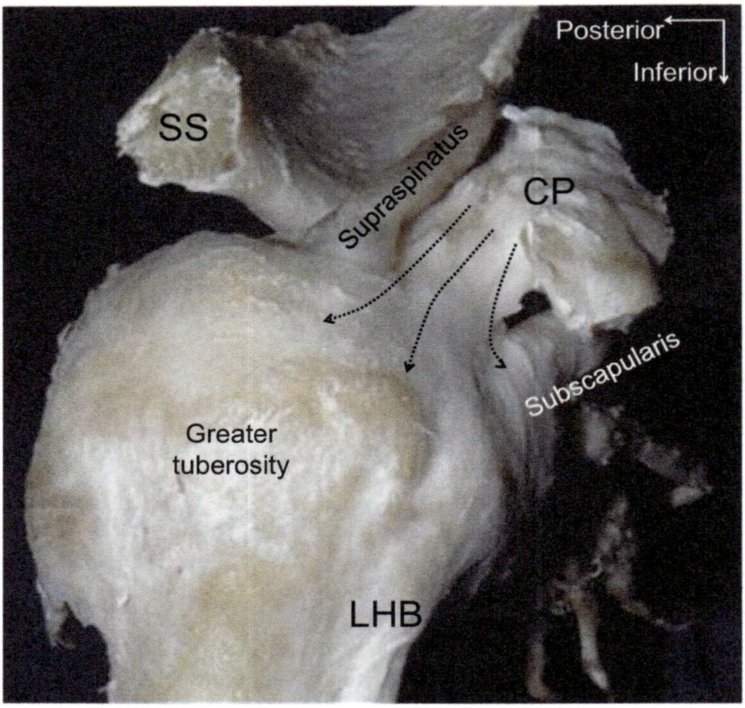

Fig. 1.13 Expansion of the coracohumeral ligament (*CHL*). Right shoulder viewed from lateral side. Scapular spine (*SS*) was cut and muscular tissue of supraspinatus and subscapularis was removed. The CHL originates from the coracoid process (*CP*) (*black dotted arrows*): it covers a broad area of the surface of the subscapularis and supraspinatus tendon. *LHB* long head of biceps

spreads fibers over the rotator interval to the posterior portion of the greater tuberosity as previously described, and the other part extends fibers to envelop the cranial part of the subscapularis muscle (Fig. 1.13) [11]. Moreover, the superficial layer tightly covers a broad area of the anterior surface of the latter, seamlessly continues to the subscapularis fascia, and tightly covers a broad area of the anterior surface of the subscapularis muscle.

As already described, at the lateral portion, the subscapularis tendon has a tendinous floor under the long head of the biceps tendon. The superior glenohumeral ligament (SGHL) and the CHL run spinally and finally attach to the tendinous slip of the subscapularis insertion [12]. Just above the intertubercular groove, the SGHL and CHL attach to the surface of the tendinous slip of the subscapularis insertion and support the long head of the biceps from the anteroinferior side (Fig. 1.14). When viewed from the inferior side of the coracoid process, the CHL attachment is composed of a narrow anteromedial part and a broad lateral part. The anteromedial part of the CHL attaches to the anterior edge of the inferior surface of the coracoid process. The lateral part attaches to the lateral one-third area of the inferior surface of the horizontal limb of the process (Fig. 1.15).

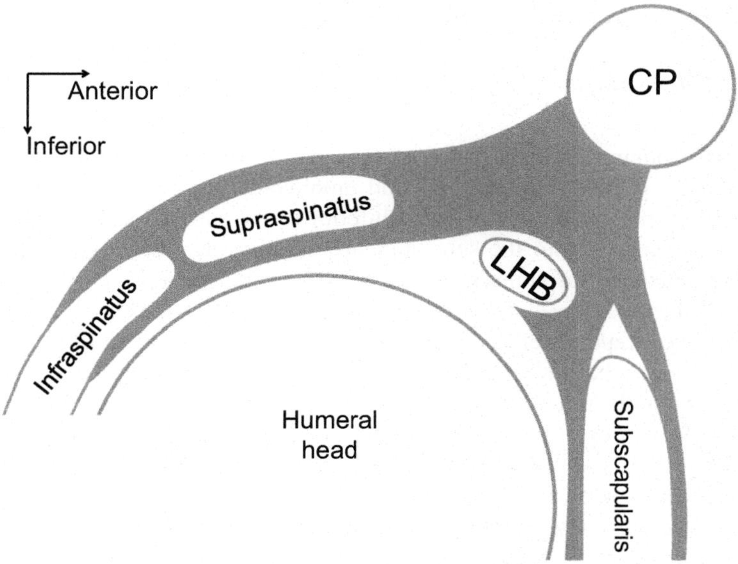

Fig. 1.14 Schematic illustration of anterior and posterior parts of the coracohumeral ligament (*CHL*). CHL (*gray area*) extends laterally from the base of the coracoid process (*CP*). The anterior CHL likely holds the subscapularis muscle and anchors the muscle to the coracoid process in a manner similar to that of the posterior CHL enveloping the supraspinatus and infraspinatus. The CHL and the superior glenohumeral ligament (*SGHL*) also function as a sustainer of the long head of the biceps tendon (*LHB*)

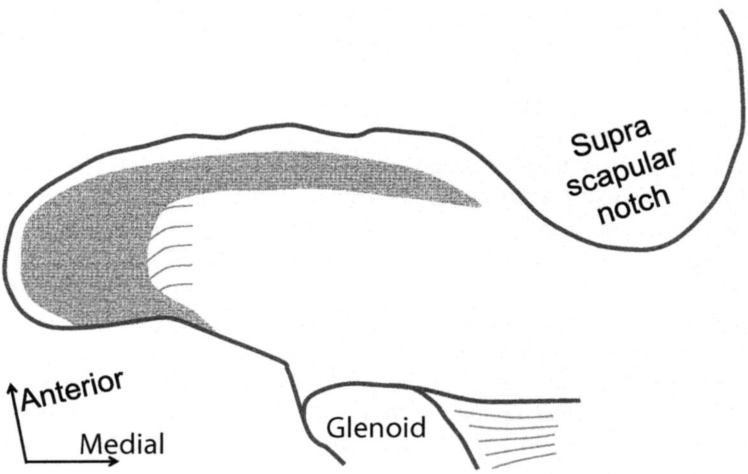

Fig. 1.15 Schematic illustration of dimensions of the coracohumeral ligament (*CHL*) on inferior surface of coracoid process. Inferior surface of right coracoid process is shown. Typical attachment of the CHL shown as *gray area*

1.4 Nerves Around the Shoulder Joint

1.4.1 The Suprascapular Nerve

The suprascapular nerve is a branch of the superior trunk of the brachial plexus. It runs laterally, deep to the trapezius and omohyoid, and enters the supraspinous fossa through the suprascapular notch inferior to the superior transverse scapular ligament. It runs deep to the supraspinatus, supplies it, passes the spinoglenoid notch to reach the infraspinous fossa, and innervates it. The suprascapular nerve has the potential to be exposed to various stresses during its course along the posterior aspect of the scapula before finally innervating the infraspinatus. Although a number of studies have reported a variety of causes of suprascapular nerve entrapment, several authors have reported that one of the main etiological factors of the suprascapular neuropathy is the morphological variation of the suprascapular notch. Rengachary et al. [13, 14] proposed that the variation in shape could be a risk factor for suprascapular nerve entrapment. They also described that the nerve direction of the suprascapular nerve changes from craniocaudal to anteroposterior at the suprascapular notch and concluded that "the sling effect" caused by this direction change could be a potential risk factor for suprascapular nerve neuropathy. Based on their report, several publications have discussed the morphological differences in the suprascapular notch in terms of the diagnosis and treatment of suprascapular nerve neuropathy. However, in the previous reports, the configuration of the suprascapular notch was analyzed only by the anteroposterior view, whereas in fact the approach direction of the suprascapular nerve to the inlet of the suprascapular notch is consistently craniocaudal and mediolateral.

In the recent study, the suprascapular notch was observed in the nerve approach direction in relationship to the suprascapular nerve. When the inlet of the suprascapular notch was observed from the anteroposterior view, the subscapularis lies just anterior to the suprascapular notch and the superior part of the subscapularis covers the suprascapular notch (Fig. 1.16) [15]. When the inlet of the suprascapular notch is observed from the craniocaudal and mediolateral view, it is recognized to be a triangular space that is bordered by the medial wall of the coracoid process as the lateral plane, the deep fascia of the subscapularis as the anterior plane, and the superior transverse scapular ligament as the posterior plane. The sagittal section of the scapula showed that the suprascapular nerve ran along the superior part of the supraspinous fossa underneath the supraspinatus muscle, to reach the spinoglenoid notch (Fig. 1.17). The suprascapular nerve appears to run posterior to the superior part of the subscapularis. This suprascapular nerve course corresponds to the approach direction of the suprascapular nerve. From the posteroanterior view, the superior transverse scapular ligament covers the superior part of the suprascapular notch (Fig. 1.18a). Although the craniocaudal width of the superior transverse scapular ligament varies among samples, the superior transverse scapular ligament forms a plane resembling a sheet-like structure rather than a cord-like one. The plane containing the superior transverse scapular ligament is nearly parallel to the direction of the suprascapular nerve and the superior bony aspect of the scapula. This plane of

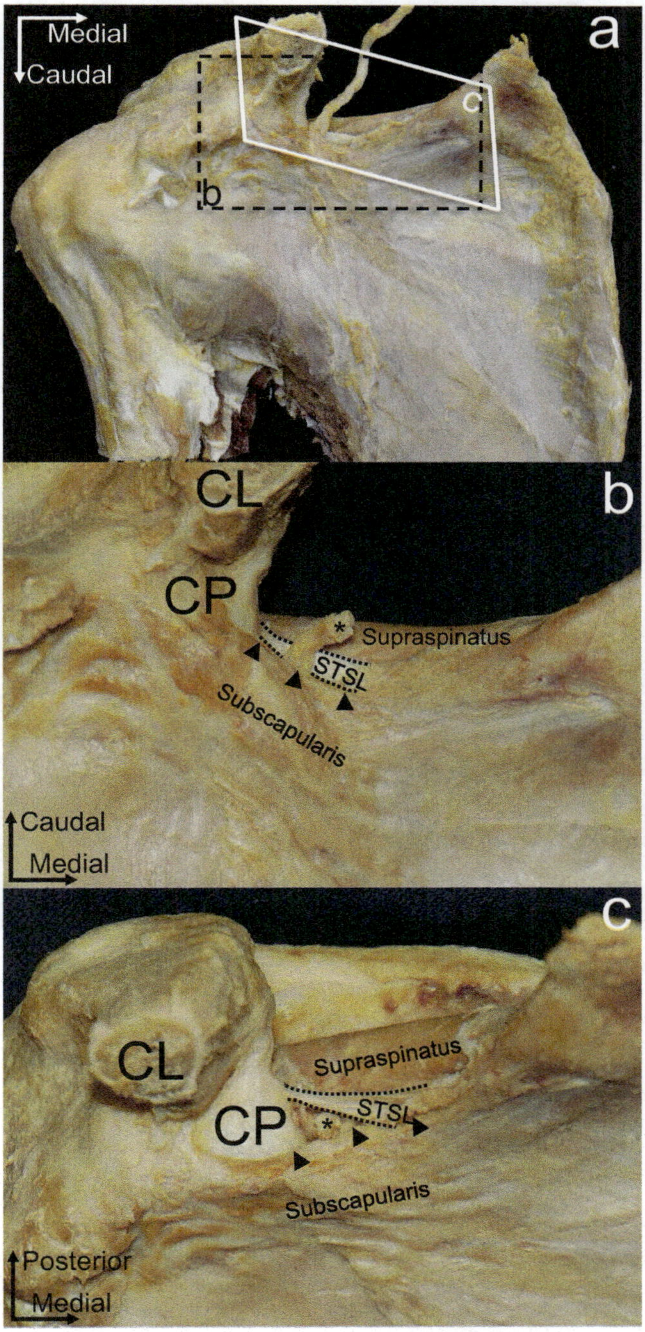

Fig. 1.16 Two views of suprascapular nerve entering the suprascapular notch. (**a**) Anterior view of right shoulder. Anteroposterior view (*black-dotted square*) is magnified in (**b**); craniocaudal and mediolateral view (*white parallelogram*) is magnified in (**c**). (**b**) Superior part of the subscapularis

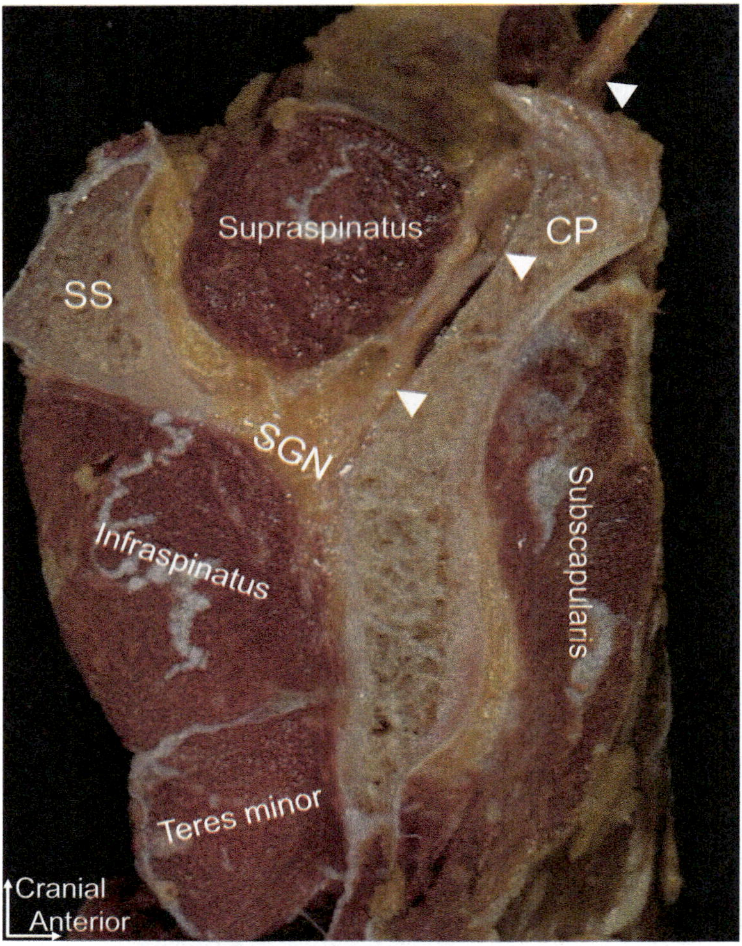

Fig. 1.17 Course of the suprascapular nerve (*arrowheads*) from the suprascapular notch to the spinoglenoid notch (*SGN*) in the sagittal section of the scapula. The suprascapular nerve runs along the superior part of the supraspinous fossa underneath the supraspinatus muscle to reach SGN. *CP* coracoid process, *SS* scapular spine. (From Tasaki et al. [15])

Fig. 1.16 (continued) (*arrowheads*) covers the suprascapular notch. (**c**) The inlet of the nerve running space of the suprascapular nerve (*asterisk*) at the suprascapular notch is surrounded by three planes: the medial wall of the coracoid process (*CP*) as the lateral plane, deep fascia of the subscapularis (*arrow heads*) as the anterior plane, and the superior transverse scapular ligament (*STSL*) as the posterior plane. *CL* clavicle. (From Tasaki et al. [15])

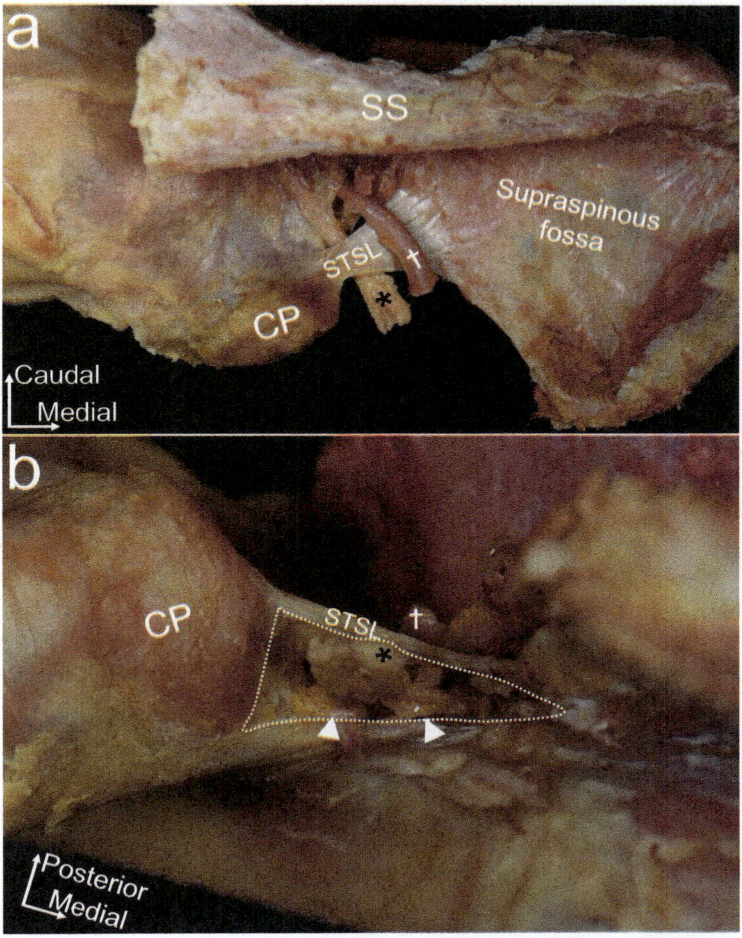

Fig. 1.18 Spatial relationships between suprascapular notch, superior transverse scapular ligament (*STSL*), and suprascapular nerve (*asterisk*). The muscles around the suprascapular nerve were removed. (**a**) Posterior view. (**b**) View from running direction of suprascapular nerve. *Dotted area* indicates nerve running space at the inlet of the suprascapular notch, which space was bordered by STSL and the superior surface of the supraspinous fossa (*arrowheads*). *CP* coracoid process, *cross* suprascapular artery. (From Tasaki et al. [15])

the superior transverse scapular ligament acts as a posterior wall of the suprascapular nerve space (Fig. 1.18b). The identification of the suprascapular nerve space can be confirmed by observation from the craniocaudal and mediolateral view. No part of the nerve running course of the suprascapular nerve interferes with the plane of the superior transverse scapular ligament. The inlet of the suprascapular notch seems to be reasonable to ensure the nerve running space rather than harmful. As for clinical relevance, regarding suprascapular nerve neuropathy, there has been no evidence of compression of the suprascapular nerve localized in the suprascapular notch except for a ganglion or abnormal mass. If imaging of the suprascapular notch using three-dimensional computed tomography or arthroscopy could be analyzed from the craniocaudal and mediolateral view, these might provide clues to reveal the etiology of suprascapular nerve neuropathy.

1.4.2 The Axillary Nerve

The axillary nerve originates from the posterior cord of the brachial plexus. At first, it is lateral to the radial nerve, posterior to the axillary artery, and anterior to the subscapularis. At the lower border of the subscapularis, it curves inferior to the joint capsule of the shoulder with the posterior circumflex humeral vessels. The axillary nerve transverses a quadrangular space bounded above by the teres minor, below by the teres major, medially by the long head of triceps, and laterally by the surgical neck of the humerus. The axillary nerve has the distinctive characteristic of surrounding the humerus from posterior to anterior. It divides into the anterior branch and the posterior branch, and is distributed to the deltoid muscle, teres minor muscle, and the skin on the posterolateral aspect of the shoulder (Fig. 1.19). The

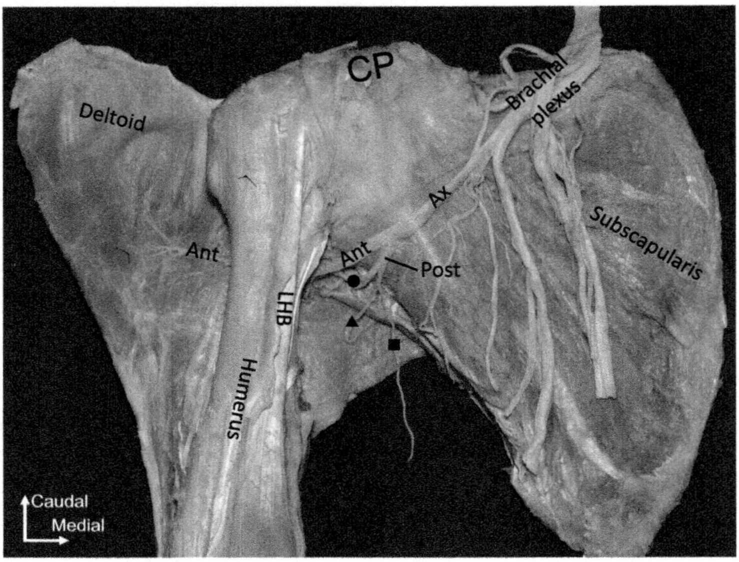

Fig. 1.19 Overall view of the division of the axillary nerve in an anterior view of the right shoulder. Deltoid muscle is detached and reflected laterally. Axillary nerve (*Ax*) originates from brachial plexus and bifurcates into the anterior branch (*Ant*) and the posterior branch (*Post*) at the inferolateral part of the subscapularis muscle. The anterior branch runs anteriorward from behind the humerus and supplies branches to the anterior and middle parts of the deltoid muscle. The posterior branch trifurcates into the branch to the teres minor muscle (*black circle*), the branch to the posterior part of the deltoid muscle (*black triangle*), and the superior lateral brachial cutaneous nerve (*black square*). *CP* coracoid process. (From Nasu et al. [17])

axillary nerve also has an articular branch that arises from the origin of the axillary nerve and enters the inferior part of the shoulder joint capsule [16]. The recent study reveals the presence of additional branches that innervate structures around the shoulder joint [17]. The thin branches from the anterior branch of the axillary nerve are distributed to the subacromial bursa and the area around the long head of the biceps tendon. The branches from the main trunk of the axillary nerve or the branch to the teres minor muscle are distributed to the inferoposterior part of the shoulder joint. As clinical implications, symptoms of the anterior or lateral aspect of the shoulder that had been considered to originate from the suprascapular nerve might be related to the thin branches from the axillary nerve.

References

1. Clark JM, Harryman DT 2nd (1992) Tendons, ligaments, and capsule of the rotator cuff. Gross and microscopic anatomy. J Bone Joint Surg Am 74(5):713–725
2. Minagawa H, Itoi E, Konno N, Kido T, Sano A, Urayama M, Sato K (1998) Humeral attachment of the supraspinatus and infraspinatus tendons: an anatomic study. Arthroscopy 14(3):302–306
3. Mochizuki T, Sugaya H, Uomizu M, Maeda K, Matsuki K, Sekiya I, Muneta T, Akita K (2008) Humeral insertion of the supraspinatus and infraspinatus. New anatomical findings regarding the footprint of the rotator cuff. J Bone Joint Surg Am 90(5):962–969
4. Clemente C (1985) Osteology, and muscles and fasciae of the upper limb. In: Gray's anatomy, 30th American edition. Lea & Febiger, Philadelphia, pp 233–234
5. Nozaki T, Nimura A, Fujishiro H, Mochizuki T, Yamaguchi K, Kato R, Sugaya H, Akita K (n.d.) The anatomic relationship between the morphology of the greater tubercle of the humerus and the insertion of the infraspinatus tendon. J Shoulder Elbow Surg. doi:S1058-2746(14)00537-0 [pii] 10.1016/j.jse.2014.09.038 [doi]
6. Kato A, Nimura A, Yamaguchi K, Mochizuki T, Sugaya H, Akita K (2012) An anatomical study of the transverse part of the infraspinatus muscle that is closely related with the supraspinatus muscle. Surg Radiol Anat 34(3):257–265. doi:10.1007/s00276-011-0872-0[doi]
7. Arai R, Sugaya H, Mochizuki T, Nimura A, Moriishi J, Akita K (2008) Subscapularis tendon tear: an anatomic and clinical investigation. Arthroscopy 24(9):997–1004. doi:10.1016/j.arthro.2008.04.076, S0749-8063(08)00359-9 [pii]
8. Nimura A, Akita K, Sugaya H (2015) Rotator cuff. In: Bain GI, Itoi E, Di Giacomo G, Sugaya H (eds) Normal and pathological anatomy of the shoulder. Springer, Berlin. doi:10.1007/978-3-662-45719-1
9. Nimura A, Kato A, Yamaguchi K, Mochizuki T, Okawa A, Sugaya H, Akita K (2012) The superior capsule of the shoulder joint complements the insertion of the rotator cuff. J Shoulder Elbow Surg 21(7):867–872. doi:10.1016/j.jse.2011.04.034, S1058-2746(11)00203-5 [pii]
10. Kim HM, Dahiya N, Teefey SA, Middleton WD, Stobbs G, Steger-May K, Yamaguchi K, Keener JD (2010) Location and initiation of degenerative rotator cuff tears: an analysis of three hundred and sixty shoulders. J Bone Joint Surg Am 92(5):1088–1096. doi:10.2106/JBJS.I.00686, 92/5/1088 [pii]
11. Arai R, Nimura A, Yamaguchi K, Yoshimura H, Sugaya H, Saji T, Matsuda S, Akita K (2014) The anatomy of the coracohumeral ligament and its relation to the subscapularis muscle. J Shoulder Elbow Surg. doi:10.1016/j.jse.2014.02.009, S1058-2746(14)00119-0 [pii]
12. Arai R, Mochizuki T, Yamaguchi K, Sugaya H, Kobayashi M, Nakamura T, Akita K (2010) Functional anatomy of the superior glenohumeral and coracohumeral ligaments and the

subscapularis tendon in view of stabilization of the long head of the biceps tendon. J Shoulder Elbow Surg 19(1):58–64. doi:10.1016/j.jse.2009.04.001, S1058-2746(09)00194-3 [pii]
13. Rengachary SS, Burr D, Lucas S, Brackett CE (1979) Suprascapular entrapment neuropathy: a clinical, anatomical, and comparative study. Part 3: comparative study. Neurosurgery 5 (4):452–455
14. Rengachary SS, Burr D, Lucas S, Hassanein KM, Mohn MP, Matzke H (1979) Suprascapular entrapment neuropathy: a clinical, anatomical, and comparative study. Part 2: anatomical study. Neurosurgery 5(4):447–451
15. Tasaki A, Nimura A, Mochizuki T, Yamaguchi K, Kato R, Sugaya H, Akita K (2014) Anatomic observation of the running space of the suprascapular nerve at the suprascapular notch in the same direction as the nerve. Knee Surg Sports Traumatol Arthrosc. doi:10.1007/s00167-014-3129-8
16. Gardner E (1948) The innervation of the shoulder joint. Anat Rec 102(1):1–18
17. Nasu H, Nimura A, Yamaguchi K, Akita K (2014) Distribution of the axillary nerve to the subacromial bursa and the area around the long head of the biceps tendon. Knee Surg Sports Traumatol Arthrosc. doi:10.1007/s00167-014-3112-4

Chapter 2
Biomechanics

Nobuyuki Yamamoto and Eiji Itoi

Abstract For advances in any field of medicine, we need basic research as well as clinical research. Biomechanics, which is a category of basic research, has a long history and has developed with modern robotic, measurement, or image techniques. This chapter presents an up-to-date overview of biomechanical research on the shoulder. We focus on some pertinent topics discussed in recent meetings or articles and herein introduce the latest biomechanical studies, especially the matter at hand regarding the pathophysiology or surgical procedure described in recently published articles. Also, we selected the articles that had great clinical relevance and would give the readers useful information when considering the diagnosis, treatment, and surgical indication. Basic knowledge about shoulder biomechanics, which can be found in other books or review articles, is not described in this chapter; rather, new findings published for the past 10 years are presented. We believe this chapter would be useful for surgeons in daily practice.

Keywords Biomechanics • Stability • Pathophysiology • Surgical procedure

2.1 Shoulder Instability

2.1.1 Multidirectional Instability

The contribution of intraarticular pressure of the glenohumeral joint to the inferior stability of the shoulder has been extensively studied [1, 2], and it is generally accepted that intraarticular pressure is an important inferior stabilizer of the shoulder with the arm in adduction [3, 4] (Fig. 2.1a, b). In shoulders with multidirectional instability (MDI), the joint volume is increased [5], and the joint capsule is lax and thin. It is assumed that capsular redundancy in shoulders with MDI decreases the sucking strength created by the negative pressure, which in turn becomes less effective in stabilizing the shoulder inferiorly. Yamamoto et al. [6] biomechanically

N. Yamamoto (✉) • E. Itoi
Department of Orthopaedic Surgery, Tohoku University School of Medicine, 1-1 Seiryo-machi, Aoba-ku, Sendai, Miyagi 980-8574, Japan
e-mail: koyomoe@med.tohoku.ac.jp

K. Tamai et al. (eds.), *Advances in Shoulder Surgery*,
DOI 10.1007/978-4-431-55988-7_2

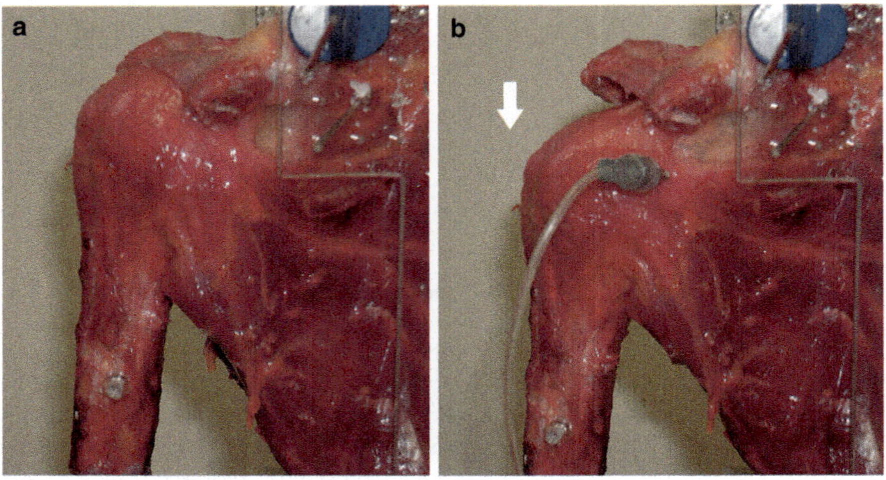

Fig. 2.1 (**a**) Before venting the capsule. (**b**) The humerus displaced inferiorly after venting the capsule

clarified the relationship between the joint volume and intraarticular pressure. They reported that the volume of the intact shoulder was decreased to 42 % (58 % reduction) by anterior and posterior imbrication. By this volume reduction, the negative values of intraarticular pressure increased. It is most likely that the response of intraarticular pressure to the external load improved by decreasing the joint volume, and thereby inferior displacement was stabilized. This finding indicated the relationship between intraarticular pressure and inferior stability.

Since the report by Neer and Foster [7], excellent clinical outcomes of inferior capsular shift procedure have been reported. It has become the standard operative treatment for MDI. Recently, arthroscopic capsular plication has been performed for MDI, and there have been many reports describing its excellent results [8]. Ponce et al. [9] quantified the relationship between the amount of shoulder capsule plication and the degree of joint volume reduction in a MDI model. Also, they identified the number of arthroscopic plication stitches required to reduce the joint volume equal to that of an open inferior capsular shift and compared volume reductions between suture anchor and capsular plication stitches. Their results indicated that a 1-cm capsular plication stitch resulted in a 10 % volume reduction of the joint, and five simple capsular plication stitches resulted in a volume reduction equivalent to an open capsular shift. It is easily expected that the restriction of range of motion would occur after capsular plication. To avoid constraining the joint, Shapiro et al. [10] proposed an arthroscopic capsular plication in line with the fibers of the inferior glenohumeral ligament. They demonstrated, in a biomechanical study using an anterior instability model, that a 10-mm capsular plication in line with the fibers of the inferior glenohumeral ligament reduced capsular laxity without overtightening the joint.

2.1.2 Remplissage Procedure

There are several treatment options to manage a large Hill-Sachs lesion that engages with the glenoid rim. The remplissage procedure, which has a tenodesis effect of the infraspinatus tendon, is one of these [11–14]. The remplissage procedure has rapidly gained popularity because it is an arthroscopic technique and is relatively easily performed. However, does the remplissage procedure really contribute to stability? Looking at the surgical indication of this procedure described in recent reports, it seems to be becoming wider. Several biomechanical studies have been reported investigating the effect of the remplissage procedure on stability. Some studies support the effectiveness of this procedure but some do not. Grimberg et al. [15] compared Bankart repair with and without remplissage procedure. In cadaveric shoulders with Bankart and Hill–Sachs lesions, Bankart repair with remplissage procedure restored joint stability compared to Bankart repair alone. Elkinson et al. [16] also reported that the remplissage procedure enhanced stability.

On the other hand, some investigators indicated that the remplissage procedure did not contribute to stability. Argintar et al. [17] investigated the effects of the remplissage procedure combined with Bankart repair on the range of motion, translation, and shoulder kinematics. They demonstrated that the addition of the remplissage procedure had no significant effect on the range of motion or translation, but altered the shoulder kinematics: at maximum external rotation at 60° abduction, the humeral head shifted posterior-inferiorly with the remplissage procedure. Elkinson et al. [18] created two sizes (moderate and large) of Hill–Sachs lesions and demonstrated that an addition of remplissage procedure resulted in little additional benefit to a Bankart repair in specimens with a 15 % Hill–Sachs lesion but it enhanced stability and prevented engagement in specimens with a 30 % Hill–Sachs lesion. Thus, to prove the contribution of the remplissage procedure to stability, we need further high-level evidence clinical studies.

The Latarjet procedure, humeral head allograft, and partial resurfacing arthroplasty have been also reported as treatment options to manage large Hill–Sachs lesions that engage with the glenoid rim. Degen et al. [19] performed a biomechanical comparison of the remplissage procedure to the Latarjet procedure in terms of capsular stiffness that was calculated from load-displacement curve, range of motion, and frequency of dislocation. Both procedures proved effective in reducing the frequency of dislocation in a 25 % Hill-Sachs defect model, although neither procedure altered capsular stiffness. This study supports the use of both the remplissage and Latarjet procedures. Giles et al. [20] compared three surgical procedures (remplissage, humeral head allograft, and partial resurfacing arthroplasty) for large Hill–Sachs lesions. The remplissage procedure improved stability and eliminated engagement but caused reductions in the range of motion. The humeral head allograft and partial resurfacing arthroplasty reestablished intact range of motion, but partial resurfacing arthroplasty could not prevent engagement. They concluded that the effects of these techniques are not equivalent.

The remplissage procedure is a procedure that has a tenodesis effect of the infraspinatus tendon. Thus, it is expected that the range of motion, especially external rotation and horizontal extension, are restricted after this procedure. Omi et al. [21] assessed the effects of the remplissage procedure for small and large Hill–Sachs lesions on the range of motion. This procedure for a large Hill–Sachs lesion caused significant restrictions in the range of abduction and external rotation with the humerus in both adduction and abduction. It also caused significant restrictions in both external rotation and extension motions in the apprehension position. Thus, we need to be careful when performing the remplissage procedure in throwing athletes.

2.1.3 Latarjet Procedure

Recently, coracoid transfer procedures have gained popularity again. Because recent reports [22, 23] have shown that postoperative arthritis can be avoided by appropriate positioning of a coracoid bone graft, and the clinical results of this procedure for shoulders with a large glenoid defect or Hill–Sachs lesion and for contact or collision athletes have been reported to be excellent compared to those of arthroscopic Bankart repair. There seem to be two coracoid transfer procedures (the Bristow and Latarjet procedures), that are frequently used to address a large glenoid defect. Giles et al. [24] compared the biomechanical effects of these two procedures and reported that both procedures have equivalent stabilizing effects in unstable shoulders without glenoid defect. However, the Latarjet procedure conferred superior stabilization in shoulders with a large (30 %) glenoid defect. In another study that compared the effects of these two procedures, Nourissat et al. [25] assessed the effect of the position of the bone graft on anterior and inferior stability. They showed that positioning the bone graft so that it lies on the anterior glenoid can decrease anterior displacement of the humeral head and inferior translation, especially in adduction and external rotation for anterior displacement and in abduction and external rotation for inferior displacement.

Clinicians believed that the stabilizing mechanism of the Latarjet procedure was the "sling effect" of the subscapularis or conjoint tendon [22, 26, 27], the "bone-block effect" [28], or the combination of tendinous, ligamentous, and bony effects [29, 30]. Its main stabilizing mechanism was demonstrated to be the sling effect at both the end-range and the mid-range positions by Yamamoto et al. [31]. At the end-range position, 76–77 % of the stability was attributed to the sling effect (Fig. 2.2); the remaining 23–24 % was contributed to the suturing of the coracoacromial ligament. In the mid-range position, the contribution of the sling effect was 51–62 %. Reconstruction of the glenoid concavity contributed the remaining 38–49 % (Fig. 2.3).

Bhatia et al. [32] investigated glenohumeral contact areas, contact pressures, and peak forces after the creation of a large glenoid defect and subsequent bone augmentation with a coracoid graft or an allograft. They concluded that reconstruction of anterior glenoid defects with an allograft may allow improved joint congruity and lower peak force within the glenohumeral joint than Latarjet reconstruction at 60° of abduction and the abduction and external rotation position.

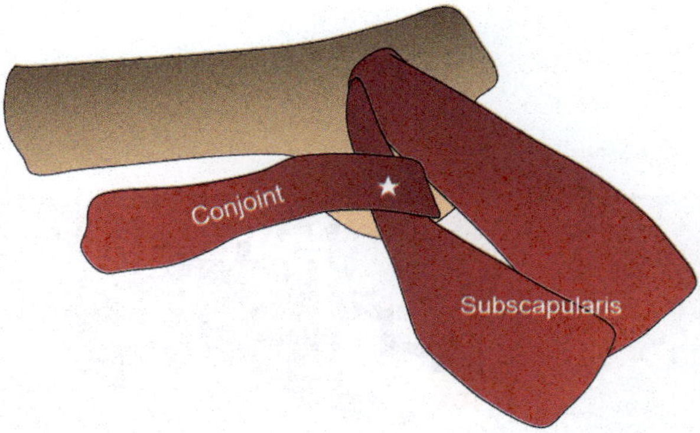

Fig. 2.2 Schematic illustration of the sling effect. The sling effect was provided by the subscapularis and conjoint tendons. The split subscapularis tendon provided muscle stability, working as a barrier because the intersection (⋆) of the conjoint tendon added tension to the inferior portion of the subscapularis

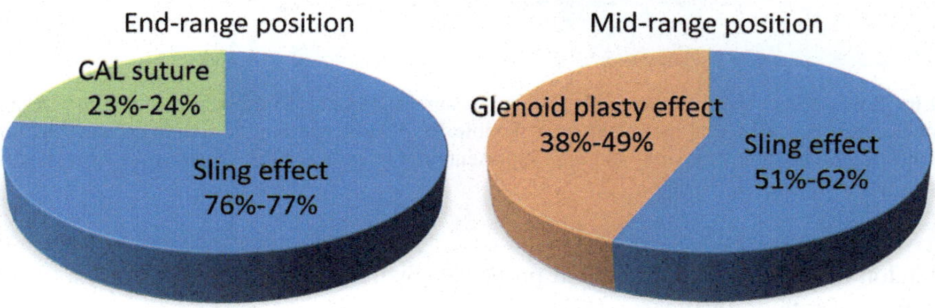

Fig. 2.3 Stabilizing mechanism of the Latarjet procedure. At the end-range position, 76–77 % of the stability was contributed by the sling effect and the remaining 23–24 % by the suturing of the coracoacromial ligament. In the mid-range position, the contribution of the sling effect was 51–62 %. Reconstruction of the glenoid concavity contributed the remaining 38–49 %. CAL suture, suturing the coracoacromial ligament (capsular flap); glenoid plasty effect, reconstruction of the glenoid concavity

2.2 Rotator Cuff Tendon

2.2.1 Physiological Condition and Tear

The supraspinatus tendon consists morphologically of two subregions, anterior and posterior. The anterior subregion is thick and tubular and the posterior is thin and strap like. Matsuhashi et al. [33] compared the structural and mechanical properties of the anterior and posterior subregions of the supraspinatus tendon. The ultimate stresses were 22.1 MPa in the anterior subregion and 11.6 MPa in the posterior one. They recognized that the anterior and posterior subregions of the supraspinatus

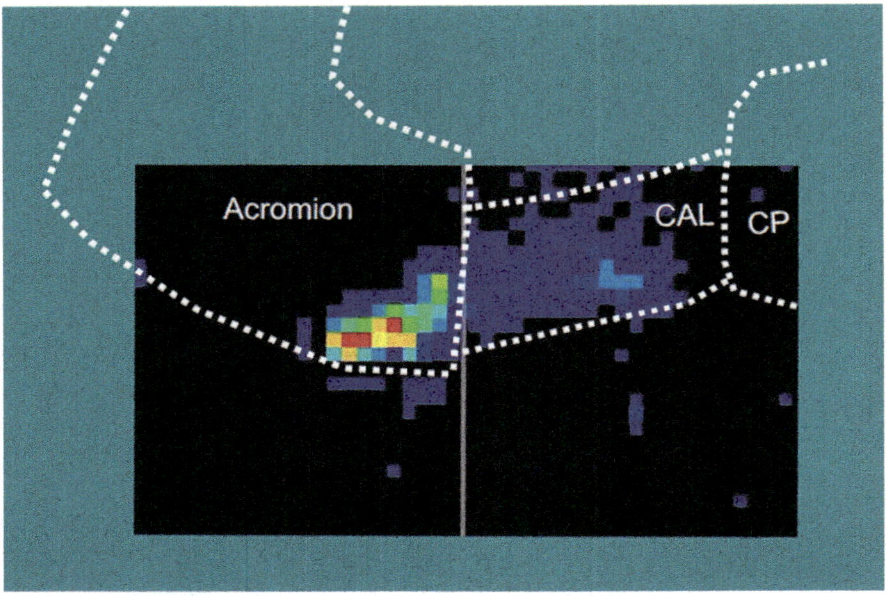

Fig. 2.4 Contact pressure beneath the coracoacromial arch. Contact pressure beneath the coracoacromial arch was measured by a flexible force sensor during various motions. The *red* color represents high pressure, and *blue* represents low pressure. *CAL* coracoacromial ligament, *CP* coracoid process

tendon have different mechanical properties, which might be related to one of the causes of rotator cuff tears.

It is well known that subacromial impingement is a common cause of shoulder pain. On the other hand, there are several biomechanical and clinical reports describing that the coracoacromial ligament contacts with the cuff tendons to restrict superior humeral head migration during motion in normal shoulders [34, 35]. Yamamoto et al. [36] evaluated this contact phenomenon quantitatively by measuring contact pressure beneath the coracoacromial arch, hypothesizing that physiological contact beneath the coracoacromial arch occurred in normal shoulders (Fig. 2.4). This study showed that contact phenomenon of the coracoacromial arch was observed during all motions. They surmised that physiological contact beneath the coracoacromial arch might be present in normal shoulders, and this repetitive contact of the coracoacromial ligament might lead to its degenerative change and proliferative acromial spurs.

With the advent of arthroscopic surgeries, more partial subscapularis tears are being recognized during surgery. Which size of partial subscapularis tears should be treated surgically? Because the biomechanical effects of partial subscapularis tears are not yet clarified, there is no consensus regarding their treatment. Yoo et al. [37] clarified the effect of various subscapularis tears (one fourth subscapularis tear; one half subscapularis tear; one half subscapularis and complete supraspinatus tear; supraspinatus repair; and supraspinatus and subscapularis repair) with the arm in 0°, 30°, and 60° of abduction. They concluded that additional repair of a partial subscapularis tear with supraspinatus tear did not affect external rotation or glenohumeral kinematics.

2.2.2 Transosseous-Equivalent Rotator Cuff Repair

The surgical techniques for rotator cuff tears has been developed from a single-row to a double-row technique. Recently, the transosseous-equivalent (TOE) repair has been widely used because surgeons believe that the TOE provides a stronger initial fixation and a better footprint coverage compared to a single-row or double-row technique. Park et al. [38] biomechanically demonstrated that the TOE repair improved contact area and pressure between the tendon and footprint when compared with a double-row technique. Spang et al. [39], in a sheep model, studied that two double-row techniques, the one with corkscrew suture anchors for the medial row and insertion anchors for the lateral row and the other with insertion anchors for both the medial and lateral rows, both provided excellent biomechanical profiles. There are some modifications of TOE repair. Among them, whether to tie the medial sutures is still controversial. There are some clinical reports describing that a failure of the medial rotator cuff occurred at the site of medial-row mattress sutures [40]. To avoid retear at the medial row, some do not tie the sutures at the medial row. Maguire et al. [41] evaluated the biomechanical behavior of four variants of the TOE repair. The groups tested were (1) knotted standard transosseous-equivalent (standard TOE), transosseous-equivalent with two medial mattress stitches; (2) knotted double transosseous-equivalent (double TOE), four medial mattress stitches; (3) untied transosseous-equivalent with medial FT anchors (untied TOE with FT), two medial mattress stitches without knots; and (4) untied transosseous-equivalent with push-type anchors (untied TOE with push-type anchors), two medial mattress stitches without knots. The contact area of the footprint was measured with an electronic pressure film. They reported that the TOE repair with four stitches tied in the medial row and maximal lateral suture strand utilization (double TOE) outperformed all other repairs in terms of failure load, tendon–bone contact, and gapping characteristics. The presence of knots in the medial row did not change tendon fixation with respect to failure load, contact area, and gapping characteristics.

Several reports have clarified that although the medial tendon is reruptured, the footprint healing remains intact after TOE repair [42]. They claimed that the failure might be caused by the tension overload in the medial suture–tendon interface or possible necrosis of the cuff at the medial row caused by the strong pressure from the TOE construct. The TOE technique is expected to provide a strong initial fixation. At the same time, this rigid fixation may make the tendon less flexible and less extensible. We probably need the strong fixation for the first several months after surgery until the healing is completed. Once the healing is completed, the strong fixation is no longer necessary. Instead, normal flexibility and extensibility are more desirable. Nagamoto et al. [43] demonstrated that the TOE technique may increase the strain gap between the normal tendon and the repaired tendon, resulting in stress concentration along the medial row. The results revealed that the strain at the footprint of the tendon was extremely small, whereas the strain of the tendon at the medial row increased significantly after the TOE technique with the medial sutures tied. This increased difference in strain may lead to stress concentration at the medial row, which might be a cause of the medial reruptures observed after the TOE technique. Tying the medial row sutures seems to increase the strain difference between the proximal and distal portions of the repaired tendon.

2.3 Acromioclavicular Joint

The acromioclavicular (AC) joint capsule is quite thin, but has considerable ligamentous support; there are four AC ligaments: superior, inferior, anterior, and posterior. Several biomechanical studies have showed that horizontal stability of the AC joint is mediated by the AC ligaments whereas vertical stability is mediated by the coracoclavicular (CC) ligaments. The stabilizing mechanism of the AC joint has been extensively studied but the kinematics of the AC joint has not been clarified yet. Sahara et al. [44], in an in vivo study, analyzed the three-dimensional (3D) kinematics of the AC joint during abduction motion using 3D Magnetic Resonance (MR) images. They found that the clavicle translated most posteriorly (-1.9 ± 1.3 mm) at 90° of abduction and most anteriorly (1.6 ± 2.7 mm) at maximum abduction in the anteroposterior direction, which may be caused by the influence of the surrounding muscles (deltoid or trapezius). At 90° of abduction, the anterior component of the traction force of the deltoid muscle may have become smaller than the posterior component of the traction force of the superior trapezius, causing the clavicle to translate posteriorly. At maximum abduction, the anterior component of the traction force of the trapezius muscle may have become larger than the posterior component of the superior trapezius, causing the clavicle to translate anteriorly. We need to know this laxity of the AC joint when fixing the AC joint by using the fixation devices such as plates.

2.4 Shoulder Problems in Overhead Athletes

Baseball players, especially pitchers, who undergo superior labrum anteroposterior (SLAP) repair often have difficulty returning to their previous level of performance. Laughlin et al. [45], in an in vivo study using a 3D motion analysis system, compared pitching biomechanics between a group of collegiate and professional pitchers with a history of a SLAP tear and a control group of pitchers with no history of surgery. They found that pitchers with a history of SLAP repair produce less horizontal abduction, external rotation, and forward trunk tilt during pitching than do pitchers with no history of injury. This study showed that external rotation at 90°, horizontal abduction, and forward trunk tilt should be the primary objectives in rehabilitation after SLAP repair for pitchers to return to their previous level.

The restriction of internal rotation in abduction is believed to be one of the causes of shoulder pain in overhead athletes. Some pointed out that this reduced internal rotation might come from the posterior capsule tightness because the superoanterior migration of the humeral head occurred during shoulder flexion [46, 47]. Muraki et al. [48] measured contact pressure on the coracoacromial arch during various arm motions to clarify whether the existence of the posterior tightness increased the force of contact between the coracoacromial arch and humeral head. Posterior capsule tightness was demonstrated to increase contact pressure during flexion. The peak contact pressure was observed close to the end range of flexion. These findings are useful to understand the contribution of posterior capsule tightness to subacromial contact.

References

1. Cooper RA, Brems JJ (1992) The inferior capsular-shift procedure for multidirectional instability of the shoulder. J Bone Joint Surg Am 74:1516–1521
2. Gibb TD, Sidles JA, Harryman DT II, McQuade KJ, Matsen FA III (1991) The effect of capsular venting on glenohumeral laxity. Clin Orthop Relat Res 268:120–127
3. Itoi E, Motzkin NE, Browne AO, Hoffmeyer P, Morrey BF, An KN (1993) Intraarticular pressure of the shoulder. Arthroscopy 9:406–413
4. Kumar VP, Balasubramaniam P (1985) The role of atmospheric pressure in stabilizing the shoulder: an experimental study. J Bone Joint Surg Br 67:719–721
5. Jerosch J, Castro WH (1990) Shoulder instability in Ehlers–Danlos syndrome: an indication for surgical treatment? Acta Orthop Belg 56:451–453
6. Yamamoto N, Itoi E, Tuoheti Y, Seki N, Abe H, Minagawa H, Shimada Y, Okada K (2006) The effect of the inferior capsular shift on shoulder intra-articular pressure: a cadaveric study. Am J Sports Med 34(6):939–944
7. Neer CS, Foster GR (1980) Inferior capsular shift for involuntary inferior and multidirectional instability of the shoulder. J Bone Joint Surg Am 62:897–908
8. Barkatali BM, Lea M, Aster A, Marynissen H (2014) Arthroscopic medial capsular plication using the suture anchor technique. Knee Surg Sports Traumatol Arthrosc 22(10):2513–2517
9. Ponce BA, Rosenzweig SD, Thompson KJ, Tokish J (2011) Sequential volume reduction with capsular plications: relationship between cumulative size of plications and volumetric reduction for multidirectional instability of the shoulder. Am J Sports Med 39(3):526–531
10. Shapiro TA, Gupta A, McGarry MH, Tibone JE, Lee TQ (2012) Biomechanical effects of arthroscopic capsulorrhaphy in line with the fibers of the anterior band of the inferior glenohumeral ligament. Am J Sports Med 40(3):672–680
11. Boileau P, O'Shea K, Vargas P, Pinedo M, Old J, Zumstein M (2012) Anatomical and functional results after arthroscopic Hill–Sachs remplissage. J Bone Joint Surg Am 94:618–626
12. Haviv B, Mayo L, Biggs D (2011) Outcomes of arthroscopic "remplissage:" capsulotenodesis of the engaging large Hill–Sachs lesion. J Orthop Surg Res 6:29

13. Koo SS, Burkhart SS, Ochoa E (2009) Arthroscopic double pulley remplissage technique for engaging Hill–Sachs lesions in anterior shoulder instability repairs. Arthroscopy 25:1343–1348
14. Nourissat G, Kilinc AS, Werther JR, Doursounian L (2011) A prospective, comparative, radiological, and clinical study of the influence of the "remplissage" procedure on shoulder range of motion after stabilization by arthroscopic Bankart repair. Am J Sports Med 39:2147–2152
15. Grimberg J, Diop A, Ghosn RB, Lanari D, Canonne A, Maurel N (2014) Bankart repair versus Bankart repair plus remplissage: an in vitro biomechanical comparative study. Knee Surg Sports Traumatol Arthrosc 24(2):374–380
16. Elkinson I, Giles JW, Boons HW, Faber KJ, Ferreira LM, Johnson JA, Athwal GS (2013) The shoulder remplissage procedure for Hill–Sachs defects: does technique matter? J Shoulder Elbow Surg 22(6):835–841
17. Argintar E, Heckmann N, Wang L, Tibone JE, Lee TQ (2014) The biomechanical effect of shoulder remplissage combined with Bankart repair for the treatment of engaging Hill–Sachs lesions. Knee Surg Sports Traumatol Arthrosc 24(2):585–592
18. Elkinson I, Giles JW, Faber KJ, Boons HW, Ferreira LM, Johnson JA, Athwal GS (2012) The effect of the remplissage procedure on shoulder stability and range of motion: an in vitro biomechanical assessment. J Bone Joint Surg Am 94(11):1003–1012
19. Degen RM, Giles JW, Johnson JA, Athwal GS (2014) Remplissage versus latarjet for engaging Hill–Sachs defects without substantial glenoid bone loss: a biomechanical comparison. Clin Orthop Relat Res 472(8):2363–2371
20. Giles JW, Elkinson I, Ferreira LM, Faber KJ, Boons H, Litchfield R, Johnson JA, Athwal GS (2012) Moderate to large engaging Hill–Sachs defects: an in vitro biomechanical comparison of the remplissage procedure, allograft humeral head reconstruction, and partial resurfacing arthroplasty. J Shoulder Elbow Surg 21(9):1142–1151
21. Omi R, Hooke AW, Zhao KD, Matsuhashi T, Goto A, Yamamoto N, Sperling JW, Steinmann SP, Itoi E, An KN (2014) The effect of the remplissage procedure on shoulder range of motion: a cadaveric study. Arthroscopy 30(2):178–187
22. Walch G, Boileau P (2000) Latarjet-Bristow procedure for recurrent anterior instability. Tech Shoulder Elbow Surg 1(4):256–261
23. Edwards TB, Boulahia A, Kempf JF, Boileau P, Nemoz C, Walch G (2002) The influence of rotator cuff disease on the results of shoulder arthroplasty for primary osteoarthritis: results of a multicenter study. J Bone Joint Surg Am 84(12):2240–2248
24. Giles JW, Degen RM, Johnson JA, Athwal GS (2014) The Bristow and Latarjet procedures: why these techniques should not be considered synonymous. J Bone Joint Surg Am 96 (16):1340–1348
25. Nourissat G, Delaroche C, Bouillet B, Doursounian L, Aim F (2014) Optimization of bone-block positioning in the Bristow-Latarjet procedure: a biomechanical study. Orthop Traumatol Surg Res 100(5):509–513
26. Burkhart SS, De Beer JF, Barth JR, Cresswell T, Roberts C, Richards DP (2007) Results of modified Latarjet reconstruction in patients with anteroinferior instability and significant bone loss. Arthroscopy 23(10):1033–1041
27. Arrigoni P, Huberty D, Brady PC, Weber IC, Burkhart SS (2008) The value of arthroscopy before an open modified latarjet reconstruction. Arthroscopy 24(5):514–519, Epub 2008 Feb 01
28. Weaver JK, Derkash RS (1994) Don't forget the Bristow-Latarjet procedure. Clin Orthop Relat Res 308:102–110
29. Patte D, Bernageau J (1988) Epaules douloureuses par accidents d'instabilités inapparents (EDI). Rev Chir Orthop 74:259–263, suppl. II
30. Patte D (n.d.) Traitement chirurgical des instabilités de l'épaule Luxations récidivantes de l'épaule. EMC Paris, 44–265. 4-5-04

31. Yamamoto N, Muraki T, An KN, Sperling JW, Cofield RH, Itoi E, Walch G, Steinmann SP (2013) The stabilizing mechanism of the latarjet procedure: a cadaveric study. J Bone Joint Surg Am 95(15):1390–1397
32. Bhatia S, Van Thiel GS, Gupta D, Ghodadra N, Cole BJ, Bach BR Jr, Shewman E, Wang VM, Romeo AA, Verma NN, Provencher MT (2013) Comparison of glenohumeral contact pressures and contact areas after glenoid reconstruction with latarjet or distal tibial osteochondral allografts. Am J Sports Med 41(8):1900–1908
33. Matsuhashi T, Hooke AW, Zhao KD, Goto A, Sperling JW, Steinmann SP, An KN (2014) Tensile properties of a morphologically split supraspinatus tendon. Clin Anat 27(5):702–706
34. Wiley AM (1991) Superior humeral dislocation. A complication following decompression and debridement for rotator cuff tears. Clin Orthop Relat Res 263:135–141
35. Burns WC II, Whipple TL (1993) Anatomic relationships in the shoulder impingement syndrome. Clin Orthop Relat Res 294:96–102
36. Yamamoto N, Muraki T, Sperling JW, Steinmann SP, Itoi E, Cofield RH, An KN (2010) Contact between the coracoacromial arch and the rotator cuff tendons in nonpathologic situations: a cadaveric study. J Shoulder Elbow Surg 19(5):681–687
37. Yoo JC, McGarry M, Jun BJ, Scott J, Lee TQ (2014) The influence of partial subscapularis tendon tears combined with supraspinatus tendon tears. J Shoulder Elbow Surg 23(6):902–908
38. Park MC, ElAttrache NS, Tibone JE, Ahmad CS, Jun B, Lee TQ (2007) Part I: footprint contact characteristics for a transosseous-equivalent rotator cuff repair technique compared with a double-row repair technique. J Shoulder Elbow Surg 16(4):461–468
39. Spang JT, Buchmann SN, Brucker PU, Kouloumentas P, Obst T, Schröder M, Burgkart R, Imhoff AB (2009) A biomechanical comparison of 2 transosseous-equivalent double-row rotator cuff repair techniques using bioabsorbable anchors: cyclic loading and failure behavior. Arthroscopy 25(8):872–879
40. Kim KC, Shin HD, Cha SM, Park JY (2014) Comparisons of retear patterns for 3 arthroscopic rotator cuff repair methods. Am J Sports Med 42(3):558–565
41. Maguire M, Goldberg J, Bokor D, Bertollo N, Pelletier MH, Harper W, Walsh WR (2011) Biomechanical evaluation of four different transosseous-equivalent/suture bridge rotator cuff repairs. Knee Surg Sports Traumatol Arthrosc 19(9):1582–1587
42. Rhee YG, Cho NS, Parke CS (2012) Arthroscopic rotator cuff repair using modified Mason–Allen medial row stitch: knotless versus knot-tying suture bridge technique. Am J Sports Med 40(11):2440–2447
43. Nagamoto H, Kawakami J, Yamamoto N, Shiota Y, Mineta M, Itoi E (2015) Strain of the tendon after tranosseous equivalent repair: a cadaveric study presented at the Orthopaedic Research Society meeting, Las Vegas, 28 March–1 April 2015
44. Sahara W, Sugamoto K, Murai M, Tanaka H, Yoshikawa H (2006) 3D kinematic analysis of the acromioclavicular joint during arm abduction using vertically open MR. J Orthop Res 24 (9):1823–1831
45. Laughlin WA, Fleisig GS, Scillia AJ, Aune KT, Cain EL Jr, Dugas JR (2014) Deficiencies in pitching biomechanics in baseball players with a history of superior labrum anterior-posterior repair. Am J Sports Med 42(12):2837–2841
46. Burkhart SS, Morgan CD, Kibler WB (2003) The disabled throwing shoulder: spectrum of pathology. Part I: pathoanatomy and biomechanics. Arthroscopy 19:404–420
47. Grossman MG, Tibone JE, McGarry MH, Schneider DJ, Veneziani S, Lee TQ (2005) A cadaveric model of the throwing shoulder: a possible etiology of superior labrum anterior-to-posterior lesions. J Bone Joint Surg Am 87:824–831
48. Muraki T, Yamamoto N, Zhao KD, Sperling JW, Steinmann SP, Cofield RH, An KN (2012) Effects of posterior capsule tightness on subacromial contact behavior during shoulder motions. J Shoulder Elbow Surg 21(9):1160–1167

Chapter 3
Kinematics and Motion Analysis

Wataru Sahara and Kazuomi Sugamoto

Abstract The shoulder girdle has a complex motion. Many researchers have taken interest in the complex motions of the shoulder and investigated it by various methodologies. We have recently been able to evaluate 3D kinematics of the shoulder with the aid of 3D motion analysis systems such as 3D motion capture system, 3D MRI, and 2D/3D registration technique. In this chapter, we summarize the advantage and disadvantage of each 3D motion analysis system and introduce the results of the shoulder kinematics previously reported.

Keywords Translation • Rotation • 3D motion capture system • 3D MRI • 2D/3D registration technique

3.1 Techniques for Analysis of Shoulder Motion

The shoulder girdle is a fundamental joint responsible for arm movement. When an upper limb is likened to a crane, the humerus is likened to the arm and the shoulder girdle to a swivel base. The shoulder girdle evolved into a complex joint with the widest range of motion for an upper limb to move into various positions. The scapula is able to widely slide on the chest wall, and the glenohumeral joint has a wide range of motion because of the decreasing coverage rate of the glenoid relative to the humeral head, which is almost one third of the articular surface of the humeral head. However, these evolutions induce less bony stability of the glenohumeral joint, and so the dynamic stabilizer such as the rotator cuff muscles

---

The online version of this chapter (doi:10.1007/978-4-431-55988-7_3) contains supplementary material, which is available to authorized users.

W. Sahara (✉)
Department of Orthopaedics, Osaka University Graduate School of Medicine, 2-2 Yamadaoka, Suita, Osaka 565-0871, Japan
e-mail: w-sahara@umin.ac.jp

K. Sugamoto
Department of Orthopaedic Biomaterial Science, Osaka University Graduate School of Medicine, Osaka, Japan

K. Tamai et al. (eds.), *Advances in Shoulder Surgery*,
DOI 10.1007/978-4-431-55988-7_3

and capsular ligaments compensate for this lesser bony stability. A correct understanding of shoulder kinematics is necessary for solving the pathogenesis and clinical condition of the shoulder problems, such as impingement syndrome, rotator cuff tears, and shoulder instability.

3.1.1 Development of Shoulder Motion Analysis

The shoulder girdle consists of the sternoclavicular, acromioclavicular, glenohumeral, and scapulothoracic joints. The integrated motions of these joints make three-dimensional complicated movements. Many researchers have taken interest in shoulder motions and investigated these by various methodologies. Codman [1] described in his textbook that understanding of the shoulder motions is difficult by palpation of the bony landmarks or X-rays. In 1944, Inman showed the relationship and contribution glenohumeral and scapulothoracic joins during arm elevation in roentgenographic observations, which is famous as the scapulohumeral rhythm [2]. Since then, X-ray has been one of the methods for in vivo motion analysis of the shoulder. On the other hand, many researchers have observed the cadaveric anatomy. The anatomic findings described by Kapandji have given us very useful information about the motion and morphology of the joints [3]. However, these methods and findings have the disadvantage that these are nonphysiological or two-dimensional (2D) motions.

The modalities such as computed tomography (CT) and magnetic resonance imaging (MRI) were developed following X-rays; these provide cross-sectional images of the joints and soft tissues. Some authors have investigated the kinematics of the labrum or capsulolabral complex during axial rotation with adducted or abducted position of the arm using MRI or MR arthrography [4–7]. Then, a few researchers performed kinematic analysis using cine-MRI during sequentially active motions of the arm [8, 9]. However, these 2D assessments of glenohumeral joint motion cannot sufficiently characterize three-dimensional (3D) motion of a joint that has six degrees of freedom including three translations and three rotations.

3.1.2 3D Motion Analysis System

Recently, the development of many medical imaging systems and computers has enabled analyzing 3D motion analysis of the shoulder. The 3D motion analysis systems mainly include the 3D motion capture system, 3D MRI, and 2D/3D registration technique.

In the analysis by the 3D motion capture system, the 3D electromagnetic tracking sensors or the optical markers are mounted on the skin of bony landmarks, and the motions of a joint are analyzed by tracking of these sensors. In 1973, the International Society of Biomechanics (ISB; web site https://isbweb.org/) was founded and recommended a standardized protocol for the kinematic analysis of the shoulder; for example, anatomic landmarks, definition of the local coordinate systems, and expression of the 3D motions [10]. Recently, high-speed video cameras permit analyzing high-speed motions, such as throwing motions [11]. This system offers several advantages. More rapid, even real-time, results can be repeatedly obtained. The arm movement is not restricted in the analyzing environments. On the other hand, this system has some disadvantages. The capture system may require the specific space in which it is operated, depending on camera field of view or magnetic distortion. Skin-mounted sensors are highly susceptible to palpation error of the bony landmarks and skin movement artifact, especially for the scapula. de Groot reported that the palpation error was less than 3°, the motoric noise was approximately 3° to 6°, and the intersubject variability was 5° to 10° [12]. Karduna et al. and Ludewig et al. demonstrated that the rotational errors of the scapular motion was less than 5° below 120° of the arm elevation whereas these errors were increased over 120° of the elevation because of skin movement artifact [13, 14]. In addition, the humeral sensor is typically mounted on a circular cuff around the upper arm. Hamming et al. [15] reported that the cuff errors were acceptable during elevation of the arm, but that these showed significantly larger errors during the axial rotation of the arm, running up to 30°. As the other disadvantage, these systems are incapable of visualizing the morphology of bones and joints. Thus, they are superior in assessing the rotational motions of the joint, but they do not provide the morphological relationship of the joint, that is, translation and contact area.

The techniques of acquisition of 3D MR images and creating of 3D surface bone models enabled precise analysis of joint motions, including morphology. In addition, the voxel-based registration technique was developed that provides 3D motion by superimposing a segmented MRI in a position on that in the other image. This technique has high accuracy with less than 0.5 mm of translational error and less than 0.5° of rotational error [16], and it has been applied to 3D kinematic analyses for in vivo human joints, such as wrist, elbow, knee, spine, and shoulder [16–24]. It has some advantages, such as high accuracy and visual understanding of joint motion. However, it has some disadvantages, such as the long time of acquisition of 3D MR images in several positions, cumbersome processing of the segmentation and registration, and the restriction of the arm position by the MRI gantry.

Recently, another technique, called the 2D/3D registration technique, was developed. In 1996, Banks and colleagues estimated the 3D positions of the femoral and tibial components after total knee arthroplasty (TKA) by superimposing the 3D surface of the components on the 2D contours of fluoroscopic images using this method [25]. Single-plane fluoroscopy [26] was previously used, but biplane fluoroscopy can now be used in kinematic analysis for patients after TKA. Then, this technique as applied to subjects without a prosthesis by creating 3D surface bone models instead of that of the prosthesis, has been used for many human joints [27–29]. In vitro validation studies for the glenohumeral joint showed that translational and rotational errors were less than 0.5 mm and 1° for in-plane motion, but these errors were 1.5–5 mm and 2°–4° for out-of-plane motion using the single-plane images [30, 31], and that the translational errors were less than 0.5 mm and the rotational errors were less than 0.6° using the biplane images [31–33]. This technique has some advantages, being capable of kinematic analysis of dynamic motion and the morphological relationship of the joint, and disadvantages such as exposure to radiation and cumbersome processing.

3.2 Description of 3D Shoulder Motion

The 3D motion of an object is often expressed using the Euler angle system and the screw axis method.

3.2.1 Euler Angles System

The Euler angles represent three translations and three rotations to describe the orientation of a local coordinate system (LCS) relative to another one. In the description of rotational parameters using the Euler angles, an object is first rotated around an axis (first rotation), then rotated around an axis rotated after the first rotation (second rotation), and finally rotated around an axis rotated after the second rotation (third rotation). For instance, when the rotational sequence consists of a first rotation around the y-axis, a second rotation around the x-axis, and a third rotation around the z-axis, this sequence is expressed as Y-X'-Z'' (Fig. 3.1). The kinds of rotational sequences are called classic Euler angles when using the first and third rotations around the same axes (e.g., Y-X'-Y''), and those of sequences are called Cardan angles when using all rotations around the different axes (e.g., Y-X'-Z''). As a note of caution, the sequence of rotations affects the results of rotational parameters [34].

The International Shoulder Group (ISG: http://www.internationalshouldergroup.org/), which is a subgroup of ISB, has recommended researchers to use the same bony landmarks, the same LCS of each bone, and the same rotational sequences as a standardized protocol for the description of shoulder motions (Fig. 3.2 and Tables 3.1 and 3.2) [10]. However, this description has a major problem, the gimbal lock problem. When the second rotation is ±90° using the Cardan angles (e.g., Y-X′-Z″) and when the second rotation is 0° or 180° using the classic Euler angles (e.g., Y-X′-Y″), the first and third rotations may be unstable because the first and third rotations occur around axes close to each other. This problem would not occur using the Cardan angles for the description of rotations of the clavicle and the scapula because the second rotations of these bones do not reach 90°. However, the gimbal lock problem would occur when the elevation angle of the humerus (second rotation) is close to 0° or 180° using the Euler angles for description of rotation of the humerus [35]; this means that the rotational results of the plane of elevation and axial rotation would be doubtful when the arm is positioned at the side or at

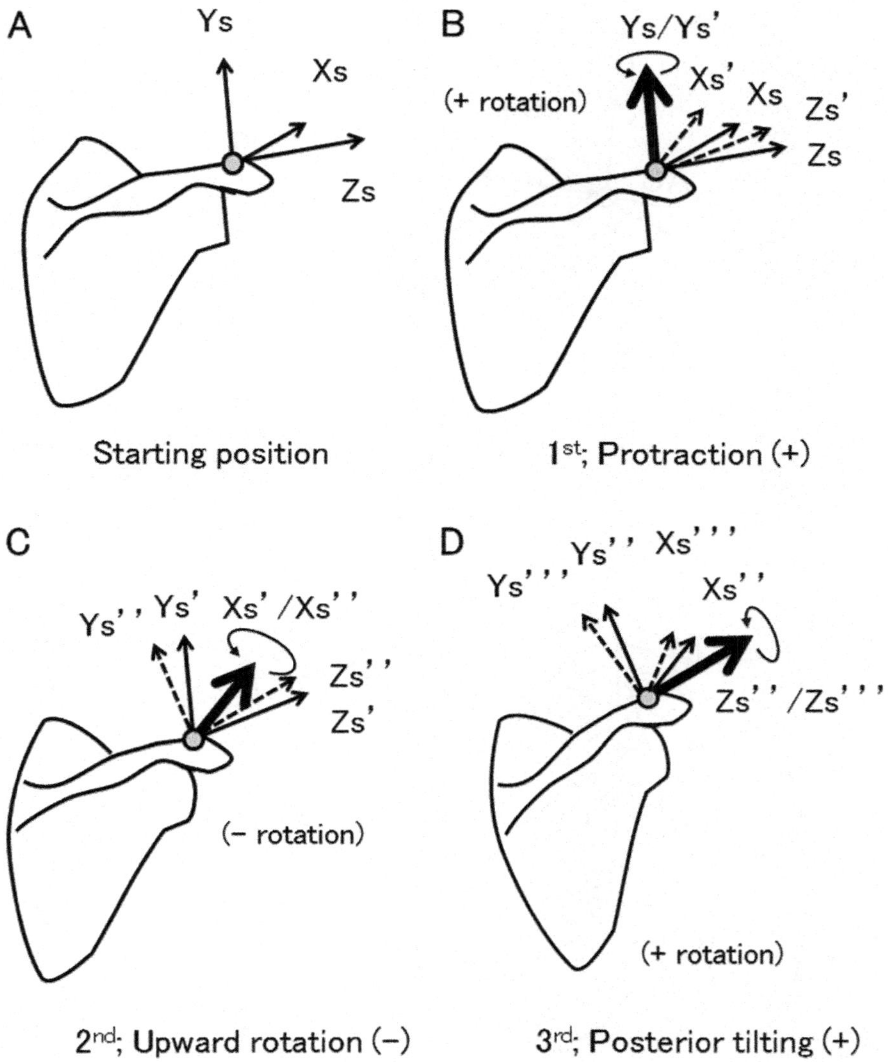

Fig. 3.1 Posterior view of right shoulder. Three-dimensional (3D) rotations around each axis of local coordinate system (LCS) of the scapula. Scapular rotation is described by the Cardan angles, Ys-Xs′-Zs″ sequence

maximum elevation. Some authors used the Cardan angles (Xh, adduction/abduction; Zh′, flexion/extension; Yh″, internal/external rotation) for the description of the humeral rotations at the glenohumeral and humerothoracic joints [36, 37]. Authors should pay attention to effects of the gimbal lock problem when the second rotation (Zh) is close to 90°, that is, the forward flexion using the Cardan angles. Senk and Cheze [38] recommended this rotational sequences for the

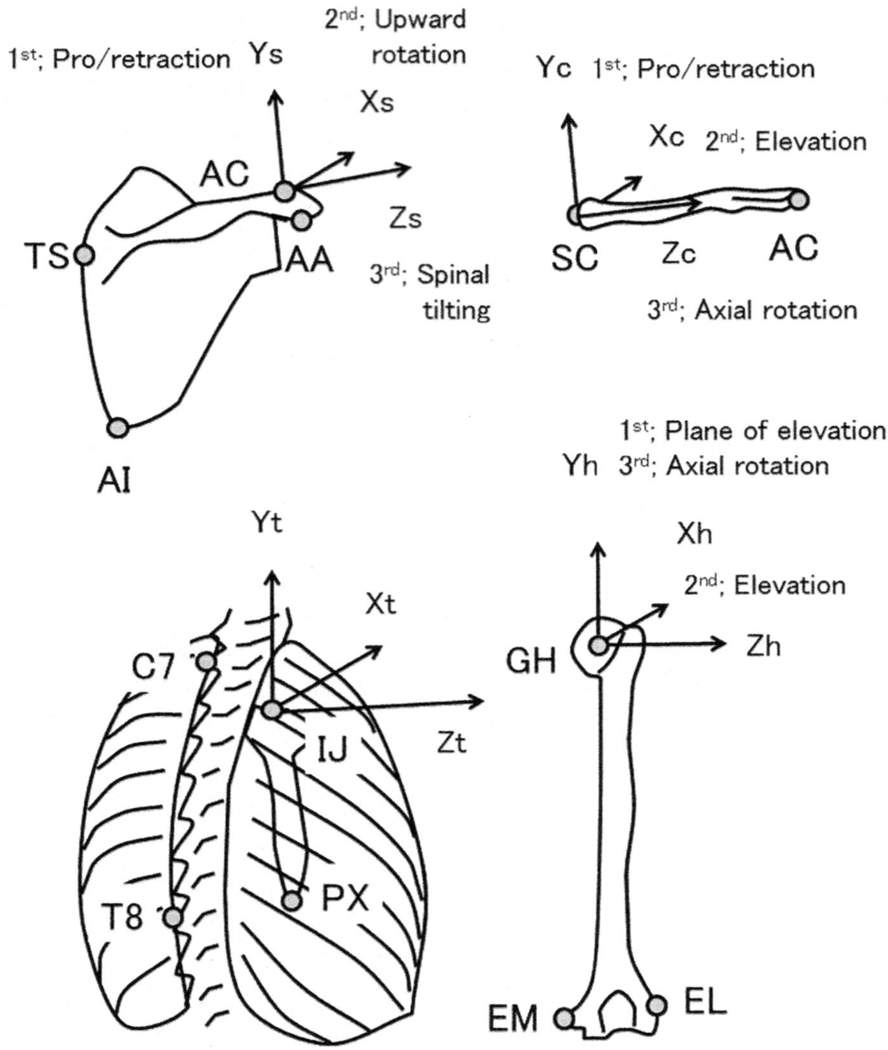

Fig. 3.2 Posterior view of right shoulder. Anatomic bony landmarks and definition of local coordinate systems

description of the glenohumeral joint and reported the results were less affected and agreed much more with the clinical angles compared with the other rotational sequences.

Table 3.1 Definition of local coordinate systems (LCS)

LCS	Axis	Definition
Thorax	Bony landmarks	IJ, incisura jugularis
		PX, processus xiphoideus
		C7, processus spinosus of 7th cervical vertebra
		T8, processus spinosus of 8th thoracic vertebra
	Origin	IJ
	Xt	Perpendicular to Yt and Zt, pointing forward
	Yt	Vector from the midpoint between PX and T8 to the midpoint between IJ and C7, pointing upward
	Zt	Perpendicular to the plane fitted to the points IJ, C7, and the midpoint between PX and T8, pointing to the right
Clavicle	Bony landmarks	SC, sternoclavicular joint
		AC, acromioclavicular joint
	Origin	SC
	Xc	Perpendicular to Zc and Yt (thoracic *y*-axis), pointing forward
	Yc	Perpendicular to Xc and Zc, pointing upward
	Zc	Vector from SC to AC, pointing laterally
Scapula	Bony landmarks	AC, acromioclavicular joint
		TS, trigonum spinae scapulae
		AI, angulus inferior
		AA, angulus acromialis
	Origin	AC
	Xs	Perpendicular to the plane consisting of AA, AI, and TS, pointing forward, i.e., perpendicular to the scapular plane
	Ys	Perpendicular to Xs and Zs, pointing upward
	Zs	Vector from TS to AA, pointing laterally
Humerus	Bony landmarks	GH, glenohumeral rotation center, estimated by regression or motion recordings
		EM, medial epicondyle
		EL, lateral epicondyle
	Origin	GH
	Xh	Perpendicular to the plane fitted to the points GH, EL, and EM, pointing forward
	Yh	Vector from the midpoint between EM and EL to GH, pointing upward
	Zh	Perpendicular to Xh and Yh, pointing laterally

3.2.2 *Screw Axis (Helical Axis)*

The displacement of an object in 3D space has a screw axis, and the movement can be decomposed into a rotation about and a translation along this screw axis, which is called the screw axis or helical axis [39]. This description method is clinically useful for the determination of the rotational axis and a rotation angle about this axis at the glenohumeral joint [40, 41]. Sahara et al. [42] reported that the

Table 3.2 Definition of order of rotations

LCS	Order	Axis	Terminology
Clavicle	1st	Yc	Protraction/retraction
	2nd	Xc	Depression/elevation
	3rd	Zc	Posterior/anterior (backward/forward) axial rotation
Scapula	1st	Ys	Protraction/retraction
	2nd	Xs	Downward/upward (medial/lateral) rotation
	3rd	Zs	Posterior/anterior spinal tilting
Humerus (classic Euler angles)	1st	Yh	Plane of elevation (+, anterior plane; −, posterior plane)
	2nd	Xh	Depression (lowering)/elevation angle
	3rd	Yh	Internal/external rotation
Humerus (Cardan angles)	1st	Xh	Adduction/abduction
	2nd	Zh	Flexion/extension
	3rd	Yh	Internal/external rotation

The former terminology means plus and the latter means minus
For the description of the humeral rotations, the classic Euler angle is recommended by the ISB [10] and the Cardan angle is recommended by Senk and Cheze [38]

acromioclavicular joint has a unique motion by calculating a position and a rotation of the screw axis at this joint as we see later in this chapter.

3.3 Shoulder Motion

3.3.1 Arm Elevation

Arm elevation, which is one of the most important movements in daily living, has been extensively studied. The motions of the arm elevation are commonly analyzed during the arm elevation in the sagittal plane (forward elevation, flexion), the coronal plane (the frontal plane, abduction), and the scapular plane (scapular abduction, scaption). This scapular plane is often defined as the 30–45° anterior plane to the coronal plane [35, 43, 44].

3.3.1.1 Scapulohumeral Rhythm in Arm Elevation

The movements of arm elevation have been evaluated by X-ray during the elevation in the coronal or scapular planes. In 1944, Inman [2] described that the ratio between the glenohumeral (GH) and scapulothoracic (SH) joints, called the scapulohumeral rhythm (SH rhythm), had a constant ratio of 2:1 above 60°of forward flexion and above 30° of abduction. Conversely, the ratio was unstable because the muscular contraction around both humerus and scapula might be unstable below these angles of elevation, which is called the setting phase. Subsequently, many researchers studied the SH rhythm. Poppen and Walker [43] reported the SH rhythm was 5:4. Freedman [45] reported this ratio became larger in the end range of elevation. Giphart et al. [46] evaluated the SH rhythm using the 2D/3D registration technique and stated that the SH rhythm ratios were different for planes of the arm elevation; the ratio was 2:1 for abduction, 1.6:1 for scaption, and 1.1:1 for forward flexion.

3.3.1.2 Motion of the Scapula in Arm Elevation

The scapula is important as the controller and stabilizer of the arm. The scapular motion is regulated by many muscles around it. The superior and inferior trapezius, the inferior part of serratus anterior, and the pectoralis minor act during upward rotation of scapula. The levator scapulae, rhomboids, and latissimus dorsi act during downward rotation. The serratus anterior and pectoralis minor act during protraction. The rhomboid, middle trapezius, and latissimus dorsi act during retraction. Many researchers have been interested in these complex motions and the function of the scapula.

Roentgenographic examinations showed the glenoid faced slightly downward at rest and the scapula rotated upward 50°–60° between 0° and 150° or maximum elevation [2, 43, 47]. Studies using the 3D electromagnetic device revealed that the upward rotation of the scapula started from 0° to 20° at rest, and totally rotated 50°–60° in all three planes of the arm elevation, that is, the sagittal, scapular, and frontal planes [34, 44, 48, 49]. Scapular protraction started from 30° to 40° at rest, gradually increased to 40°–50° at approximately 100° of forward flexion, and decreased to 15°–40°. Scapular protraction ranged from 30° to 40° during the scaption (the scapular plane abduction), which was smaller than that in forward flexion. The scapular protraction ranged from 25° to 30°during abduction, which was smaller than that during scaption. The spinal tilting of the scapula started from −10° to +5° (+ means posterior tilting) at rest, and gradually increased 20°–30° in all three planes of the arm elevation.

Some authors reported that scapular motion altered in various conditions. McClure et al. [44] compared scapular motions between elevating and lowering, and reported upward rotation of the scapula was slightly greater in lowering than in elevating. Other researchers [49, 50] stated that the protraction and posterior tilting of the scapula were larger in lowering. Comparison between dominant and nondominant sides did not show any significant differences [51, 52]. There are some reports about the effects of aging. Comparing between children and adults, children had significantly more anterior tilting and larger upward rotation of the scapula [53, 54]. Endo et al. [55] investigated the influence of aging for healthy adults and reported that the posterior tilting and the upward rotation decreased as a consequence of aging. Talkhani et al. [56] concluded that although the total range of elevation angle decreased with increasing age, the SH rhythm did not change. Then, studies for scapular kinematics on the effect of arm loading revealed that the upward rotation increased in the early range of elevation, decreased in middle range, or did not change [28, 57, 58]. Investigating the effect of elevation velocity, Michiels et al. [59] showed the ratio of SH rhythm was slightly larger in slow-speed elevation than in high speed (slow, 2.03 versus fast, 1.89). Sugamoto et al. [60] reported that the ratio stayed constant at 2.3 in low-speed elevation but that in high-speed elevation decreased from 2.7 to 1.7 with increasing elevation.

3.3.1.3 Motion at the Glenohumeral Joint in Arm Elevation

3.3.1.3.1 Rotation at the Glenohumeral Joint in Arm Elevation

The coupling motion of the humerus and scapula is not only the SH rhythm but the external rotation in the GH joint during the arm elevation. Codman [1] stated that external rotation of the humerus was required in abduction and internal rotation was required in forward flexion. Conversely, in the cadaveric study reported by Browne et al. [61], external rotation was required during arm elevation in any plane anterior to the scapular plane, and internal rotation was required for increased elevation posterior to the scapular plane.

Recently, the 3D motion analysis system was applied for in vivo kinematics of coupling motion at the GH joint. Many authors used the rotational sequence of the Euler angles recommended by the ISB (Y-X′-Y″) [46, 48]. However, the parameters of the plane of elevation and the axial rotation at the GH joint may be unstable below 20° of GH elevation angle, that is, approximately 30° of the arm elevation angle, as previously stated. In the report of Meskers et al., the plane of elevation and the axial rotation at the GH joint varied with wide ranges below 30° of arm elevation angle [the plane of elevation ranged from −50° to +150° (+ means anterior), and the axial rotation ranged from −100° to +30° (+ means internal rotation)] [48]. Recently, some authors [30, 38, 49, 62] recommended and used the Cardan angles (Y-X′-Z″) for description of the GH motions because of the smaller effect of the gimbal lock problem (Table 3.2). Phadke et al. [62] compared the rotational parameters using between the Euler angles and the Cardan angles, and reported that the plane of elevation and axial rotation showed approximately 15° and more than 20° of differences below 30° of arm elevation angle, respectively. Ludewig et al. [49] and Phadke at al. [62] directly measured the movements of the bones by insertion of pins and decomposed the rotational parameters using the Cardan angles. The GH elevation angle started from 0° to 10° and linearly increased to 85°–90° in all three planes of elevation. Flexion/extension began from 0° to 10° (+ means the flexion and anterior plane of elevation), increased to +30° at 70° of the forward flexion of the arm, and decreased to +15° at 140° of elevation angle. That value stayed constant approximately 5° during scaption, which means the humerus moved parallel to the scapular plane. The flexion/extension decreased to −20° at 80° of abduction of the arm, and increased to 0° at 140° of abduction. These findings indicated that the humerus aligns parallel to the scapular plane at the end of the arm elevation in all planes. The axial rotation started at more external positions at start of the elevation in the order to flexion, scaption, and abduction (15°, 35°, and 50°, respectively); that linearly increased during forward flexion. During scaption, that steeply increased until 40° of arm elevation and gradually increased after that. During the abduction, that increased to 65° at 40° of arm elevation, and decreased after that. The axial rotation reached 55°–65° externally at 140° of arm elevation in all planes. These results of three humeral rotations showed the interesting finding that the humerus relative to the scapula reached almost the same position at the end of arm elevation in any plane.

3.3.1.3.2 Translation at Glenohumeral Joint in Arm Elevation

The glenohumeral joint corresponds to the hip joint as compared to the low extremities. The hip joint consists of the acetabulum of the pelvis and the femoral head, which is a ball-and-socket joint. The glenohumeral joint is also assumed to be a ball-and-socket joint, but it may allow some degrees of translations because the bony stability is slightly poor. Many researchers have taken interest in the degree and pattern of translations at the GH joint during arm elevation.

Poppen and Walker [43] investigated the translations at the GH joint during scaption using the X-ray and stated that the superior translation of the humeral head was initially 3 mm below 30° of elevation and varied only 1 mm over 30° of elevation. It is considered that the muscular activity centered the humeral head relative to the glenoid below 30° of elevation, which is called the setting phase, as previously stated. Beaulieu et al. [63] evaluated the 2D coronal images during arm abduction using the vertically open MRI; the humeral head moved superiorly less than 3 mm relative to the glenoid.

Graichen et al. [64] and Sahara et al. [65] evaluated the GH movements during arm abduction using 3D open MRI and reported similar results. The humeral head translated inferiorly from +1.6–2 mm to +0.4–0.8 mm with increasing the abduction angle. It also translated anteriorly from 0–1.6 mm to +2–2.5 mm at 90° of abduction and posteriorly −1.4–0.1 mm at 150° of abduction. Graichen et al. [64] stated that the humeral head was more centered with 1 mm of variation under the condition of muscular activity. Nishinaka et al. [27] and Matsuki et al. [30] investigated the GH movements using the 2D/3D single-plane fluoroscopy registration algorithm and Giphart et al. [46] evaluated that using the biplane fluoroscopy. In the reports evaluated by the single-plane fluoroscopy, Nishinaka et al. reported the humeral head translated from −1.7 to 0 mm superiorly with increasing the arm elevation, and Matsuki et al. stated the humeral head started from −2.7 mm, translated 2.1 mm superiorly between 0° and 105° of elevation, and translated 0.9 mm inferiorly between 105° and the maximum elevation. The investigation by Giphart et al. [46] showed the superoinferior and anteroposterior translations using the biplane fluoroscopy during forward flexion, scaption, and abduction of the arm. In the superoinferior direction, the excursions (difference between maximum and minimum translations) had no significant difference among the abduction, scaption, and forward flexion (4.2 mm, 2.5 mm, and 3.0 mm, respectively), but the humeral head translated from the superior to inferior direction during abduction. In the anteroposterior direction, the excursions for all three elevations had significant differences from each other (5.1 mm, 3.6 mm, and 2.4 mm for abduction, scaption, and forward flexion, respectively). Considering these findings together, the translation for abduction may be larger and that for scaption may be smaller, although these studies were different in measurement accuracy, definition of the local coordinate system, and repeatability of the arm elevations.

3.3.1.3.3 Contact Area at Glenohumeral Joint in Arm Elevation

It has been interesting and very difficult to know the contact area between the humeral head and the glenoid in the various positions of the arm. Nobuhara [66] directly measured the contact area using cadaveric specimens and obtained the mapping of the contact areas during various glenohumeral motions (Fig. 3.3). Soslowsky et al. [67] and Warner et al. [68] also reported patterns similar to the results of Nobuhara in regard to the mapping of contact area during the glenohumeral elevation. They showed that the contact area started from the inferior part of the humeral head, shifted through the center, and ended at the superior part, and that the contact area of the glenoid face was minimum at 0° of elevation and became maximum at 120° or 180° of elevation. Therefore, these findings suggest

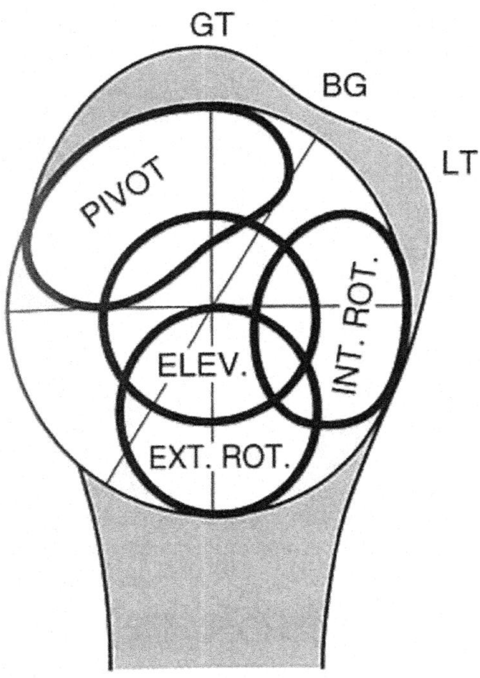

Fig. 3.3 Contact areas of the humeral head to the glenoid in various positions of the arm [66]

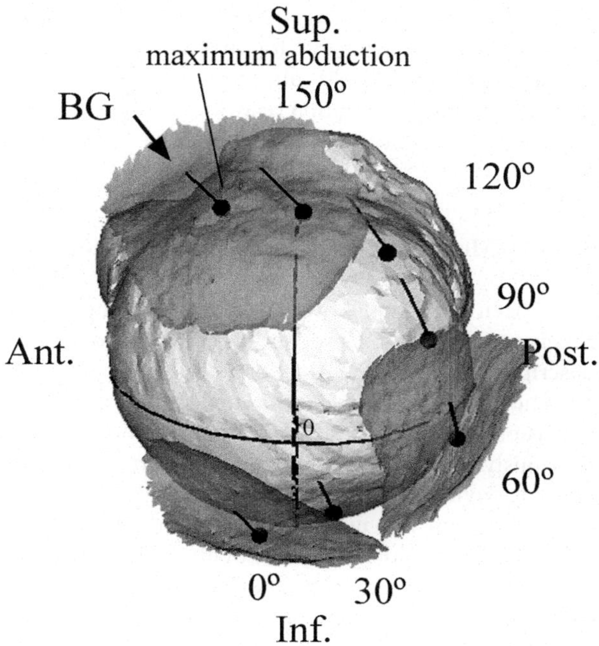

Fig. 3.4 Tracking of the glenoid movement relative to the humeral head. The semitransparent gray ellipse is the glenoid at 0°, 60°, and maximum abduction [65]

that the higher elevation of the arm may be more functional and stable position because the glenohumeral surface contact is maximum. Sahara et al. [65] used open MRI to investigate in vivo 3D motions of the glenoid relative to the humeral head during the arm abduction. They described that the glenoid started from the inferior part of the humeral head at 0° of abduction, shifted posteriorly until 60° of abduction, moved superiorly until 120° of abduction, and then moved anteriorly close the bicipital groove at 180° of abduction (Fig. 3.4 and Video 3.1).

3.3.1.3.4 Kinematics of Subacromial Space in Arm Elevation

In 1972, Neer [69] described the concept of the impingement syndrome, and many researchers have considered that the phenomenon is part of the pathogenesis of rotator cuff tears. Weiner and Macnab [70] measured the acromiohumeral interval (AHI) using X-rays, and indicated that it varied between 7 and 13 mm in normal subjects and that narrowing of this interval of less than 5 mm should be considered compatible with rotator cuff tears. Recently, some evaluated the 3D closest points in the subacromial space during arm elevation. Graichen et al. [71] reported that the 3D distance between the anterior surface of the acromion and the greater tuberosity of the humerus was minimized at 90° of abduction and external rotation. Giphart et al. [72] also described those were minimum at 83° of scaption and 97° of forward flexion. Some authors more recently stated a physiological contact under the coracoacromial arch in the normal shoulder and evaluated the deformity of the coracoacromial arch using ultrasound [73, 74]. Yanai et al. [73] revealed the physiological impingement for in vivo normal shoulders and reported that the impingement forces at 90° abduction with internal rotation, and at 90° of forward flexion with internal rotation (Hawkins test position), were significantly larger than those at 90° of abduction with neutral and external rotations.

3.3.1.4 Motion of Humerus in Arm Elevation

It has been interesting how much range of coupling motion of the humerus occurs relative to the trunk. However, it is difficult to avoid the gimbal lock problem for description of humeral rotations using the Euler angles because the humeral elevation angle varied from 0° to 180° in classic Euler angles and the flexion/extension of humerus reached 90° during forward flexion in the Cardan angles, as previously mentioned. The previous reports [35, 48] evaluated by a 3D magnetic tracking device using the classic Euler angles showed that the plane of elevation for forward flexion was unstable under 60° of elevation angle and stayed at 60°–80° over 60° of elevation. The plane of elevation for abduction stayed at approximately 0° under 120° of elevation and became unstable over that elevation angle. The external rotation occurred during both planes of elevation. For forward flexion, axial rotation was unstable under 30° of arm elevation and was almost constant in 40° of external rotation over that elevation angle. For abduction, the humerus rotated externally to 50° of external rotation at 120° of elevation, and rotated internally over that elevation angle. Xu et al. [75] created an external frame for the positioning of the various shoulder postures, which were designed to be consistent with the description of the Euler angles recommended by the ISB. They compared the three rotations of the humerus by the 3D motion tracking system and by definition of the frame. The angle difference was minimized at 30° of the arm elevation and the average was 24° below 90° of elevation, but the difference was larger than 40° over 120° of elevation angle. Researchers should pay attention to the mismatch between the clinical rotations of the humerus and the rotations described using the Euler angles.

An approach called the globe system was modified to easily understand the clinical situation based on the Euler angles recommended by the ISB [76]. In this system, the humeral rotations relative to the trunk were described in terms of latitudes and longitudes along a globe in a specified sequence. The axial rotation of humerus was defined as an angle between the latitude and the forearm in 90° of elbow flexion. On the other hand, Masuda et al. [77] proposed another description for axial rotation of the humerus called the nonsingular angle. The axial rotation of humerus, φ, was defined as $\varphi = \gamma_{h1} \cos \beta + \gamma_{h2}$, where γ_{h1} was indicated as the plane of elevation, β was indicated as the elevation angle, and γ_{h2} was indicated as the axial rotation using the classic Euler angles. This nonsingular angle of the axial rotation has an advantage in that its value is also stable below 30° of arm elevation, which is called the gimbal lock position.

3.3.1.5 Motion of the Clavicle in Arm Elevation

In the evaluation using X-ray reported by Inman et al., the clavicular elevation increased 4° for every 10° of the arm elevation below 90° of the arm elevation, but did not change above 90° [2]. In the investigation by insertion of pins into the clavicle of a living subject, the posterior axial rotation of the clavicle began to gradually increase above 50° of arm elevation and ended at 40° in the maximum elevation.

In the reports evaluated by the 3D skin-mounted electromagnetic sensors, the clavicular elevations were 10° and 15° for forward flexion and abduction, respectively, and the clavicular retractions were 30° for both arm elevations [48]. However, the clavicle axial rotation cannot be measured directly, as this system tracks only two bony landmarks: the acromioclavicular and sternoclavicular joints. Therefore, the authors assumed that the axial rotations of the clavicle mainly moved at the sternoclavicular joint and then estimated by minimizing the rotations at the acromioclavicular joint. Thus, the posterior axial rotations were 60° for both arm elevations in their reports. Some authors recently measured the 3D movements of the clavicle including the axial rotation by insertion of pins into the bones [44, 49]. Although the angle of arm elevation ranged from 15° to 140° because of restriction of the motions by the pins, the elevation, retraction, and posterior axial rotation of the clavicle increased 6°, 23°, and 30° during forward flexion, respectively. Regarding the differences of elevation planes of the arm, the clavicular elevation for the abduction were larger for the flexion and scaption, the clavicular retraction were sequentially larger for abduction, scaption, and flexion, and the posterior axial rotations had no significant difference. Sahara et al. [78] evaluated the clavicular motions using the 3D open MRI, and reported similar results, that the clavicular elevation, retraction, and posterior axial rotation were 10°, 30°, and 30°, respectively.

3.3.1.6 Motion in the Acromioclavicular Joint in Arm Elevation

Inman et al. [2] evaluated angles between the clavicle and the scapular spine during the forward flexion and abduction using X-ray. The angles mainly increased between 30° and 135° of both arm elevations and totally increased 20°. The evaluation of the 3D motions at the acromioclavicular joint (AC joint) using 3D skin-mounted electromagnetic sensors showed that the upward rotation of the scapula relative to the clavicle was approximately 0° for forward flexion and abduction, the protraction was 20° for both elevations, and the spinal tilting was estimated at 0°, as previously mentioned [48]. Recent 3D measurements by the insertion of pins reported the upward rotation, protraction, and posterior spinal tilting increased 11°, 8°, and 19° during the forward flexion, respectively [49]. The protraction only had significant differences among the planes of arm elevation, and that for flexion was larger than for the scaption and abduction. Sahara et al. [78] reported similar results evaluated by the 3D open MRI. These findings suggested that the AC joint has a quite large rotation during arm elevation.

Regarding translations at the AC joint, previous cadaveric studies showed that the AC joint had 7–10 mm and 4–6 mm of anteroposterior and superoinferior translations, respectively [79–81]. Sahara et al. [42] and Seo et al. [82] evaluated translations in the AC joint during arm abduction using open MRI and 3D CT, respectively. They reported the similar results of translations: the distal clavicle translated posteriorly relative to the acromion at 60° and 90° of abduction and it translated anteriorly at the maximum abduction. The AC joint might have 3–6 mm of excursion in the anteroposterior direction. On the other hand, the superoinferior translation varied within 1 mm during the abduction. Kim et al. [83] evaluated 3D motions of the AC joint for patients with AC dislocation or distal clavicular fracture treated by hook plate. They reported that the rotations of the distal clavicle relative to the acromion were 16° smaller in the operated side compared with unaffected side (11° versus 27°, respectively). The anteroposterior translations were 2.2 mm larger in the operated side (7.2 mm versus 5.1 mm, respectively). These findings suggested that the surgeons should pay attention to a quite large restriction of the physiological motions at the AC joint using the hook plane.

In an interesting report, Kapandji described the scapula rotated relative to the clavicle around the axis passing through the AC joint from cadaveric observations [3]. Sahara et al. [42] elucidated the in vivo rotational axis at the AC joint using the screw axis method. The scapula rotated 35° around a specific axis passing through the insertions of both AC and coracoclavicular (CC) ligaments on the coracoid process (Fig. 3.5 and Video 3.2). Seo et al. [82] recently demonstrated change of the CC

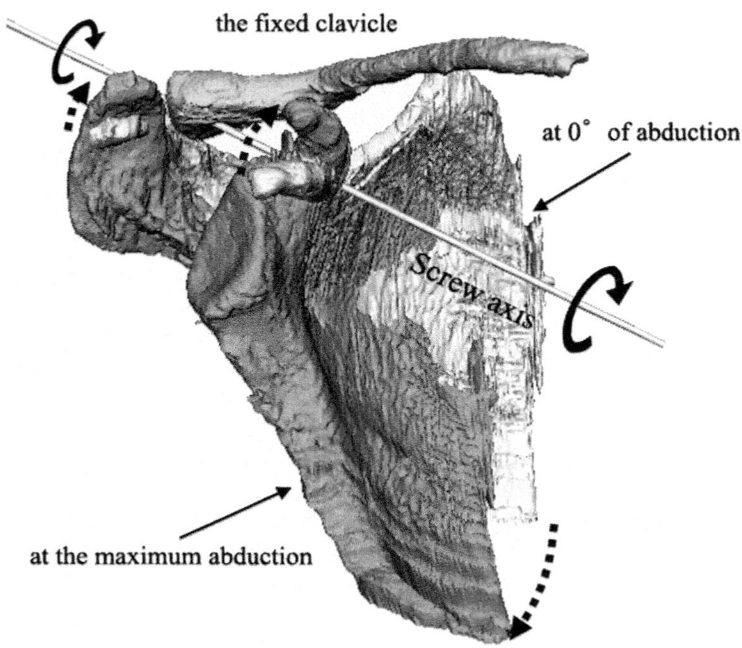

Fig. 3.5 Scapular rotation relative to the clavicle around the screw axis, passing through the acromioclavicular joint and coracoid attachment site of the coracoclavicular ligament [42]

ligament using a 3D finite-element model based on CT images. They reported that the conoid ligament was gradually elongated at 60°–120° of the arm abduction, whereas the trapezoid ligament was relatively consistent and then lax at maximum abduction. These findings suggested that the AC joint would be constrained by both AC and CC ligaments, and the scapula would rotate hanging down from the clavicle.

3.3.2 Axial Rotation with Abducted Position

The kinematics of the shoulder during axial rotation with abducted position should be important to elucidate the pathogenesis of traumatic shoulder instability and shoulder injuries in overhead sports. The knowledge about translations in the GH joint, and the functions and constraint effects of the glenohumeral ligaments, might lead to the elucidation of this pathogenesis.

3.3.2.1 Motion in Glenohumeral Joint in Abducted Rotations

Howell et al. [84] obtained axillary roentgenography in the horizontal plane of motion based on throwing motion. They reported that the humeral head was centered in the glenoid throughout the horizontal plane of motion, except the late cocking position, in normal subjects, whereas more than half of patients with shoulder anterior instability had anterior translations. Schiffern et al. [85] evaluated the translation of the humeral head during axial rotation with 35° of scapular plane abduction using open MRI. They stated that the humeral head center relative to the glenoid center was positioned 0.1 mm anteriorly in the midrange of axial rotation, but 3.1 mm posteriorly at 60° of external rotation. The measurement of translations by 3D MRI in traumatic shoulder instability also revealed a significant anterior translation of the humeral head in the affected side compared with the unaffected side at external rotation with 90° of abduction (3.6 mm versus 0.7 mm, respectively) [86]. These results suggested that external rotation with abduction would be the most adequate position for quantification of the stabilizing effect in the GH joint.

Koishi et al. [87] evaluated the contribution in rotations of the GH joint against total rotation arc during axial rotation with 90° of abduction using a wide-gantry MRI. They reported that the GH joint mainly contributed in rotations between 90° of external rotation and 60° of internal rotation with abduction.

On the other hand, an engaged Hill–Sachs lesion was reported as a risk factor for recurrence after Bankart repair. Yamamoto et al. [88] investigated tracking of the glenoid on the articular surface of the humeral head, called the glenoid track, during arm abduction with maximum external rotation in a cadaveric study to clarify the degree of the size of the Hill–Sachs lesion. Omori et al. [89] evaluated this in vivo glenoid track in healthy subjects using a wide-gantry MRI and reported their results were consistent with the cadaveric study. The glenoid track indicated a zone of contact along the rim of the humeral head, and its anterior rim was located at 84 %

of the glenoid width from the attachment site of the greater tuberosity of the rotator cuff. In their concept of the glenoid track, if the Hill–Sachs lesion is located within the glenoid track, it does not engage with the glenoid, whereas there is a risk of the engagement if the Hill–Sachs lesion extends more medially than the glenoid track.

3.4 Kinematics of Glenohumeral Ligaments

The stability of the GH joint consists of static and dynamic elements (for details, see Chap. 2, Biomechanics). The static elements are divided to contributions of the bone and soft tissues. The congruency of the GH joint [90, 91], the scapular inclination, and the intraarticular pressure [92, 93] are included in the bony elements of stability. The labrum [94–96], glenohumeral ligaments [97–99], and coracohumeral ligament (CHL) are included in the soft tissue elements. The kinematics of the soft tissues is described in this chapter.

Turkel et al. [100] inserted radiopaque markers into the glenohumeral ligaments of the cadaveric shoulders and demonstrated the kinematics of the glenohumeral ligaments during various positions of abduction and external rotation. Yang et al. [101] evaluated changes of length of glenohumeral ligaments during arm abduction in healthy subjects using open MRI and reported that the anterior and posterior bands of CHL showed maximum length at 60° and 0° of abduction, respectively. The superior, middle, and anterior band of inferior glenohumeral ligaments (SGHL, MGHL, and AB of IGHL) showed maximum length at 30°, 60°, and 120° of abduction, respectively. Shibano et al. [102] measured changes of length of AB of IGHL during axial rotation with 90° of abduction and reported that its length gradually increased from neutral rotation with abduction and was maximized at 90° external rotation with abduction. Massimini et al. [103] analyzed the kinematics of these ligaments during 0°, 45°, and 90° of abduction with neutral rotation and axial rotation with 90° of abduction using the 2D/3D biplane registration technique. They reported that the SGHL showed maximum length at 45° of abduction, the MGHL showed maximum length at 45° of abduction and maximum external rotation with 90° of abduction, and the anterior and posterior bands of IGHL showed maximum length at maximum external and internal rotations with 90° of abduction, respectively. These findings suggested that the SGHL and MGHL might contribute to joint stability in the mid-range and AB of IGHL might contribute in the end-range of motion.

References

1. Codman EA (1984) Chapter 2: Normal motions of the shoulder joint. In: The shoulder: rupture of the supraspinatus tendon and other lesions in or about the subacromial bursa. G. Miller & Co. Medical Publishers, Inc, New York, pp 32–64

2. Inman VT, Saunders JB, Abbott LC (1944) Observations of the function of the shoulder joint. J Bone Joint Surg 26:1–30
3. Kapandji IA (1985) Chapter 1: the shoulder. In: Ogishima H, Shimada T (eds) The physiology of the joints, vol 1, 5th edn. Ishiyaku Publishers, Inc, Tokyo, pp 10–77
4. Rafii M, Firooznia H, Golimbu C et al (1986) CT arthrography of capsular structures of the shoulder. AJR Am J Roentgenol 146:361–367
5. Coumas JM, Waite RJ, Goss TP et al (1992) CT and MR evaluation of the labral capsular ligamentous complex of the shoulder. AJR Am J Roentgenol 158:591–597
6. Sans N, Richardi G, Railhac JJ et al (1996) Kinematic MR imaging of the shoulder: normal patterns. AJR Am J Roentgenol 167:1517–1522
7. Tokuda O, Kunihiro Y, Matsunaga N (2002) Kinematic MRI of the normal shoulder using a specially designed positioning device. J Comput Assist Tomogr 26:849–854
8. Bonutti PM, Norfray JF, Friedman RJ et al (1993) Kinematic MRI of the shoulder. J Comput Assist Tomogr 17:666–669
9. Allmann KH, Uhl M, Gufler H et al (1997) Cine-MR imaging of the shoulder. Acta Radiol 38:1043–1046
10. Wu G, van der Helm FC, Veeger HE et al (2005) ISB recommendation on definitions of joint coordinate systems of various joints for the reporting of human joint motion. Part II: shoulder, elbow, wrist and hand. J Biomech 38:981–992
11. Takagi Y, Oi T, Tanaka H et al (2014) Increased horizontal shoulder abduction is associated with an increase in shoulder joint load in baseball pitching. J Shoulder Elbow Surg 23:1757–1762
12. de Groot JH (1997) The variability of shoulder motions recorded by means of palpation. Clin Biomech 12:461–472
13. Karduna AR, McClure PW, Michener LA et al (2001) Dynamic measurements of three-dimensional scapular kinematics: a validation study. J Biomech Eng 123:184–190
14. Ludewig PM, Behrens SA, Meyer SM et al (2004) Three-dimensional clavicular motion during arm elevation: reliability and descriptive data. J Orthop Sports Phys Ther 34:140–149
15. Hamming D, Braman JP, Phadke V et al (2012) The accuracy of measuring glenohumeral motion with a surface humeral cuff. J Biomech 45:1161–1168
16. Ishii T, Mukai Y, Hosono N et al (2004) Kinematics of the upper cervical spine in rotation: in vivo three-dimensional analysis. Spine 29:E139–E144
17. Moritomo H, Goto A, Sato Y et al (2003) The triquetrum-hamate joint: an anatomic and in vivo three-dimensional kinematic study. J Hand Surg [Am] 28:797–805
18. Goto A, Moritomo H, Murase T et al (2004) In vivo elbow biomechanical analysis during flexion: three-dimensional motion analysis using magnetic resonance imaging. J Shoulder Elbow Surg 13:441–447
19. Moritomo H, Murase T, Goto A et al (2006) In vivo three-dimensional kinematics of the midcarpal joint of the wrist. J Bone Joint Surg Am 88:611–621
20. Oka K, Doi K, Suzuki K et al (2006) In vivo three-dimensional motion analysis of the forearm with radioulnar synostosis treated by the Kanaya procedure. J Orthop Res 24:1028–1035
21. Fujii R, Sakaura H, Mukai Y et al (2007) Kinematics of the lumbar spine in trunk rotation: in vivo three-dimensional analysis using magnetic resonance imaging. Eur Spine J 16:1867–1874
22. Fujimori T, Iwasaki M, Nagamoto Y et al (2012) Kinematics of the thoracic spine in trunk rotation: in vivo 3-dimensional analysis. Spine 37:E1318–E1328
23. Fujimori T, Iwasaki M, Nagamoto Y et al (2012) Three-dimensional measurement of intervertebral range of motion in ossification of the posterior longitudinal ligament: are there mobile segments in the continuous type? J Neurosurg Spine 17:74–81
24. Nagamoto Y, Ishii T, Iwasaki M et al (2012) Three-dimensional motion of the uncovertebral joint during head rotation. J Neurosurg Spine 17:327–333
25. Banks SA, Hodge WA (1996) Accurate measurement of three-dimensional knee replacement kinematics using single-plane fluoroscopy. IEEE Trans Biomed Eng 43:638–649

26. Yamazaki T, Watanabe T, Nakajima Y et al (2004) Improvement of depth position in 2-D/3-D registration of knee implants using single-plane fluoroscopy. IEEE Trans Med Imaging 23:602–612
27. Nishinaka N, Tsutsui H, Mihara K et al (2008) Determination of in vivo glenohumeral translation using fluoroscopy and shape-matching techniques. J Shoulder Elbow Surg 17:319–322
28. Kon Y, Nishinaka N, Gamada K et al (2008) The influence of handheld weight on the scapulohumeral rhythm. J Shoulder Elbow Surg 17:943–946
29. Matsuki K, Matsuki KO, Mu S et al (2011) In vivo 3-dimensional analysis of scapular kinematics: comparison of dominant and nondominant shoulders. J Shoulder Elbow Surg 20:659–665
30. Matsuki K, Matsuki KO, Yamaguchi S et al (2012) Dynamic in vivo glenohumeral kinematics during scapular plane abduction in healthy shoulders. J Orthop Sports Phys Ther 42:96–104
31. Zhu Z, Massimini DF, Wang G et al (2012) The accuracy and repeatability of an automatic 2D-3D fluoroscopic image-model registration technique for determining shoulder joint kinematics. Med Eng Phys 34:1303–1309
32. Bey MJ, Zauel R, Brock SK et al (2006) Validation of a new model-based tracking technique for measuring three-dimensional, in vivo glenohumeral joint kinematics. J Biomech Eng 128:604–609
33. Massimini DF, Warner JJ, Li G (2011) Non-invasive determination of coupled motion of the scapula and humerus: an in-vitro validation. J Biomech 44:408–412
34. Karduna AR, McClure PW, Michener LA (2000) Scapular kinematics: effects of altering the Euler angle sequence of rotations. J Biomech 33:1063–1068
35. Stokdijk M, Eilers PH, Nagels J et al (2003) External rotation in the glenohumeral joint during elevation of the arm. Clin Biomech 18:296–302
36. Ludewig PM, Cook TM (2000) Alterations in shoulder kinematics and associated muscle activity in people with symptoms of shoulder impingement. Phys Ther 80:276–291
37. Rundquist PJ, Anderson DD, Guanche CA et al (2003) Shoulder kinematics in subjects with frozen shoulder. Arch Phys Med Rehabil 84:1473–1479
38. Senk M, Cheze L (2006) Rotation sequence as an important factor in shoulder kinematics. Clin Biomech 21:S3–S8
39. Kinzel GL, Hall AS Jr, Hillberry BM (1972) Measurement of the total motion between two body segments. I. Analytical development. J Biomech 5:93–105
40. Panjabi MM, Krag MH, Goel VK (1981) A technique for measurement and description of three-dimensional six degree-of-freedom motion of a body joint with an application to the human spine. J Biomech 14:447–460
41. Morrey BF, Itoi E, An KN (1998) Biomechanics of the shoulder. In: Rockwood CA, Matsen FA (eds) The shoulder, vol 1, 2nd edn. WB Saunders Company, Philadelphia, pp 233–276
42. Sahara W, Sugamoto K, Murai M et al (2006) 3D kinematic analysis of the acromioclavicular joint during arm abduction using vertically open MRI. J Orthop Res 24:1823–1831
43. Poppen NK, Walker PS (1976) Normal and abnormal motion of the shoulder. J Bone Joint Surg Am 58:195–201
44. McClure PW, Michener LA, Sennett BJ et al (2001) Direct 3-dimensional measurement of scapular kinematics during dynamic movements in vivo. J Shoulder Elbow Surg 10:269–277
45. Freedman L, Munro RR (1966) Abduction of the arm in the scapular plane: scapular and glenohumeral movements. A roentgenographic study. J Bone Joint Surg Am 48:1503–1510
46. Giphart JE, Brunkhorst JP, Horn NH et al (2013) Effect of plane of arm elevation on glenohumeral kinematics: a normative biplane fluoroscopy study. J Bone Joint Surg Am 95:238–245
47. Bagg SD, Forrest WJ (1988) A biomechanical analysis of scapular rotation during arm abduction in the scapular plane. Am J Phys Med Rehabil 67:238–245

48. Meskers CG, Vermeulen HM, de Groot JH et al (1998) 3D shoulder position measurements using a six-degree-of-freedom electromagnetic tracking device. Clin Biomech 13:280–292
49. Ludewig PM, Phadke V, Braman JP et al (2009) Motion of the shoulder complex during multiplanar humeral elevation. J Bone Joint Surg Am 91:378–389
50. Borstad JD, Ludewig PM (2002) Comparison of scapular kinematics between elevation and lowering of the arm in the scapular plane. Clin Biomech 17:650–659
51. Yoshizaki K, Hamada J, Tamai K et al (2009) Analysis of the scapulohumeral rhythm and electromyography of the shoulder muscles during elevation and lowering: comparison of dominant and nondominant shoulders. J Shoulder Elbow Surg 18:756–763
52. Yano Y, Hamada J, Tamai K et al (2010) Different scapular kinematics in healthy subjects during arm elevation and lowering: glenohumeral and scapulothoracic patterns. J Shoulder Elbow Surg 19:209–215
53. Dayanidhi S, Orlin M, Kozin S et al (2005) Scapular kinematics during humeral elevation in adults and children. Clin Biomech 20:600–606
54. Habechian FA, Fornasari GG, Sacramento LS et al (2014) Differences in scapular kinematics and scapulohumeral rhythm during elevation and lowering of the arm between typical children and healthy adults. J Electromyogr Kinesiol 24:78–83
55. Endo K, Yukata K, Yasui N (2004) Influence of age on scapulo-thoracic orientation. Clin Biomech 19:1009–1013
56. Talkhani IS, Kelly CP (2001) Movement analysis of asymptomatic normal shoulders: a preliminary study. J Shoulder Elbow Surg 10:580–584
57. McQuade KJ, Smidt GL (1998) Dynamic scapulohumeral rhythm: the effects of external resistance during elevation of the arm in the scapular plane. J Orthop Sports Phys Ther 27:125–133
58. de Groot JH, van Woensel W, van der Helm FC (1999) Effect of different arm loads on the position of the scapula in abduction postures. Clin Biomech 14:309–314
59. Michiels I, Grevenstein J (1995) Kinematics of shoulder abduction in the scapular plane on the influence of abduction velocity and external load. Clin Biomech 10:137–143
60. Sugamoto K, Harada T, Machida A et al (2002) Scapulohumeral rhythm: relationship between motion velocity and rhythm. Clin Orthop 401:119–124
61. Browne AO, Hoffmeyer P, Tanaka S et al (1990) Glenohumeral elevation studied in three dimensions. J Bone Joint Surg Br 72:843–845
62. Phadke V, Braman JP, LaPrade RF et al (2011) Comparison of glenohumeral motion using different rotation sequences. J Biomech 44:700–705
63. Beaulieu CF, Hodge DK, Bergman AG et al (1999) Glenohumeral relationships during physiologic shoulder motion and stress testing: initial experience with open MR imaging and active imaging-plane registration. Radiology 212:699–705
64. Graichen H, Stammberger T, Bonel H et al (2000) Glenohumeral translation during active and passive elevation of the shoulder: a 3D open-MRI study. J Biomech 33:609–613
65. Sahara W, Sugamoto K, Murai M et al (2007) The three-dimensional motions of glenohumeral joint under semi-loaded condition during arm abduction using vertically open MRI. Clin Biomech 22:304–312
66. Nobuhara K (2012) Biomechanics of the shoulder. In: Nobuhara K (ed) The shoulder: its function and clinical aspects, 4th edn. Igaku-Shoin Ltd, Tokyo, pp 47–83
67. Soslowsky LJ, Flatow EL, Bigliani LU et al (1992) Quantitation of in situ contact areas at the glenohumeral joint: a biomechanical study. J Orthop Res 10:524–534
68. Warner JJ, Bowen MK, Deng XH et al (1998) Articular contact patterns of the normal glenohumeral joint. J Shoulder Elbow Surg 7:381–388
69. Neer CS 2nd (1972) Anterior acromioplasty for the chronic impingement syndrome in the shoulder: a preliminary report. J Bone Joint Surg Am 54:41–50
70. Weiner DS, Macnab I (1970) Superior migration of the humeral head. A radiological aid in the diagnosis of tears of the rotator cuff. J Bone Joint Surg Br 52:524–527

71. Graichen H, Bonel H, Stammberger T et al (1999) Subacromial space width changes during abduction and rotation: a 3-D MR imaging study. Surg Radiol Anat 21:59–64
72. Giphart JE, van der Meijden OA, Millett PJ (2012) The effects of arm elevation on the 3-dimensional acromiohumeral distance: a biplane fluoroscopy study with normative data. J Shoulder Elbow Surg 21:1593–1600
73. Yanai T, Fuss FK, Fukunaga T (2006) In vivo measurements of subacromial impingement: substantial compression develops in abduction with large internal rotation. Clin Biomech 21:692–700
74. Yamamoto N, Muraki T, Sperling JW et al (2010) Contact between the coracoacromial arch and the rotator cuff tendons in nonpathologic situations: a cadaveric study. J Shoulder Elbow Surg 19:681–687
75. Xu X, McGorry RW, Lin JH (2014) The accuracy of an external frame using ISB recommended rotation sequence to define shoulder joint angle. Gait Posture 39:662–668
76. Doorenbosch CA, Harlaar J, Veeger DH (2003) The globe system: an unambiguous description of shoulder positions in daily life movements. J Rehabil Res Dev 40:147–155
77. Masuda T, Ishida A, Cao L et al (2008) A proposal for a new definition of the axial rotation angle of the shoulder joint. J Electromyogr Kinesiol 18:154–159
78. Sahara W, Sugamoto K, Murai M et al (2007) Three-dimensional clavicular and acromioclavicular rotations during arm abduction using vertically open MRI. J Orthop Res 25:1243–1249
79. Fukuda K, Craig EV, An KN et al (1986) Biomechanical study of the ligamentous system of the acromioclavicular joint. J Bone Joint Surg Am 68:434–440
80. Debski RE, Parsons IM 3rd, Fenwick J et al (2000) Ligament mechanics during three degree-of-freedom motion at the acromioclavicular joint. Ann Biomed Eng 28:612–618
81. Debski RE, Parsons IM 4th, Woo SL et al (2001) Effect of capsular injury on acromioclavicular joint mechanics. J Bone Joint Surg Am 83:1344–1351
82. Seo YJ, Yoo YS, Noh KC et al (2012) Dynamic function of coracoclavicular ligament at different shoulder abduction angles: a study using a 3-dimensional finite element model. Arthroscopy 28:778–787
83. Kim YS, Yoo YS, Jang SW et al (2015) In vivo analysis of acromioclavicular joint motion after hook plate fixation using three-dimensional computed tomography. J Shoulder Elbow Surg. doi:10.1016/j.jse.2014.12.012
84. Howell SM, Galinat BJ, Renzi AJ et al (1988) Normal and abnormal mechanics of the glenohumeral joint in the horizontal plane. J Bone Joint Surg Am 70:227–232
85. Schiffern SC, Rozencwaig R, Antoniou J et al (2002) Anteroposterior centering of the humeral head on the glenoid in vivo. Am J Sports Med 30:382–387
86. von Eisenhart-Rothe RM, Jager A, Englmeier KH et al (2002) Relevance of arm position and muscle activity on three-dimensional glenohumeral translation in patients with traumatic and atraumatic shoulder instability. Am J Sports Med 30:514–522
87. Koishi H, Goto A, Tanaka M et al (2011) In vivo three-dimensional motion analysis of the shoulder joint during internal and external rotation. Int Orthop 35:1503–1509
88. Yamamoto N, Itoi E, Abe H et al (2007) Contact between the glenoid and the humeral head in abduction, external rotation, and horizontal extension: a new concept of glenoid track. J Shoulder Elbow Surg 16:649–656
89. Omori Y, Yamamoto N, Koishi H et al (2014) Measurement of the glenoid track in vivo as investigated by 3-dimensional motion analysis using open MRI. Am J Sports Med 42:1290–1295
90. Itoi E, Lee SB, Berglund LJ et al (2000) The effect of a glenoid defect on anteroinferior stability of the shoulder after Bankart repair: a cadaveric study. J Bone Joint Surg Am 82:35–46
91. Halder AM, Kuhl SG, Zobitz ME et al (2001) Effects of the glenoid labrum and glenohumeral abduction on stability of the shoulder joint through concavity-compression: an in vitro study. J Bone Joint Surg Am 83:1062–1069

92. Habermeyer P, Schuller U, Wiedemann E (1992) The intra-articular pressure of the shoulder: an experimental study on the role of the glenoid labrum in stabilizing the joint. Arthroscopy 8:166–172
93. Itoi E, Motzkin NE, Browne AO et al (1993) Intraarticular pressure of the shoulder. Arthroscopy 9:406–413
94. Howell SM, Galinat BJ (1989) The glenoid-labral socket. A constrained articular surface. Clin Orthop 243:122–125
95. Lazarus MD, Sidles JA, Harryman DT 2nd et al (1996) Effect of a chondral-labral defect on glenoid concavity and glenohumeral stability. A cadaveric model. J Bone Joint Surg Am 78:94–102
96. Metcalf MH, Pon JD, Harryman DT 2nd et al (2001) Capsulolabral augmentation increases glenohumeral stability in the cadaver shoulder. J Shoulder Elbow Surg 10:532–538
97. O'Connell PW, Nuber GW, Mileski RA et al (1990) The contribution of the glenohumeral ligaments to anterior stability of the shoulder joint. Am J Sports Med 18:579–584
98. Warner JJ, Deng XH, Warren RF et al (1992) Static capsuloligamentous restraints to superior-inferior translation of the glenohumeral joint. Am J Sports Med 20:675–685
99. O'Brien SJ, Schwartz RS, Warren RF et al (1995) Capsular restraints to anterior-posterior motion of the abducted shoulder: a biomechanical study. J Shoulder Elbow Surg 4:298–308
100. Turkel SJ, Panio MW, Marshall JL et al (1981) Stabilizing mechanisms preventing anterior dislocation of the glenohumeral joint. J Bone Joint Surg Am 63:1208–1217
101. Yang C, Goto A, Sahara W et al (2010) In vivo three-dimensional evaluation of the functional length of glenohumeral ligaments. Clin Biomech 25:137–141
102. Shibano K, Koishi H, Futai K et al (2014) Effect of Bankart repair on the loss of range of motion and the instability of the shoulder joint for recurrent anterior shoulder dislocation. J Shoulder Elbow Surg 23:888–894
103. Massimini DF, Boyer PJ, Papannagari R et al (2012) In-vivo glenohumeral translation and ligament elongation during abduction and abduction with internal and external rotation. J Orthop Surg Res 7:29

Chapter 4
Advanced MR Imaging of the Shoulder

Ryuji Sashi

Abstract Advanced 3-Tesla MRI can visualize normal anatomy and pathology more precisely and provides new insights. The chasing interpretation method is introduced to identify precise anatomy on high-quality MR images. The three-dimensional recognition of the shoulder MRI gives a new concept: the supra-/infraspinatus (SISP) muscle with two origins and one insertion. A paradigm shift from tear to avulsion in rotator cuff injury is required in the advanced MRI. Complete detachment of the SISP insertion causes muscular contraction: the pull-in phenomenon. The pull-in phenomenon causes overestimation of muscular atrophy on an oblique sagittal image at the glenoid level. The advanced MRI can detect inflammatory fibrosis of the joint capsule in the rotator interval fat tissue and/or axillary pouch as visible organic changes even in early or mild frozen shoulder. The information from oblique coronal, sagittal, and axial images is explained with an example of subacromial impingement.

Keywords MRI • Shoulder • Chasing interpretation • Avulsion • Muscular atrophy • Frozen shoulder

4.1 Chasing Interpretation Method to Identify the Same Structure Successively on Sequential MR Images

Advanced MRI with high quality visualizes the anatomy of the shoulder precisely. The chasing interpretation method is introduced to identify precise anatomy on high-quality MR images. This method is used to identify the same normal structures and lesions continuously on serial images. A certain structure is continuously identified as chasing it on next to next images from one to another in all the images. A muscle is serially identified from the proximal to the insertion. A ligament is also serially identified between both attachments. Repeating this process will build up the normal images of the anatomy in your brain. Not only a lesion but also adjacent normal

R. Sashi (✉)
Advanced Imaging Center, Yaesu Clinic, C-road Bldg, 2-1-18 Nihonbashi, Chuo-ku, Tokyo 103-0027, Japan
e-mail: sashi@m-satellite.jp

K. Tamai et al. (eds.), *Advances in Shoulder Surgery*,
DOI 10.1007/978-4-431-55988-7_4

structures should be identified to acquire MRI interpretation skill. The normal images built up in your brain make it possible to detect lesions correctly and speedily.

4.2 To Explain the Chasing Method on Oblique Sagittal (Obl. Sag.) T_2-Weighted Images with Fat Suppression (T_2WIFS) (Fig. 4.1 1–6)

Figure 4.1 1–6 shows Obl. Sag. T_2WIFS from the coracoid process (PC)–acromion (AC) level to the lateral level of the great tubercle (GT) of the humeral head. The intramuscular tendons (low signal) in the supraspinatus and infraspinatus muscles (SSP, ISP) are continuously identified on next to next images. The tendons in the SSP and ISP exist independently in Fig. 4.1 1–3. They come together in Fig. 4.1 4 and merge into one supra-/infraspinatus (SISP) tendon in Fig. 4.1 5. The SISP tendon inserts on the superior and middle facets (SF, MF) of the GT in Fig. 4.1 6. The tendons and muscular bellies of the SSP and ISP are retroversely identified from the insertion to the proximal on Figs. 4.6(a) to confirm their recognition. In the same way, the coracoacromial ligament (CAL) is identified on Figs. 4.1 *1–4* which causes subacromial impingement. Figures 4.1 *2–4* reveal the CAL to extend deeply beneath the AC. The coracohumeral ligament (CHL) can be identified only on Fig. 4.1 on this series. The chasing interpretation method is to identify the same structure serially on next to next images. The maximum information is obtained from the MR images by the chasing interpretation method. This method improves MRI interpretation skill to identify the normal structures as well as lesions in each case.

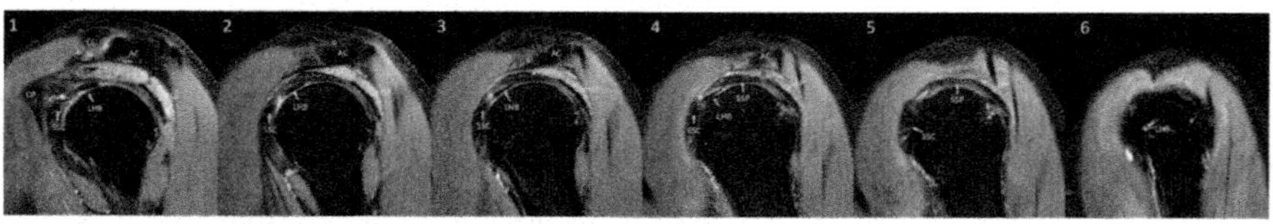

Fig. 4.1 *1–6* Oblique sagittal (Obl. Sag.). T_2WIFS from the coracoid process–acromion level to the lateral level of the great tubercle of the humeral head. *CP* coracoid process, *CL* clavicular, *AC* acromion, *CHL* coracohumeral ligament, *CAL* coracoacromial ligament, *SSP* supraspinatus tendon, *ISP* infraspinatus tendon, *SSC* subscapularis tendon, * rotator interval fat tissue, *LHB* long head of the biceps muscle, *SF* superior facet, *MF* middle facet. *1* CP and CHL, *1–3* separation of SSP and ISP, *1–4* acromion, *1–6* SSC and LHB, *2–4* CAL, *4* coming together of SSP and ISP, *5–6* SISP, *6* SF and MF

4.3 Three-Dimensional Recognition

Oblique coronal (Obl. Cor.) and oblique axial (Obl. Ax.) images should also be interpreted by the chasing interpretation method. All the structures of the shoulder should be identified on the three planes by the chasing interpretation method. Identification on the three planes makes normal and pathological three-dimensional images such as Figs. 4.2b and 4.3a, c.

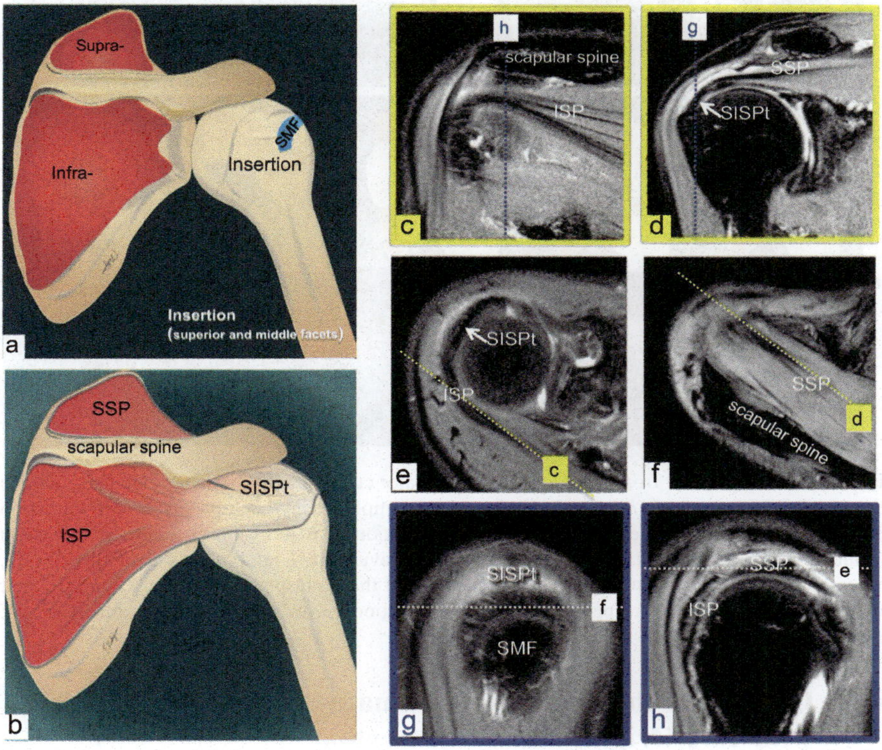

Fig. 4.2 Concept of the supra-/infraspinatus muscle (*SISP*) with two origins and one insertion. *Supra-* supraspinatus fossa, *Infra-* infraspinatus fossa, *SSP* supraspinatus muscle, *ISP* infraspinatus muscle, *SISPt* SISP tendon, *CL* clavicle, *SMF* superior and middle facets. **a** Origins and insertion of SISP; **b** SSP, ISP, SISPt, c–h T_2WIFS; **c** Obl. Cor. *yellow dotted line c* (**e**); **d** Obl. Cor. *yellow dotted line d* (**f**); **e** Obl. Ax. *white dotted line e* (**g**); **f** Obl. Ax. *white dotted line f* (**h**); **g** Obl. Sag. *blue dotted line g* (**d**); **h** Obl. Sag. *blue dotted line h* (**c**). (Illustrations **a**, **b** by T. Nakajima and R. Sashi [1])

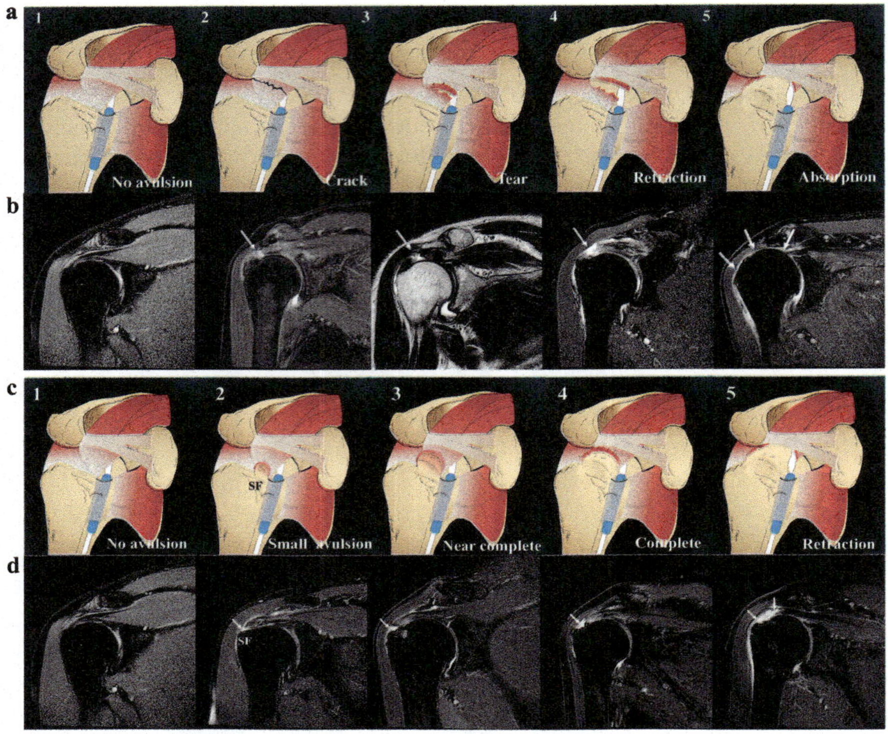

Fig. 4.3 Paradigm shift from tear to avulsion in rotator cuff injury. **a**, **b** Intertendon tear (oblique coronal T_2WIFS) (*arrow*): *1* no avulsion, *2* crack, *3* complete tear, *4* complete tear with retraction of the supraspinatus muscle, *5* absorption of the insertion. **c**, **d** Avulsion of the insertion tendon (oblique coronal T_2WIFS): *SF* superior facet, *arrow* avulsion: *1* no avulsion, *2* small avulsion, *3* near-complete tear, *4* complete tear with retraction of the supraspinatus muscle, *5* complete tear with retraction of the supraspinatus muscle. (Illustrations **a**, **c** by T. Nakajima and R. Sashi; modified from [2])

4.4 Concept of the Supra-/Infraspinatus Muscle (SISP) with Two Origins and One Insertion

Advanced MRI can visualize the intramuscular tendons of the shoulder on the T_2WI with fat suppression (FS) (Figs. 4.1 1–6, 4.2c–h). The three-dimensional recognition of the shoulder MRI gives a new concept: the SISP with two origins and one insertion (Fig. 4.2a, b) [1]. The supraspinatus and infraspinatus muscles (SSP and ISP) have large origins to almost cover the supraspinatus and infraspinatus fossae, respectively (Fig. 4.2a). The scapular spine exists between the SSP and ISP origins (Fig. 4.2b, c, f). The SSP and ISP lateral to the scapular spine neck come together to adhere together (Fig. 4.2b, h). Under the acromion, the ISP tendon turns anteriorly over the SSP tendon from behind. The two tendons contact tightly to merge into one rotator cuff (Fig. 4.2b, d, e, g). The strong contact of the SSP and ISP tendons means that functionally there is one insertion tendon (Fig. 4.2b, d, e, g). The SISP tendon

(SISPt) inserts on the superior and middle facets (SMF) of the great tubercle of the humeral head (Fig. 4.2a, g). As compared with the large origin areas, its attachment area is small (Fig. 4.2a, g), and the SISP tendon becomes thinner gradually forward toward the attachment (Fig. 4.2c, d). This gradual thinning from the SISP bellies forward to the insertion tendon reduces impingement, or friction under the coracoacromial ligament (CAL) (Fig. 4.2d). The SSP and ISP have morphologically two origins and one insertion and they work as one muscle (SISP). If the SSP and ISP contract simultaneously at the same degree, the humerus elevates to the direction of the scapular spine. In rotator cuff repair, the operation plan should include repair of the SISP tendon.

4.5 Paradigm Shift from Tear to Avulsion in Rotator Cuff Injury

4.5.1 Avulsions of the Tendon

Tears of the rotator cuff have been classified vertically from articular to bursal sides on X-ray arthrography of the shoulder. In this conventional classification, the tears are supposed to occur proximal to the attachment. Therefore, they are inter-tendon tears. Most of the inter-tendon tears are complete and communicate between the articular and bursal sides. Traumatic injury such as a fall often causes inter-tendon complete tears. The complete inter-tendon tears are observed within several months after the traumatic onset because their insertion sides will be almost absorbed in a half year (Fig. 4.3a, b). Advanced MRI of the shoulder shows clearly many small avulsions of the insertion tendon from the superior facet (SF) of the great tubercle (GT). All of these are partial tears on the conventional classification because they have no communication between the articular and bursal sides of the joint (Fig. 4.3c 2–3). Most of the small avulsions are bursal-side partial tears in the conventional classification. A paradigm shift from tear to avulsion in the rotator cuff injury is required in advanced MRI. The avulsions in the rotator cuff injury can be classified horizontally from the lateral edge to the proximal margin of the GT [2].

4.5.2 New Classification of Tendon Avulsions from the Greater Tubercle

Most tendon avulsions include the SF. These avulsions occur both spontaneously and traumatically. The bone surface of the attachment is bared even in a small avulsion. These small avulsions are classified as partial tears on the conventional classification until they completely lose their insertions of the GT. These tendon avulsions are horizontally classified into small, near-complete, complete, and full detachment with retraction (Fig. 4.3c, d 2–5). On advanced MRI, a key to diagnose rotator cuff injury is to confirm whether the supra-/infraspinatus tendon covers the SF completely [2].

4.6 Evaluation of the Rotator Muscles Atrophy

Evaluation of muscular atrophy is important before cuff repair surgery. The evaluation has usually been performed on the oblique sagittal (Obl. Sag.) image at the glenoid level (Fig. 4.4b1–4, a1–4; white broken lines). However, complete detachment of the insertion causes muscular contraction, the pull-in phenomenon that makes it difficult to estimate the muscular atrophy (Fig. 4.4a4, b4). An intact muscle–tendon should be the thinner where the more distal from a mid-belly (Fig. 4.4a1). The distal thinner portion comes to the glenoid level by the pull-in phenomenon after complete detachment (Fig. 4.4a4, b4). The pull-in phenomenon causes overestimation of muscular atrophy at the glenoid level. The evaluation is better on an Obl. Sag. image, as proximal as possible. The Obl. Sag. image near the lateral margin of the SSP origin is practical, where no strong pull-in phenomenon occurs (Fig. 4.4a4, black broken line). The lateral margin of the SSP origin locates near proximal to the suprascapular notch (SSC-n) (Fig. 4.4a4, black broken line).

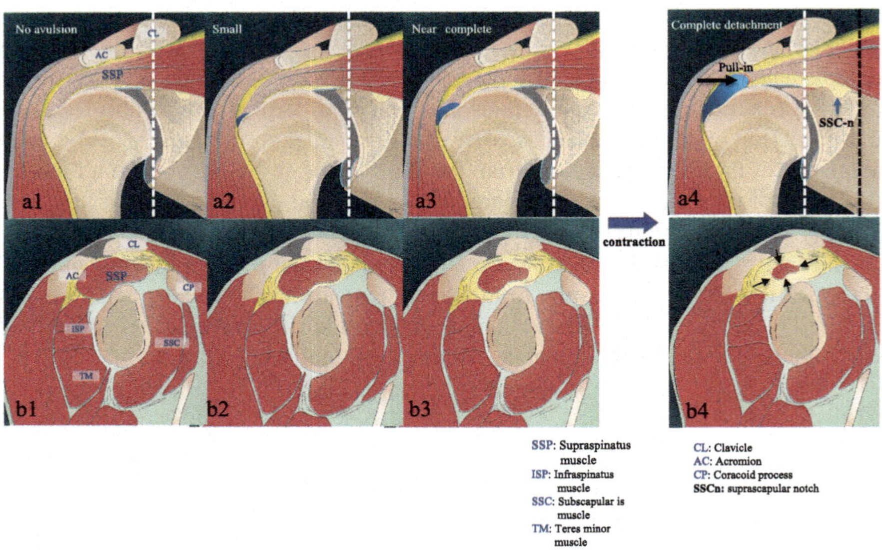

Fig. 4.4 Avulsions of the supraspinatus insertion and estimation of muscular atrophy. *CP* coracoid process, *CL* clavicular, *AC* acromion, *SSP* supraspinatus tendon, *ISP* infraspinatus tendon, *TM* teres minor, *SSC* subscapularis tendon, *white broken line* (glenoid level), *SSC-n* suprascapular notch, *black broken line* (level near lateral margin of SSP origin). **a** Oblique coronal: *1* no avulsion, *2* small avulsion, *3* near-complete avulsion, *4* complete detachment with pull-in phenomenon with retraction of the supraspinatus muscle. **b** Oblique sagittal: *1* no atrophy, *2* slight atrophy, *3* mild atrophy, *4* overestimation of muscular atrophy at the glenoid level. (Illustrations by T. Nakajima and R. Sashi; modified from [3])

The evaluation of muscular atrophy should be also done on the Obl. axial and coronal MR images in addition to sagittal images. Other important factors are disease duration, patient's age, and muscle testing [3].

4.7 MRI Findings of Frozen Shoulder (Adhesive Capsulitis)

4.7.1 Inflammatory Fibrosis of the Joint Capsule

Frozen shoulder indicates pathology that develops commonly in middle age (40 years old and later) and subsides in about 2 years. A frozen shoulder has various degrees of symptoms from only mild motion pain to severe contracture with night pain. It is not a frozen shoulder if it will not subside. It will be able to be diagnosed to have been "frozen shoulder" retrospectively only after its resolution. Frozen shoulder has been a middle-aged painful shoulder syndrome that includes various pathologies. Now advanced MRI can reveal capsulitis (inflammatory fibrosis) to explain most of the cases of middle-aged painful shoulders clinically diagnosed as frozen shoulder or periarthritis [4]. Arthroscopy shows superficial inflammatory fibrosis all over the inner joint capsule in a frozen shoulder. Advanced MRI can detect inflammatory fibrosis of the joint capsule in the rotator interval fat tissue and/or axillary pouch as strong organic changes even in early or mild frozen shoulder that has no indication for arthroscopy or open surgery (Fig. 4.5a1–2). Invasive intervention should have been performed in the fibrotic changes responsible for the symptoms. Both the rotator interval and axillary pouch work in play of the joint capsule for the range of motion (ROM). The fibrotic changes of the capsule deprive the rotator interval and/or axillary pouch of their play functions. Their fibrotic changes cause pain and contracture of the shoulder owing to volume loss of the joint cavity. The pressure of the joint cavity is negative in the normal shoulder, but it becomes positive in frozen shoulder. The positive pressure causes instability of the shoulder and hypertonia of the joint capsule and muscles. Their hypertonia causes rest and night pain in addition to motion pain.

4.7.2 MRI Findings of Frozen Shoulder

4.7.2.1 No Complete Rotator Cuff Tears and Little Opening of the Subscapular Bursa

No complete rotator cuff tears and little opening of the subscapular bursa are observed in frozen shoulder on MRI. Complete cuff tear and/or opening of the subscapular bursa decrease the joint cavity pressure to communicate with the subdeltoid bursa and/or subscapularis bursa, respectively. Inflammatory fibrosis of the joint capsule can accompany a partial tear of the rotator cuff. Muscular

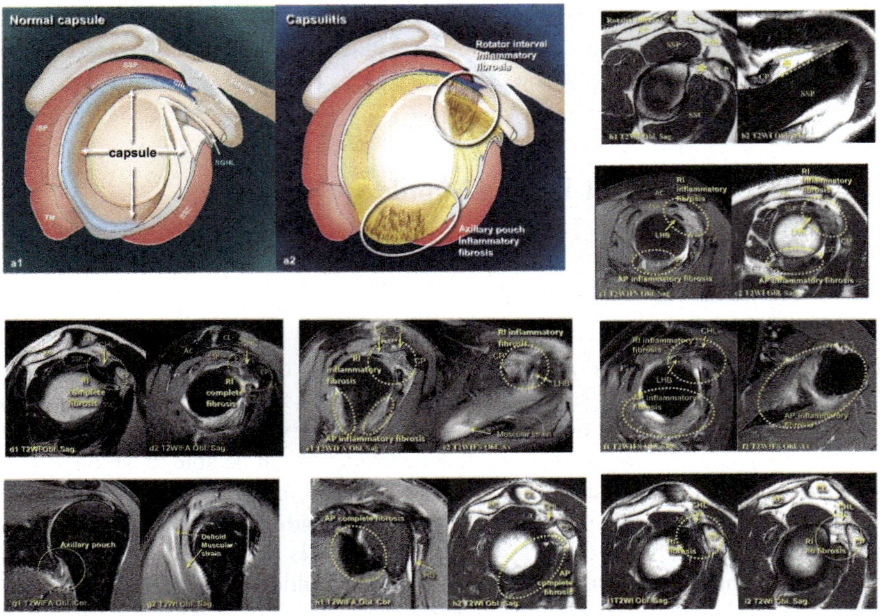

Fig. 4.5 Magnetic resonance imaging (MRI) findings of frozen shoulder (adhesive capsulitis). *CP* coracoid process, *CL* clavicular, *AC* acromion, *CHL* coracohumeral ligament, *CAL* coracoacromial ligament, *SSP* supraspinatus tendon, *ISP* infraspinatus tendon, *SSC* subscapularis tendon, * rotator interval fat tissue, *LHB* long head of the biceps muscle, *SF* superior facet, *MF* middle facet. **a1** Normal capsule, **a2** capsulitis, **b** rotator interval (*): *1* T_2WI Obl. Sag., *2* T_2WI Obl. Ax. **c** Inflammatory fibrosis: *1* T_2WIFS Obl. Sag., rotator interval (*RI*), *2* T_2WI Obl.. Sag.. **d** Complete fibrosis of rotator interval: *1* T_2WI Obl.. Sag., *2* T_2WIFS Obl. Sag. **e** Muscular strain: *1* T_2WIFS Obl. Sag., *2* T_2WIFS Obl. Ax.. **f** Inflammatory fibrosis of the axillary pouch: *1* T_2WI Obl. Sag., *2* T_2WIFS Obl. Ax.. **g** Inflammatory fibrosis of the axillary pouch and muscular strain: *1* T_2WI Obl. Cor., *2* T_2WIFS Obl. Sag.. **h** Complete fibrosis of the axillary pouch: *1* T_2WI Obl. Cor., *2* T_2WI Obl. Sag.. **i** Resolving of the frozen shoulder: *1* T_2WI Obl. Sag., *2* T_2WI Obl. Sag., 3 years later. (Illustrations **a1**, **a2** by T. Nakajima and R. Sashi)

strains are occasionally found in the frozen shoulder on T_2WI with fat suppression (FS). The muscular strain may be iatrogenic.

4.7.2.2 Inflammatory Fibrosis of the Rotator Interval Fat Tissue

The rotator interval is the joint capsule not covered with the rotator cuff but with fat tissue between the supraspinatus and subscapular muscles (Fig. 4.5b 1–2). The rotator interval works as play of the rotator cuff between the supraspinatus and subscapular muscles to give ROM of the shoulder. Fat tissue with T_2WI high signal is observed in the normal rotator interval (Fig. 4.5b1–2, *). In the early phase, inflammatory fibrosis shows vague low signal on T_2WI and high signal on the T_2WI with fat suppression (FS) (Fig. 4.5c 1–2). The signal intensities of the fibrosis come lower both on the T_2WI and T_2WIFS as completion of the fibrosis with dehydration (Fig. 4.5d 1–2, 5h 1–2, 5i 1). T_2WIFS cannot differentiate complete fibrosis from normal fat tissue because both of them are low signal (Fig. 4.5d2). Inflammatory fibrosis of the rotator interval begins from the capsule, extends fat tissue above, and involves the coracohumeral ligament (CHL) (Fig. 4.5a2, d1–2, e1, f1, i1). The inflammatory fibrosis simultaneously involves the superior glenohumeral ligament and long head of the biceps brachii muscle (LHB) (Fig. 4.5a2, c1–2, e1, f1). Involvement of these structures of the rotator interval worsens the symptoms of frozen shoulder.

4.7.2.3 Inflammatory Fibrosis of the Axillary Pouch

The axillary pouch of the joint capsule attaches medially to the glenoid neck and laterally to the humeral neck, between the subscapular and teres minor muscles. The axillary pouch works as play of the joint capsule to enable the arm elevation. Inflammatory fibrosis of the axillary pouch is observed as its thickening and high signal on the T_2WIFS (Fig. 4.5a2, c1–2, e1, f1–2, g1). The inflammatory fibrosis of the axillary pouch causes its shortening and loss of its elasticity. These changes explain motion pain, rest pain, and contraction of the shoulder. The inflammatory fibrosis of the axillary pouch tends to extend anterosuperiorly and infiltrates into the subscapular muscle (Fig. 4.5a2, e1, f1–2, h1–2). High signal of the axillary pouch on the T_2WIFS comes lower as completion of the fibrosis (Fig. 4.5h1–2, i1). The contour of the axillary pouch remains even after fibrosis completion on the T_2WIFS (Fig. 4.5h1–2).

4.7.2.4 Resolving of the Frozen Shoulder

The ratio of the rotator interval to axillary pouch inflammatory fibrosis varies depending on each case of frozen shoulder. Fibrosis of the rotator interval and/or axillary pouch (Fig. 4.5i1) diminishes much or less with resolving of the frozen shoulder (Fig. 4.5i2, 3 years later in this case).

4.8 Three MR Planes of the Shoulder and Their Information

4.8.1 Information Obtained on Each MR Plane

MR images of the shoulder are obtained on oblique coronal, sagittal, and axial planes that have different planar information. A lesion is well visualized on an adequate plane that depends on shape and size of the lesion. Each image has information of the *x–y* plane but no information as to depth (*z*-axis). The information of each MR plane is explained with an example of subacromial impingement: friction beneath the coracoacromial (CA) ligament. Every muscle decreases in its thickness from the muscular belly to the insertion tendon. The subacromial impingement can be diagnosed only on the oblique coronal plane by abnormal swelling of the supraspinatus (SSP) tendon lateral to the CA ligament (Fig. 4.6a). Fiction of the swollen SSP tendon at the CA ligament in elevation can be speculated

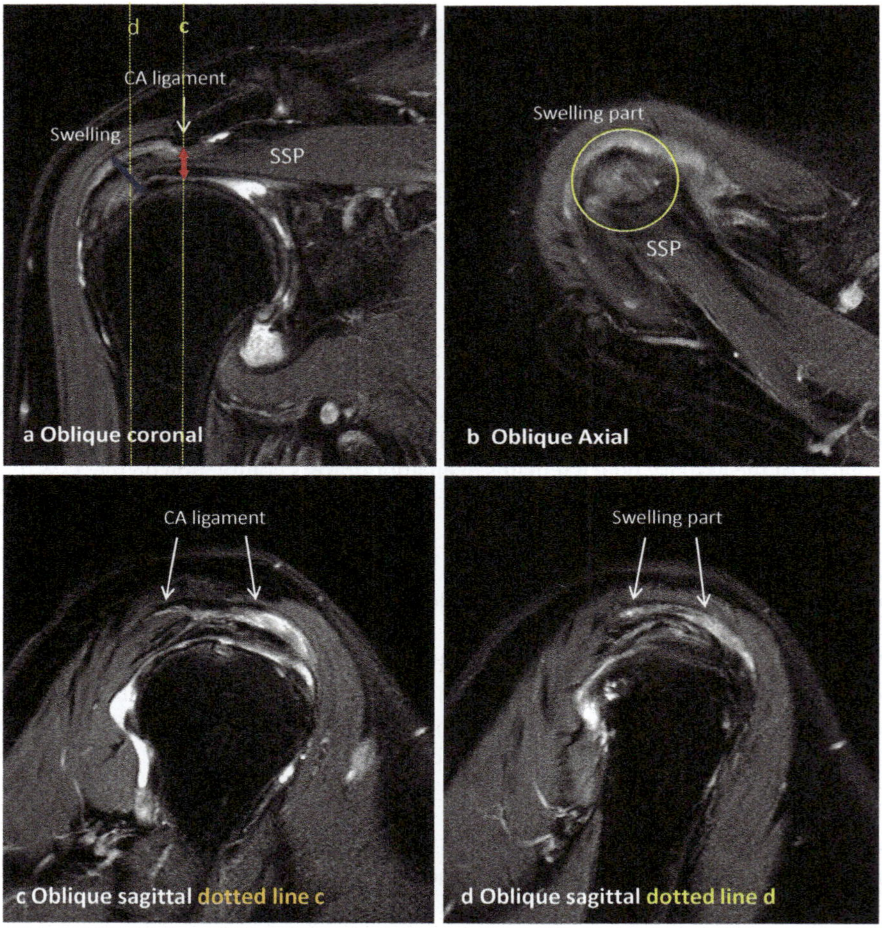

Fig. 4.6 Subacromial impingement on the three MR planes. *CA* coracoacromial, *SSP* supraspinatus muscle-tendon. T_2WIFS. **a** Oblique coronal plane. A *yellow dotted line d* shows a slice line of **d**. A *yellow dotted line c* shows a slice line of **c**. A *blue double-headed arrow* shows abnormal swelling of the SSP tendon. A *red double-headed arrow* shows the thickness of the SSP below the CA ligament. **b** Oblique axial plane. **c** Oblique sagittal plane of the *yellow dotted line c* in **a**. **d** Obl. Sag. plane of the *yellow dotted line d* in **a**

on this oblique coronal plane. The oblique axial image has no information about the SSP thickness (Fig. 4.6b). The oblique sagittal images have little information about changes of SSP thickness from the inner (Fig. 4.6c) to the lateral (Fig. 4.6d).

4.8.2 Number of Slices to Present a Lesion

The number of slices to scan a same lesion or structure is different in the oblique coronal, sagittal, and axial planes. A plane that visualizes a lesion or structure with the more slices usually has the more information about it. For example, the supraspinatus muscle is scanned with the most slices in the oblique sagittal plane and with the fewest slices in the oblique axial plane.

References

1. Sashi R (2012) Concept of the supra/infra-spinatus muscle (SISP) with two origins and one insertion. J Joint Surg 767:43–44
2. Sashi R (2011) Rotator cuff tear. In: Sashi R, Itoi E, Akita K (eds) MRI of the shoulder: all about reading skills, 2nd edn. Medical View, Tokyo, pp 58–87
3. Sashi R (2011) Pull-in phenomenon after complete tear of the supra/infara-spinatus tendon and evaluation of the muscular atrophy. In: Sashi R, Itoi E, Akita K (eds) MRI of the shoulder: all about reading skills, 2nd edn. Medical View, Tokyo, pp 66–67
4. Sashi R (2011) Axillary and rotator interval contractures. In: Sashi R, Itoi E, Akita K (eds) MRI of the shoulder: all about reading skills, 2nd edn. Medical View, Tokyo, pp 148–153

Chapter 5
Transosseous-Equivalent Arthroscopic Bankart Repair by Twin Anchor Footprint Fixation (TAFF) Technique Using JuggerKnot™ Soft Anchor

Minoru Yoneda, Naoko Mizuno, Shin-ichi Yamada, Wataru Sahara, and Tatsuo Mae

Abstract In 2004, we developed a new type of arthroscopic Bankart repair technique named the double anchor footprint fixation (DAFF), using two different suture anchors for the glenoid neck and glenoid surface anchors, to achieve a more anatomic and wider footprint fixation. As soon as the small, all-suture soft anchor was available in 2011, the twin anchor footprint fixation (TAFF) technique was developed using only the soft anchor for both the glenoid neck and glenoid surface anchors. This TAFF technique might be suitably indicated for patients with a significant ALPSA (anterior labro ligamentous periosteal sleeve avulsion) lesion or those who need capsular shift. Moreover, the specific indications of this technique are revision cases after conventional arthroscopic Bankart repair surgery, and a bony Bankart lesion with large thick bone fragments. The TAFF technique using the all-suture soft anchors is a step closer to a true transosseous suture technique, which is the conventional open procedure making a bone tunnel.

Keywords Arthroscopic Bankart repair • Footprint fixation • Soft suture anchor

---

M. Yoneda (✉)
Department of Orthopedic Surgery, Nippon Medical School, 1-1-5 Sendagi, Bunkyo-ku, Tokyo 113-8603, Japan
e-mail: yonepy2796@gmail.com

N. Mizuno
Toyonaka Municipal Hospital, Osaka, Japan

S. Yamada
JCHO Hoshigaoka Medical Center, Osaka, Japan

W. Sahara • T. Mae
Osaka University Graduate School of Medicine, Osaka, Japan

K. Tamai et al. (eds.), *Advances in Shoulder Surgery*,
DOI 10.1007/978-4-431-55988-7_5

5.1 Introduction

Arthroscopic Bankart repair on the articular surface fixation with a suture anchor is the most common technique for recurrent anterior shoulder dislocation. However, it has some disadvantages: (1) the inferior glenohumeral ligament (IGHL)–labrum complex is attached directly to the glenoid cartilage without any preparation, and (2) point fixation results from the single-row technique [1–3].

In 2004, we developed a new type of arthroscopic Bankart repair called the double anchor footprint fixation (DAFF) technique to get a more anatomic and wider footprint fixation [4–6].

The concepts of the DAFF technique are as follows:

1. Removing the cartilage of the glenoid edge to make a subchondral bone trough for increasing the healing potential
2. Spanning the sutures from glenoid neck anchors to glenoid surface anchors to make a strong footprint fixation of the labrum

In the first-generation technique, the DAFF technique used metal suture anchors, FASTak2.4 (Arthrex, Naples, FL, USA) and GII (DePuy Synthes Mitek Sports Medicine, Raynham, MA, USA), for the glenoid neck anchors and glenoid surface anchors, respectively (DAFF I). However, the glenoid surface anchors were switched to the naked Lupine Loop (DePuy Synthes Mitek Sports Medicine, Raynham, MA, USA; an absorbable PLA anchor) from the GII for the second-generation technique to prevent possible damage to humeral head cartilage by the metal anchor when it backs out of the glenoid surface (DAFF II) [7, 8]. Of the 368 shoulders with anterior glenohumeral instability that were treated by the DAFF I or II techniques from 2005 to 2011, 323 shoulders were reviewed retrospectively. The mean age at surgery was 25.5 years and the mean follow-up period was 27.6 months. At the final follow-up, the mean Rowe score improved from 37.9 preoperatively to 92.3 postoperatively, and postoperative recurrence occurred in 23 shoulders (7.1 %). Regarding the recurrence rate sorted according to sports activity, contact-collision sports was 11.6 % (18/155), limited-contact sports was 5.8 % (4/69), and non-contact sports was 2.4 % (1/41). Thus, the arthroscopic Bankart repair with the DAFF technique provides excellent clinical results [9].

In 2011, an innovative suture anchor, the JuggerKnot soft anchor (Biomet, Warsaw, IN, USA), was introduced in Japan. This anchor consists of a nonabsorbable suture material, which can be fixed in a small anchor hole 1.4 mm in diameter and reduces the likelihood of intersecting anchors. It is the optimal suture anchor for such a double anchor method placing multiple suture anchors in the small glenoid bone. Therefore, the twin anchor footprint fixation (TAFF) technique was developed by switching both glenoid neck anchors and glenoid surface anchors to the smaller JuggerKnot from the FASTak2.4 and the Lupine Loop. Although this latest technique is very similar to the DAFF technique, it was named TAFF because the same suture anchor is used for both the glenoid neck anchors and the glenoid surface anchors.

This chapter describes the arthroscopic Bankart repair by the TAFF technique using the JuggerKnot soft anchors.

5.2 Surgical Procedure of Arthroscopic Bankart Repair by TAFF Technique

5.2.1 Portal Placement

The arm is slightly abducted with traction, and lateral traction is applied or a pad is added at the axillar to make the inferior joint gap wider. Two portals are placed posteriorly and one portal anteriorly: the posterosuperolateral portal for a viewing portal (the incision is placed at one fingerbreadth lateral to the acromial posterior horn, 10–11 o'clock in height at the right shoulder, and two fingerbreadths lateral to the joint surface), the anterior portal for a working portal (the incision is placed lateral to the coracoid process, just above the tendon of the subscapularis muscle in the rotator interval and nearer the humeral head), and the posteroinferior portal for a retrieval portal (the incision is placed three fingerbreadths superior from the axilla, just above the posterior band in height, which is 7 o'clock at the right shoulder, and parallel to the joint surface) (Fig. 5.1a, b). First, mobilization and footprint preparation as described next are performed through these portals.

5.2.2 Mobilization

By viewing from the anteroinferior glenoid to the axillary area utilizing 70° arthroscope from the posterosuperolateral portal, the IGHL–labrum complex is mobilized from 2 o'clock to 6 o'clock at least (or 7 o'clock in some cases) at the right shoulder using a radiofrequency hook probe and a rasp through the anterior or the posteroinferior portal, until the inferior border of the subscapularis muscle and the tendinous insertion of the long head of the triceps can be seen (Fig. 5.2). It is important to be able to draw up the loose axillary pouch completely. Care is taken not to damage the axillary nerve and humeral circumflex artery/venous.

5.2.3 Footprint Preparation for Labrum Repair

To secure the footprint, a 4-mm-wide trough is prepared at the anterior glenoid rim from 2 o'clock to 6 o'clock (or 7 o'clock in some cases) at the right shoulder until the subchondral bone becomes exposed (Fig. 5.3a). The cartilage is ablated using a radiofrequency hook probe, and the subchondral bone of the glenoid surface and

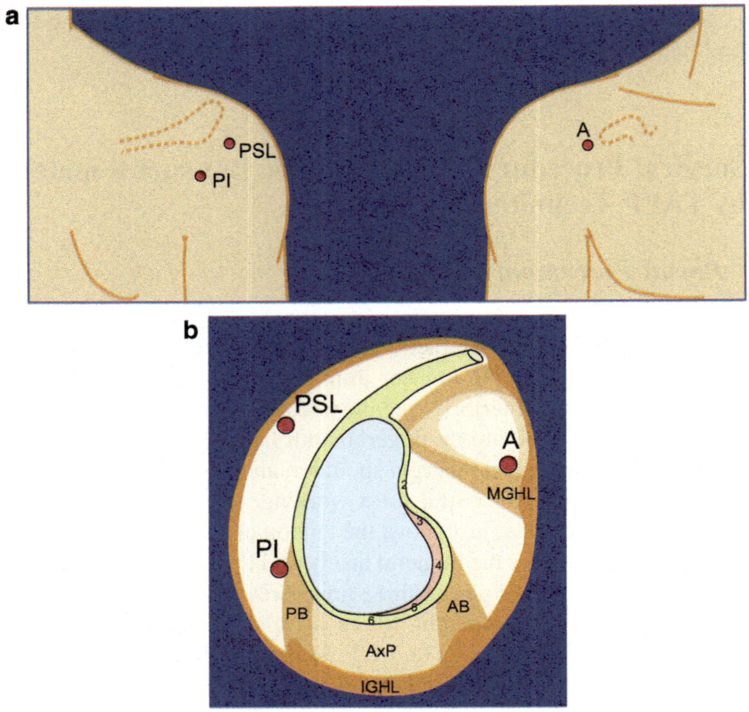

Fig. 5.1 Portal placement. *PSL* posterosuperolateral portal, *A* routine anterior portal, *PI* posteroinferior portal, *MGHL* middle glenohumeral ligament, *IGHL* inferior glenohumeral ligament, *AB* anterior band, *AxP* axillary Pouch, *PB* posterior band

neck is refreshed by 4–5 mm in width using a shaver and an abrader burr through the anterior or the posteroinferior portal (Fig. 5.3b).

5.2.4 Anteroinferior Portal Placement by Retrograde Docking Technique

An anteroinferior portal for inserting glenoid neck anchors is necessary to perform the TAFF technique. By viewing through the posterosuperolateral portal using a 70° scope, the Guide Pin (Biomet) is inserted parallel to the glenoid surface through the posteroinferior portal. With lifting up the anterior band of the IGHL laterally by the use of a switching rod inserted through the anterior portal so that the muscle belly of the subscapularis can be seen easily, the guide pin is passed through the muscle belly and pushed against the skin in the direction of 4 o'clock (Fig. 5.4a, b). Then, the anteroinferior portal is made by cutting the skin a few millimeters using a sharp-pointed knife (Fig. 5.4c) and exposing the tip of the guide pin (Fig. 5.4d, e),

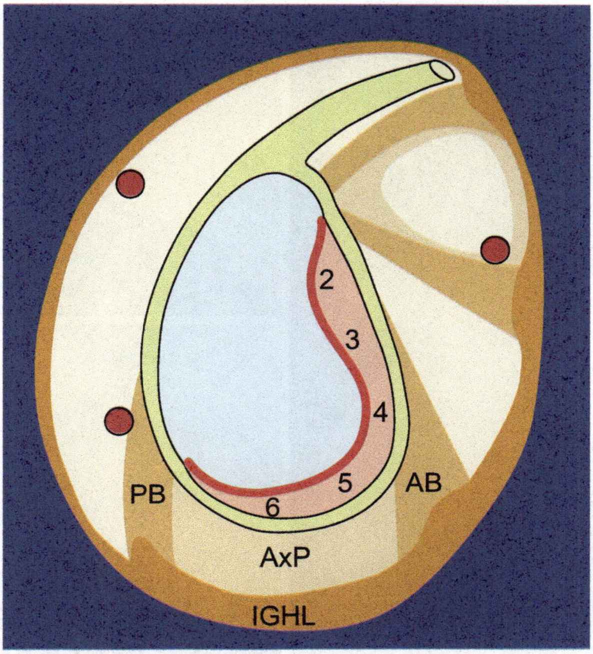

Fig. 5.2 Mobilization. The IGHL–labrum complex is fully mobilized to be able to draw up the loose axillary pouch completely. Numbers are clock time positions at right shoulder

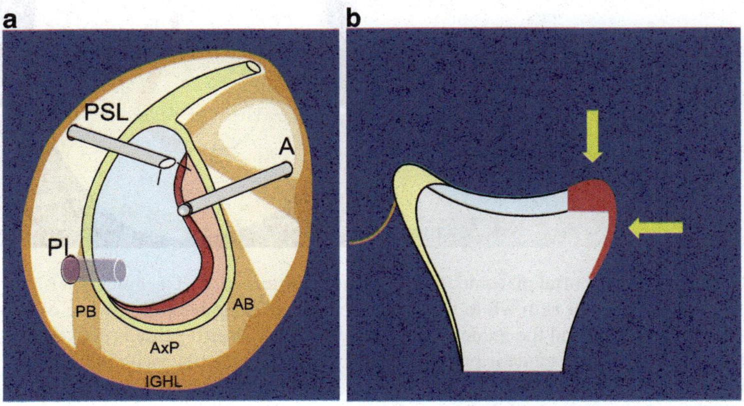

Fig. 5.3 Footprint preparation. (**a**, **b**) The *red* area is ablated and refreshed for preparing the footprint

docking the JuggerKnot drill guide on the tip of the guide pin (Fig. 5.4f, i) and pushing it into the joint space in a retrograde fashion (Fig. 5.4j, n). The postoperative incision of this portal is not so visible because the skin incision is very small and only two to four fingerbreadths medial of the axilla (Fig. 5.4o).

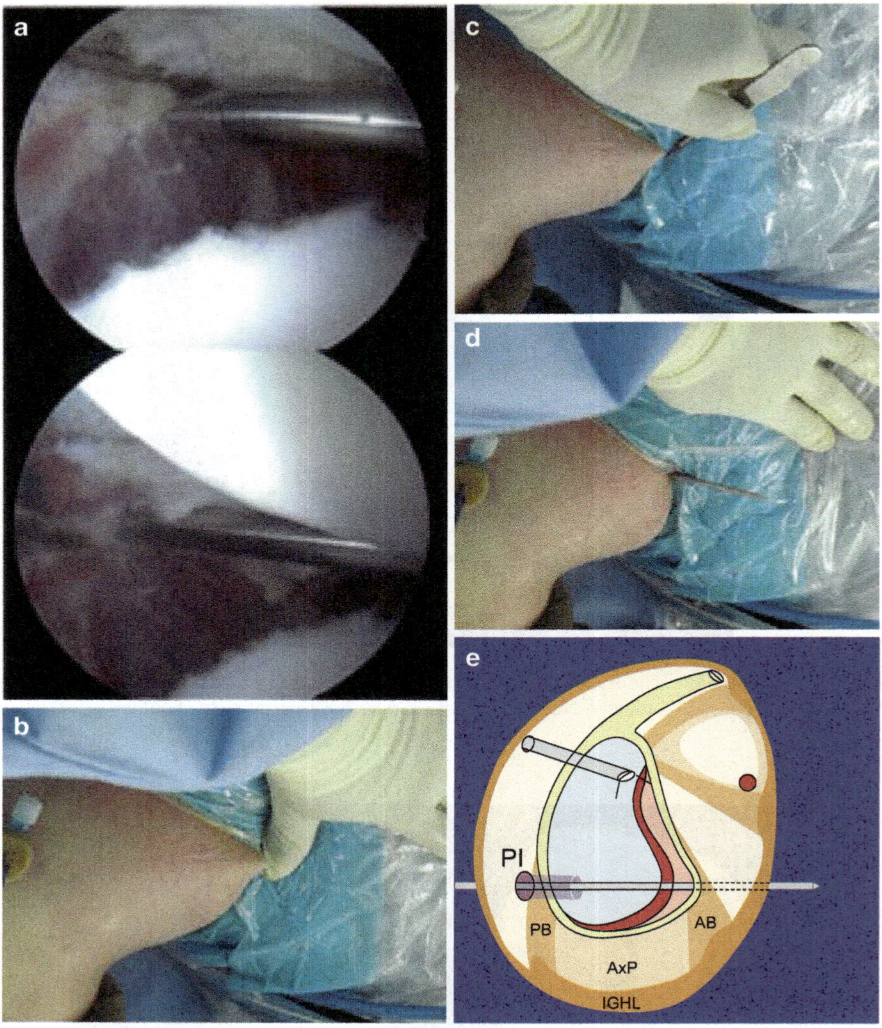

Fig. 5.4 Anteroinferior portal placement in retrograde fashion. (**a**, **b**) The guide pin is inserted and pushed against the anterior skin while lifting up the anterior band laterally by use of a switching rod. (**c**–**e**) The skin is cut and the guide pin is exposed. (**f**–**i**) The drill guide is docked on the tip of the guide pin. (**j**–**l**) The drill guide is pushed into the joint space together with the guide pin. (**m**, **n**) The guide pin is removed and the drill guide is in the anteroinferior portal. (**o**) Postoperative incision of the anteroinferior portal

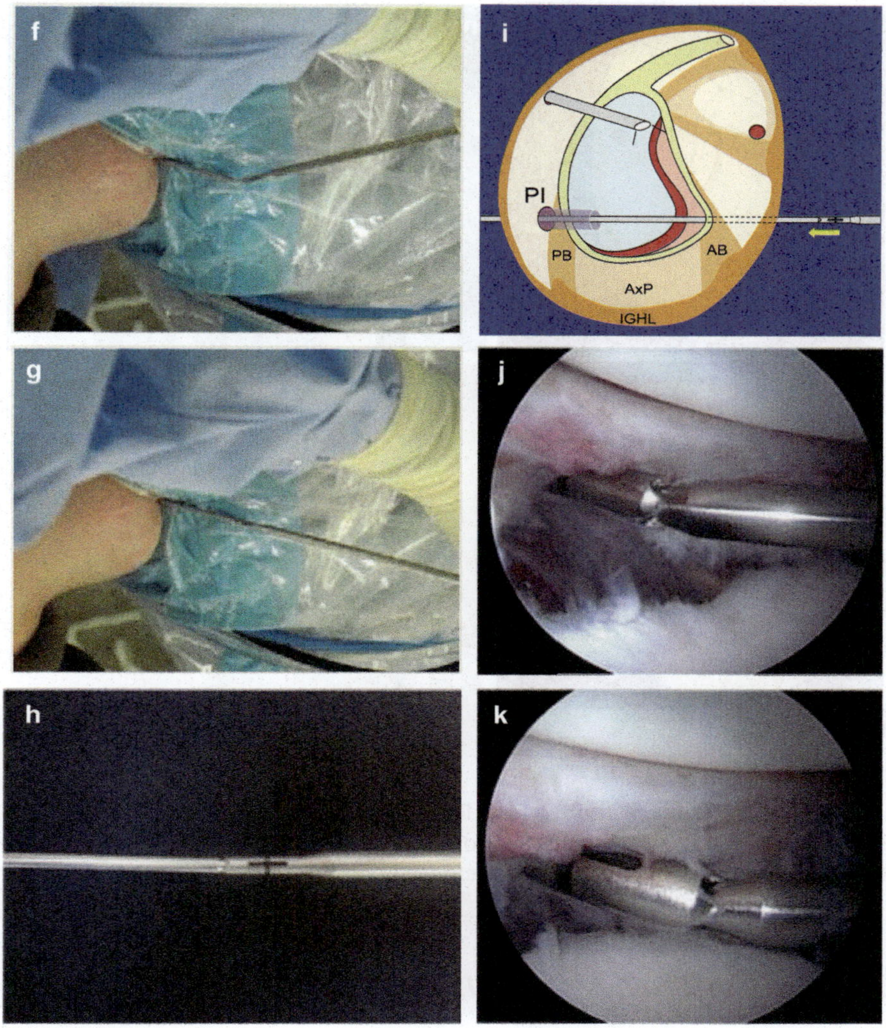

Fig. 5.4 (continued)

5.2.5 JuggerKnot Soft Anchor Insertion in the Glenoid Neck

Using the drill guide placed in the anteroinferior portal, an anchor hole is drilled in the glenoid neck 4–5 mm medial to the trough and the JuggerKnot soft anchor is inserted first at the 4:30 position (Fig. 5.5a–f). After confirming the suture sliding by pulling the suture limbs alternatively, the suture is retrieved through the posteroinferior portal.

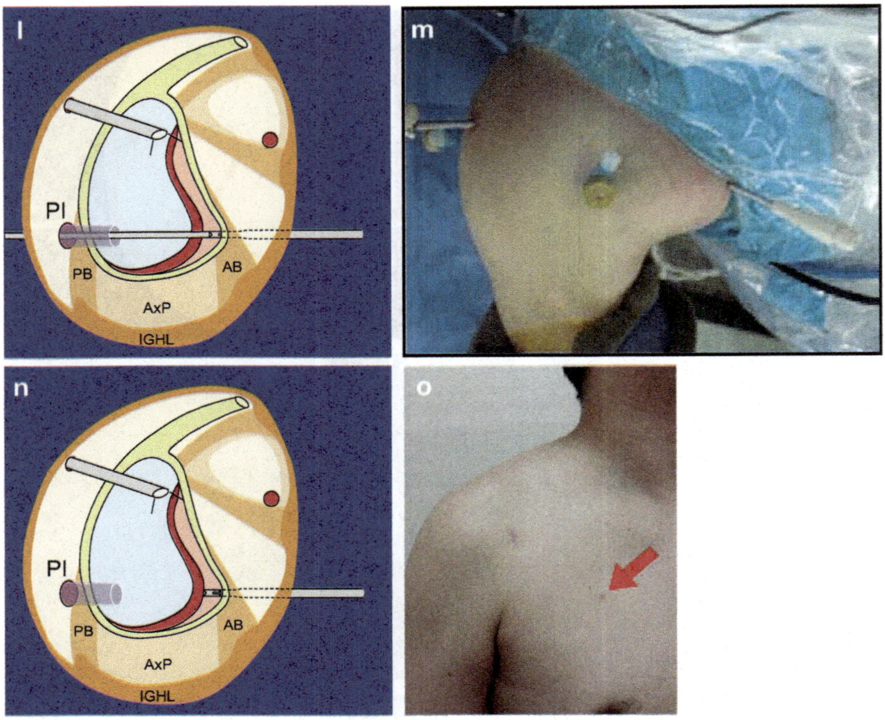

Fig. 5.4 (continued)

Then, the anchors are inserted in order of the position of 3:15 and 2:00 and their sutures are retrieved through the posteroinferior portal in the same manner (Fig. 5.5g). Finally, the drill guide is removed.

5.2.6 Mattress Suture to IGHL–Labrum Complex

One limb of the 4:30 anchor suture and both limbs of the 3:15 and 2:00 anchor sutures are retrieved through the anterior portal (Fig. 5.6a). The one limb of the 4:30 anchor suture left in the posteroinferior portal is passed through the most inferior area of the IGHL–labrum complex (axillary pouch) by hooking a 2-0 PROLENE loop to the axillary pouch using the Suture Hook (CONMED, Largo, FL, USA) through the anterior portal, retrieving the loop through the posteroinferior portal, and relaying the suture limb (Fig. 5.6b).

Then, another suture limb of the 4:30 anchor is retrieved from the anterior portal to the posteroinferior portal. With drawing up the IGHL–labrum complex by pulling the 4:30 anchor suture already passed through it, another suture limb is passed inferior to the pulling suture, and the mattress suture of the 4:30 anchor to

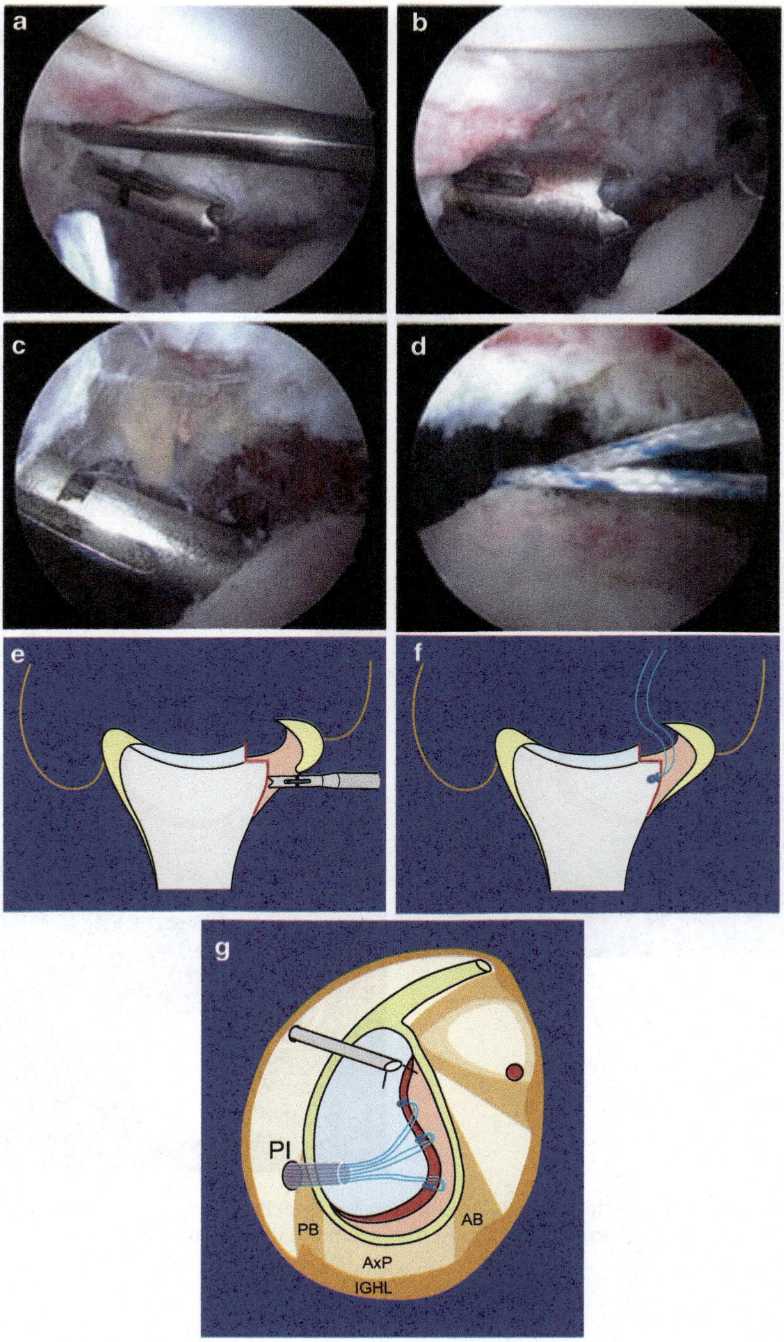

Fig. 5.5 Insertion of glenoid neck anchors through the anteroinferior portal. (**a–f**) The JuggerKnot soft anchor is inserted at 4:30 position. (**g**) Sutures are retrieved through the posteroinferior portal

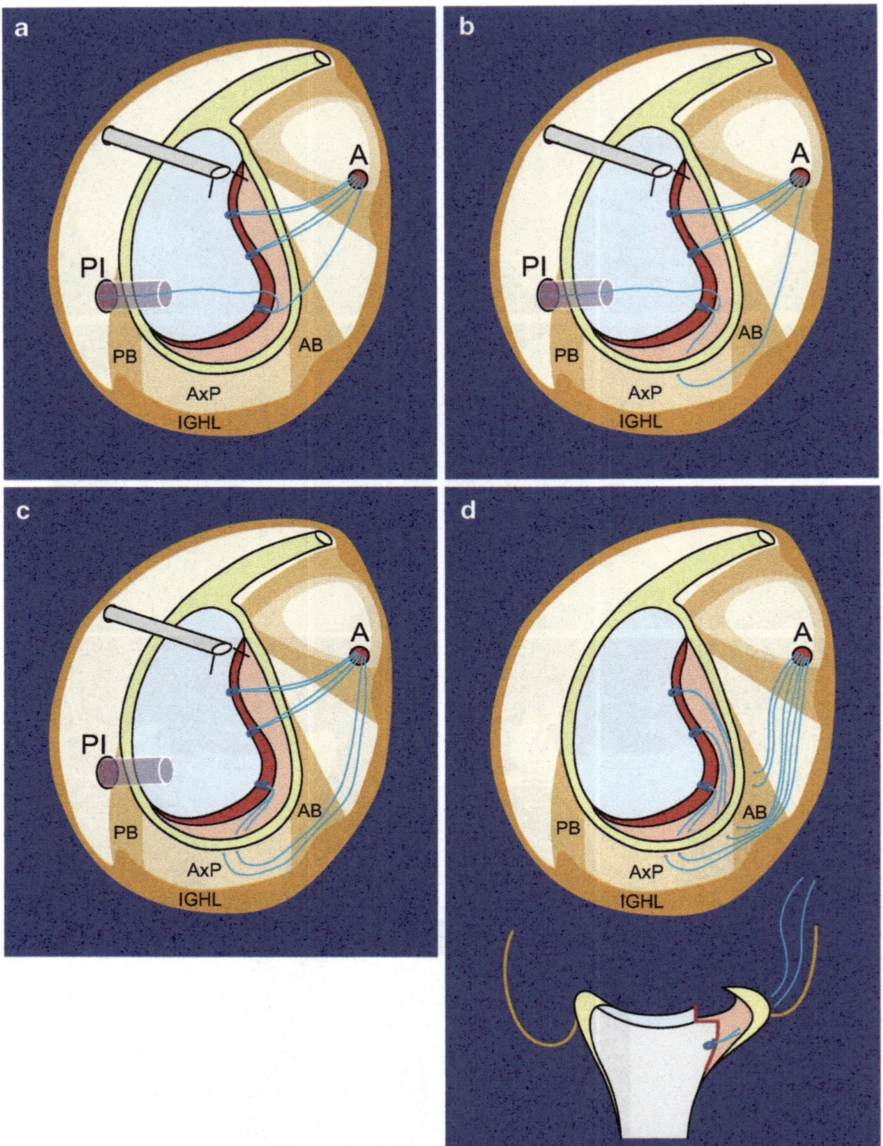

Fig. 5.6 Mattress suture to the IGHL–labrum complex. (**a–c**) Both suture limbs of the 4:30 anchor are passed through the axillary pouch. (**d**) The mattress suture of the glenoid neck anchors is completed

the axillary pouch is completed (Fig. 5.6c). It is important to confirm the suture sliding again, because it is impossible to perform the TAFF technique if the suture does not slide.

The suture of the 3:15 anchor is passed through the inferior portion of the anterior band of the IGHL and the suture of the 2:00 anchor is passed through the superior portion of the anterior band in the same manner (Fig. 5.6d).

5.2.7 JuggerKnot Anchor Insertion in the Glenoid Surface and Knot Tying

The 5-mm cannula is placed in the anterior portal with all sutures of glenoid neck anchors, which were passed through the IGHL–labrum complex, staying outside the cannula. The drill guide is inserted through the cannula, and the tip of the guide is put on the anterior edge of the cartilage at 4:30 position (Fig. 5.7a). While firmly holding the drill guide, an anchor hole is drilled and the JuggerKnot anchor is inserted. The sliding of the suture must be confirmed (Fig. 5.7b).

After retrieving one suture limb of the 4:30 glenoid neck anchor, which was passed through the IGHL–labrum complex the most inferiorly, and one suture limb of the glenoid surface anchor through the posteroinferior portal, they are tied together outside the body through the cannula (*outside knot*), and excess lengths of the suture limbs are cut (Fig. 5.7c).

Another suture limb of the glenoid neck anchor that was passed through the IGHL–labrum complex first is also retrieved through the cannula placed in the anterior portal. With pulling sutures of the 3:15 and 2:00 anchors passed through the IGHL–labrum complex, the remaining sutures of the 4:30 anchors are pulled alternatively to slide the outside knot into the joint space (Fig. 5.7d).

The outside knot can be placed at the lateral side of the labrum by pulling the suture of the glenoid neck anchor first and the suture of the glenoid surface anchor next, and the sutures should be firmly pulled enough to draw up the IGHL–labrum complex onto the footprint (Fig. 5.7e). This technique of making a knot outside the body and sliding into the joint space by pulling another limb of sutures is named the outside knot and slide-in (OKAS) technique, and the reason why the suture has to slide is to perform this OKAS technique. In addition, when this technique is performed, the traction to widen the axilla is relaxed and the humeral head is reduced posteriorly.

Finally, the remaining sutures of the 4:30 anchors are tied up at the lateral side of the labrum by the Revo knot (non-sliding knot) through the cannula in the anterior portal (Fig. 5.7f). If it is difficult to tie the knot at the 4:30 position from the anterior portal, the knot can be tied from the posteroinferior portal, taking care to place the knot at the lateral side of the labrum.

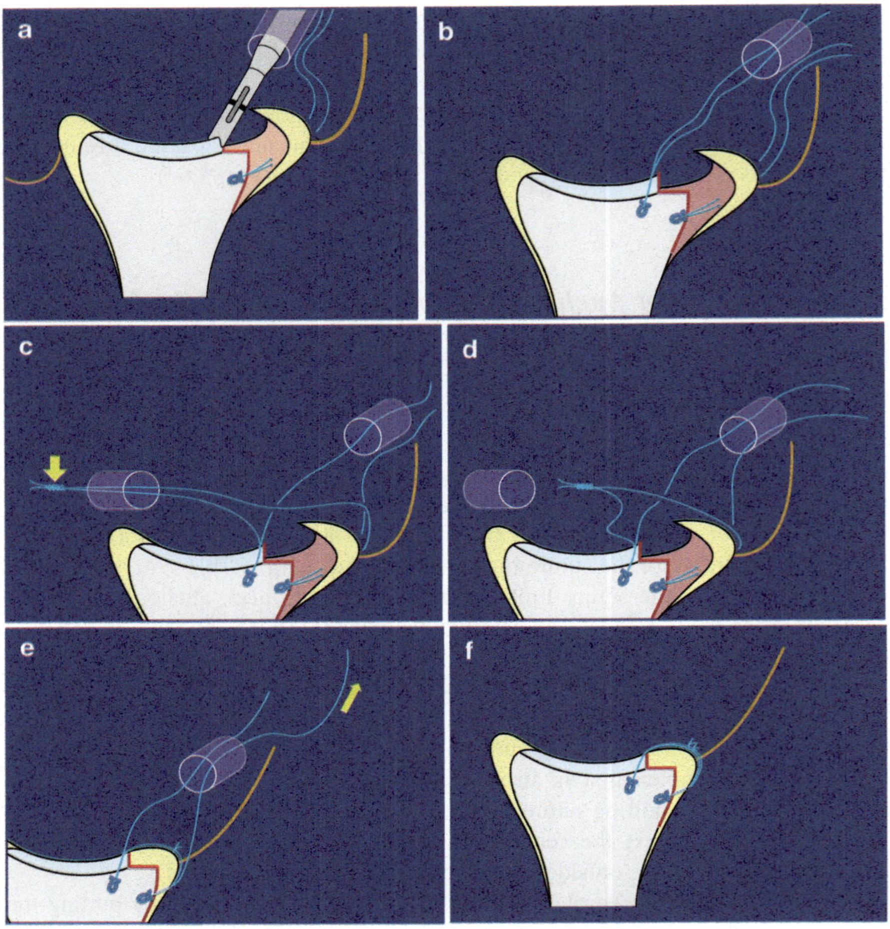

Fig. 5.7 Insertion of glenoid surface anchors through the anterior portal and knot tying. (**a**, **b**) The JuggerKnot soft anchor is inserted at the 4:30 position. (**c**) One suture limb from the glenoid neck anchor and one from the glenoid surface anchor are tied together outside the posteroinferior portal. (**d**, **e**) The outside knot is slipped into the joint space by pulling the remaining suture limbs alternatively through the anterior portal. (**f**) The remaining suture limbs are tied by the revo knot. (**g**) The triple TAFF is completed. An additional single-row suture is shown at 1:00 position. (**h**) Three-dimensional computer tomography (3D-CT) after 6 months postoperatively. These paired anchor holes look like drill holes made by the open transosseous suture method

The IGHL–labrum complex is firmly attached onto the footprint by tying knots at 3:15 and then 2:00 positions in the same manner, tying the outside knot through the posteroinferior portal and the revo knot through the anterior portal, and the triple TAFF is completed. The single-row suture is added at 1:00 position as needed to firmly attach the labrum [the anterior capsule or the middle glenohumeral

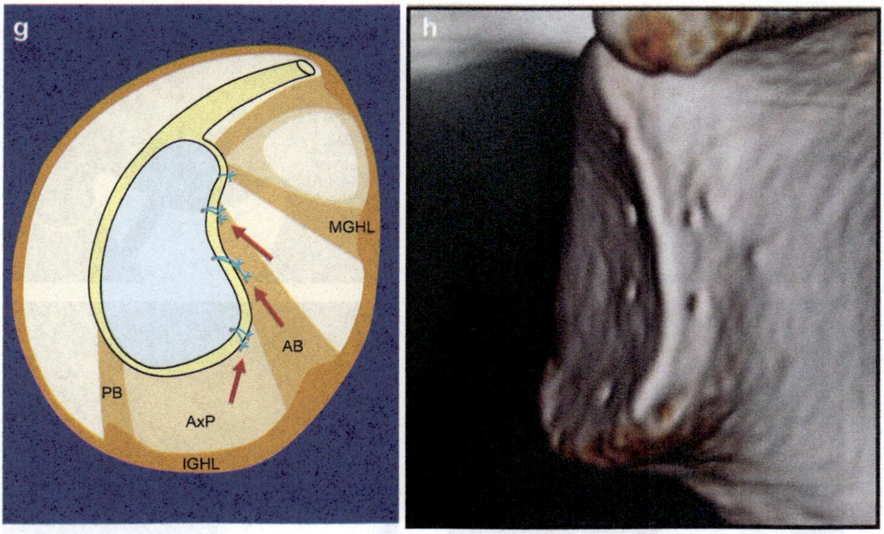

Fig. 5.7 (continued)

ligament (MGHL)] to the trough (Fig. 5.7g, h). If the IGHL–labrum complex is broad and well developed, TAFF may be performed at four places (the quadruple TAFF).

5.3 Surgical Indication of TAFF Technique

The TAFF technique not only ensures footprint fixation, but also has the advantage of being able to pass multiple sutures of the glenoid neck anchors through the IGHL–labrum complex using the mattress suture method, and to lift and draw it up strongly toward the glenoid surface by pulling the sutures of the glenoid neck anchors.

In general, this TAFF technique might be suitably indicated for patients with a significant ALPSA (anterior labroligamentous periosteal sleeve avulsion) lesion with the labrum displaced medially and inferiorly, which requires lifting up and holding the IGHL–labrum complex completely after mobilization, or those who need capsular shift as advocated by Ahmad et al., based on their cadaveric study, that the double-row suture bridge technique is effective for such significant ALPSA lesions [5].

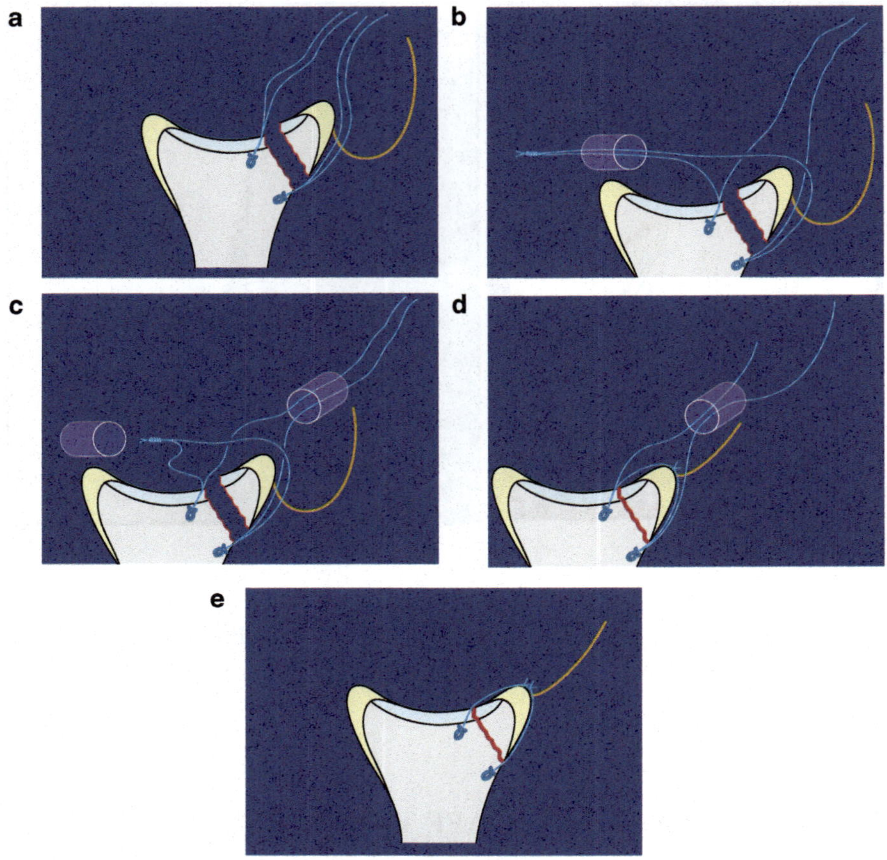

Fig. 5.8 Repair of bony Bankart lesion with large and thick bone fragment. (**a**–**e**) Bony Bankart repair by the TAFF technique. (**f**) Preoperative 3D-CT of patient with the bony Bankart lesion. (**g**) Before operation. (**h**) Just after operation by the TAFF technique. (**i**) The second look after 3 months postoperatively

Moreover, the specific indications of this technique are as follows:

1. Revision cases after conventional arthroscopic Bankart repair
2. Bony Bankart lesion with a large thick bone fragment (Fig. 5.8a–i).

In particular, this technique is very effective for bony Bankart repair [10].

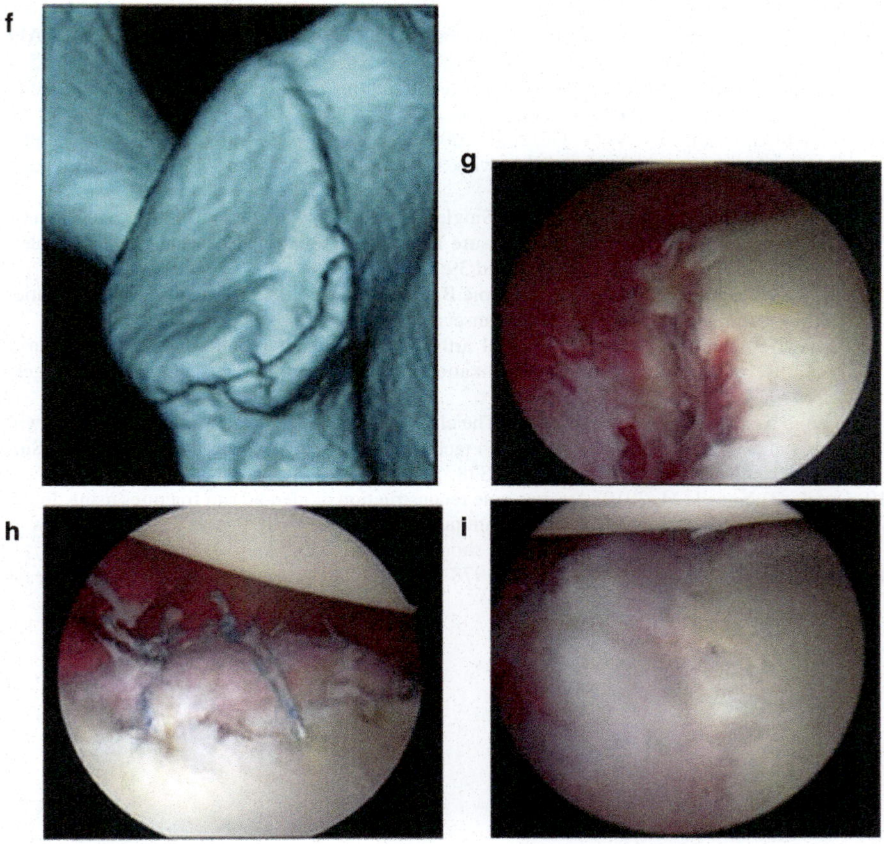

Fig. 5.8 (continued)

5.4 Conclusion

The TAFF using the JuggerKnot soft anchor is the cutting-edge technique for Bankart repair. The TAFF technique using all-suture anchors is a step closer to a true transosseous suture technique, which is a conventional open procedure making a bone tunnel [1, 11].

References

1. Tamai K, Higashi A, Tanabe T et al (1999) Recurrences after the open Bankart repair: a potential risk with use of suture anchors. J Shoulder Elbow Surg 8:37–41
2. Kim SH, Yoo JC, Ahn JM et al (2005) Arthroscopically repaired Bankart lesions and the effect of two different arm position on immediate postoperative evaluation with magnetic resonance arthrography. Arthroscopy 21:867–874

3. Sahara W, Yoneda M, Yamada S et al (2014) Stabilizing effect after arthroscopic Bankart repair evaluated by ABER-MRI: comparison among single-row fixation, DAFF and TAFF techniques (in Japanese). JOSKAS (Jpn Orthop Soc Knee Arthrosc Sports Med) 39:54–55
4. Yoneda M (2005) Arthroscopic Bankart repair in the next generation: trying for secure footprint fixation (in Japanese). Kansetsugeka 24:37–48
5. Ahmad CS, Galano GJ, Vorys GC et al (2009) Evaluation of glenoid capsulolabral complex insertional anatomy and restoration with single- and double-row capsulolabral repairs. J Shoulder Elbow Surg 18:948–954
6. Kim DS, Yoon YS, Chung HJ (2011) Single-row versus double-row capsulolabral repair: a comparative evaluation of contact pressure and surface area in the capsulolabral complex-glenoid bone interface. Am J Sports Med 39:1500–1506
7. Mizuno N, Yoneda M (2007) Arthroscopic Bankart repair by double anchor footprint fixation (DAFF) technique (in Japanese). Katakansetsu 31:497–502
8. Yamada S, Yoneda M (2011) A novel arthroscopic Bankart repair for traumatic anterior instability by double anchor footprint fixation (DAFF) technique (in Japanese). Seikeigeka 62:767–776
9. Mizuno N, Yoneda M, Ozaki R (2014) The clinical results of arthroscopic Bankart repair with double anchor footprint fixation (DAFF) technique: the study of recurrent cases. Knee Surg Sports Traumatol Arthrosc 22(suppl 1):S78
10. Goroku T, Yoneda M (2010) Arthroscopic reconstruction of glenoid rim fractures using double anchor footprint fixation (DAFF) technique (in Japanese). In: Yoneda M (ed) Atlas of arthroscopy surgical skills; arthroscopic shoulder surgery. Bunkodo, Tokyo, pp 366–374
11. Rowe CR, Patel D, Southmayd WW (1978) The Bankart procedure: a long-term end-result study. J Bone Joint Surg Am 60:1–16

Chapter 6
Complications of Arthroscopic Surgery

Teruhiko Nakagawa

Abstract The technique of arthroscopic shoulder surgery requires extreme caution, because complications have often been reported. Serious sequelae may occur in hypoxic encephalopathy, and pulmonary embolism caused by upper limb deep vein thrombosis may result in mortality. This chapter briefly describes rare complications as well as frequent complications that have been reported to date. Also, we describe our experience with complications of arthroscopic shoulder surgery, such as deviation of the anchor, breakage of surgical instruments, burns from heated irrigation fluid from a radiofrequency device, bone absorption in areas surrounding the absorbable anchor, osteolysis of the undersurface of the acromion from knot impingement, postoperative infection and pneumothorax, and subcutaneous emphysema after arthroscopic rotator cuff repair. Especially, we had 15 patients of pneumothorax or subcutaneous emphysema after arthroscopic rotator cuff repair. The incidence of pneumothorax or subcutaneous emphysema after arthroscopic rotator cuff repair was 2.3 %. Possible causes of pneumothorax and subcutaneous emphysema include the following: (1) positive pressure on the lung from the respirator under endotracheal intubation; (2) extensive infiltration of irrigation fluid into subcutaneous tissue in the thoracic wall, thereby diminishing movement of the thorax, resulting in insufficient extension of the thorax; (3) load imposition on the thoracic region from water pressure of the perfusion pump; and (4) low-temperature burn in the thoracic region by heated irrigation fluid from using a radiofrequency device.

Keywords Complication • Arthroscopic shoulder surgery • Pneumothorax

T. Nakagawa (✉)
Department of Orthopaedic Surgery, Doai Memorial Hospital, 2-1-11 Yokoami, Sumida-ku, Tokyo 130-8587, Japan
e-mail: naka0208@oak.ocn.ne.jp

K. Tamai et al. (eds.), *Advances in Shoulder Surgery*,
DOI 10.1007/978-4-431-55988-7_6

6.1 Introduction

Arthroscopic surgery of the shoulder is minimally invasive and provides a good, as well as broad, view. This form of surgery is particularly useful for repairing rotator cuff tears (arthroscopic rotator cuff repair) and recurrent dislocation of the shoulder joint (arthroscopic Bankart repair), that is, the two main disorders handled by shoulder surgery specialists. The arthroscopic surgical technique is indispensable for the shoulder surgeon. However, this technique requires extreme caution, because complications have often been reported. It can be difficult to identify the causes of complications such as postoperative infection and intraoperative pneumothorax, and they are difficult to prevent. Serious sequelae may occur in hypoxic encephalopathy, and pulmonary embolism caused by upper limb deep vein thrombosis may result in mortality.

This chapter briefly describes rare complications as well as the frequent complications that have been reported to date. We also provide detailed descriptions of complications we have experienced in actual cases undergoing arthroscopic surgery of the shoulder.

6.2 Axillary Nerve Injury

In cases undergoing circumferential articular capsule release for the treatment of shoulder contracture, caution is required when dissecting the lower part of the articular capsule because the axillary nerve runs in its vicinity. In cases receiving arthroscopic Bankart repair, caution is also necessary to avoid damaging the axillary nerve while detaching the inferior labrum and periosteum and dissecting the articular capsule.

6.3 Suprascapular Nerve Injury

Because the suprascapular nerve runs 2 cm medially to the edge of the glenoid, caution is required during mobilization of the rotator cuff when conducting arthroscopic rotator cuff repair [1]. When resecting the ganglion that is around the scapular notch, caution should be exercised to avoid damaging the suprascapular nerve.

6.4 Musculocutaneous Nerve Injury

Preparation of a medial portal in distal area of the coracoid process may result in musculocutaneous nerve damage. Therefore, the entire procedure should be performed in a blunt manner, with the course of the musculocutaneous nerve kept in mind.

6.5 Vascular Injury

The axillary artery and the brachial plexus run medially to the coracoid process, requiring caution in the preparation of a portal. Caution should also be exercised to avoid damaging the suprascapular artery running in parallel to the suprascapular nerve and to the posterior circumflex humeral artery that runs parallel to the axillary artery.

6.6 Tendon Injury

Rotator interval is sometimes dissected using a knife when preparing an anterior portal. At this time, attention should be paid to the possibility of inadvertently cutting the long head of the biceps tendon.

6.7 Acromion Fracture

If the undersurface of the acromion is excessively scraped during subacromial decompression, acromial fracture may occur. In particular, in elderly patients with osteoporosis, applying special considerations in the following manner is also necessary: the procedure should be limited to scraping of the acromial spur alone and not extended to the undersurface of the acromion.

6.8 Humerus Fracture

Manipulation may be carried out immediately after arthroscopic capsular release in patients with shoulder contracture. At this time, excessive manipulation is contraindicated in elderly patients with osteoporosis because they are at risk of humerus fracture.

6.9 Shoulder Contracture

The shoulder joint should be immobilized for a certain period of time after tissue repair, and temporary contracture is therefore inevitable. Hurberty et al. implemented rehabilitation training after arthroscopic rotator cuff repair, and reported that surgery for shoulder contracture was performed in 4.9 % of patients, with risk factors for the postoperative stiffness being calcific tendinitis, adhesive capsulitis, single-tendon cuff repair, PASTA repair, being under 50 years of age, and having Workers' Compensation insurance [2]. We also have the impression that contracture is particularly likely to persist in patients who have undergone repair of an articular side cuff tear.

6.10 Complex Regional Pain Syndrome (CRPS)

CRPS should be suspected in patients who have swelling, numbness, and contracture in the fingers and who complain of severe shoulder pain after arthroscopic surgery of the shoulder. CRPS is a relatively common postoperative complication. Treatment consists of oral therapy with antiinflammatory analgesics and opioids and gentle range-of-motion (ROM) exercises. Swelling of the fingers and joint contracture often persist for about 3 to 6 months.

6.11 Anterior Interosseous Nerve Palsy

Difficulty in active flexion of the thumb and index finger may occur on very rare occasions, rather abruptly, 1–2 weeks after surgery. Although a causal relationship with surgery is unclear, it is possible that surgical stress is involved in the occurrence of peripheral neuritis. Oral administration of vitamin B_{12} and rehabilitation training for the thumb and index finger should be conducted. Spontaneous recovery usually occurs in 6 to 12 months, but residual paralysis can be problematic in some cases.

6.12 Upper Limb Deep Vein Thrombosis and Pulmonary Embolism

When marked swelling has occurred in the upper limb on the side where arthroscopic shoulder surgery was conducted, upper limb deep vein thrombosis should be suspected, and ultrasonography and computed tomography (CT) of the upper limb should be performed to assess the presence or absence of thrombus and its size.

Blood tests for D-dimer measurement should be conducted. When a detached blood clot travels to the pulmonary artery, it can occlude the artery, leading to chest pain, dyspnea, and polypnea. The presence/absence of pulmonary embolism should be evaluated immediately by blood gas analysis, chest X-ray examination, and contrast-enhanced CT as well as contrast-enhanced magnetic resonance imaging (MRI) of the lung. The mortality rate of pulmonary embolism is as high as about 10 %, requiring emergency care. Treatment consists of drip infusion of an anticoagulant such as heparin. If possible, the patient should be transferred to a department of cardiovascular medicine or respiratory medicine. Kuremsky reported low prevalence (0.31 %) of imaging-confirmed thromboembolic events [3].

6.13 Hypoxic Encephalopathy

Neurological ischemic symptoms such as cerebral infarction and hearing loss have been described as possibly occurring after arthroscopic shoulder surgery in the beach-chair position. Koh et al. have reported that cerebral oxygen saturation was significantly lower in patients who underwent surgery in the beach-chair position under general anesthesia than in those who had received operative treatment under interscalene block, pointing out the risk of general anesthesia in the beach-chair position [4].

In addition, Moerman et al. reported that cerebral oxygen saturation decreased by more than 20 % in 80 % of patients in response to a postural change from the supine position to the beach-chair position [5].

Caution is required to limit the angle of the sitting position to 60° or less when the beach-chair position is used.

6.14 Airway Narrowing

Perfusate infiltrates the surrounding soft tissue from the portal entry site or the subacromial space and causes edema around the shoulder. Such edema, on rare occasions, extends to the cervical region and causes airway narrowing [6]. Because of the gravity effect, airway narrowing is more likely to occur in patients who had surgery in the lateral decubitus position than in those who underwent their operations in the beach-chair position. In particular, attention should be paid to swelling around the neck when surgery is prolonged.

6.15 Deviation of the Anchor

Deviation of the anchor from the bone may be identified by X-ray examination or MRI at some time point after surgery. This deviation is more likely to occur in women of advanced age with osteoporosis. If there are symptoms such as pain or discomfort, another arthroscopic operation should be performed to remove the anchor. If there is retearing of the repaired rotator cuff, the cuff is usually repaired again with another anchors. Case 1 was a 75-year-old woman who underwent reoperation to remove a deviated CorkScrew (Fig. 6.1a, b), case 2 was a 70-year-old woman who underwent a second arthroscopic rotator cuff repair after removal of a deviated Fastin (Fig. 6.1c, d), and case 3 was a 74-year-old woman who underwent a second arthroscopic rotator cuff repair after removal of a deviated Versalok (Fig. 6.1e, f).

6.16 Breakage of Surgical Instruments

Advances in surgical instruments have allowed us to conduct more rapid and precise arthroscopic surgery of the shoulder, but breakage of instruments does occasionally occur. A broken instrument, if it remains in the patient's body

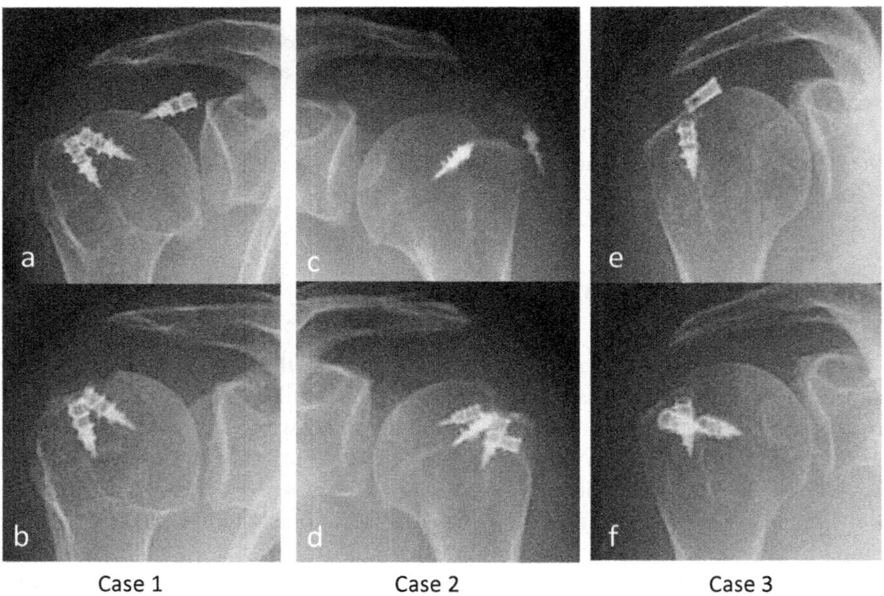

Fig. 6.1 Deviation of the anchor after arthroscopic rotator cuff repair. (**a**, **b**) Case 1. A 75-year-old woman. The deviated CorkScrew was removed by reoperation. (**c**, **d**) Case 2. A 70-year-old woman. After removal of the deviated Fastin, another arthroscopic rotator cuff repair was performed. (**e**, **f**) Case 3. A 74-year-old woman. After removal of the deviated Versalok, another arthroscopic rotator cuff repair was performed

postoperatively, may cause postoperative pain as well as legal problems. Therefore, the surgeon should endeavor to remove the broken foreign body during the surgery. If it is difficult to remove the broken foreign body, the surgeon should show the relevant X-ray image to the patient and family, and attempt to obtain their understanding by explaining the circumstances that prevent removal of the foreign body.

6.16.1 Breakage of Anchor Inserter Tip

When the inserter of the JuggarKnot was drawn, the inserter became twisted because there was resistance, which resulted in breakage of the inserter tip. Fortunately, a metal fragment was identified in the field of view (Fig. 6.2a) and could easily be removed by holding it with curette forceps (Fig. 6.2b). The metal fragment was very small (Fig. 6.2c), but might have caused injury to the articular cartilage if it had remained in the joint as a loose foreign body.

6.16.2 Breakage of Suture Punch Needle

The needle of a suture punch was broken off at the root during rotator cuff repair. The needle was embedded in the rotator cuff and could not be found under arthroscopic view. Using an image intensifier (fluoroscopic apparatus) (Fig. 6.3a), the needle in the rotator cuff was identified under fluoroscopic guidance. The rotator cuff was evaporated using VAPR (Fig. 6.3b); the needle was exposed (Fig. 6.3c) and removed with curette forceps. The rotator cuff was repaired to finish the operation.

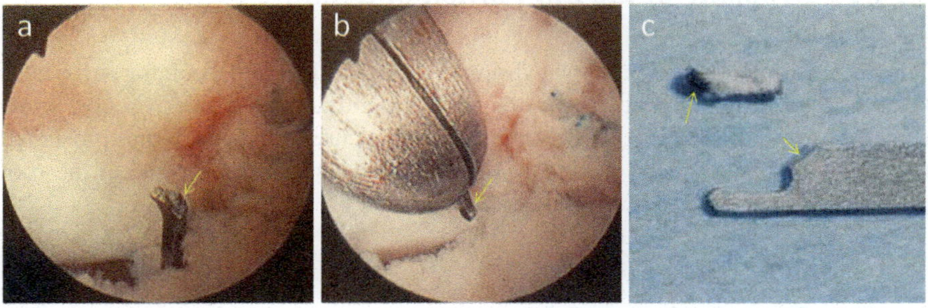

Fig. 6.2 Breakage of anchor inserter tip. (**a**) The tip of the JaggerKnot inserter was broken during arthroscopic Bankart repair, and a small metal fragment remained in the joint. (**b**) The metal fragment was held with curette forceps and removed. (**c**) Breakage of inserter tip is shown

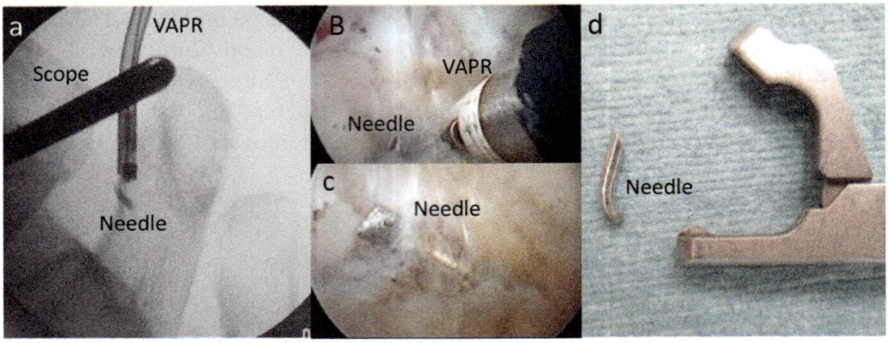

Fig. 6.3 Breakage of a suture punch needle. (**a**) Breakage of needle in the rotator cuff was confirmed under X-ray fluoroscopy, and the rotator cuff was ablated using VAPR, toward the direction of the existing needle. (**b**) A portion of the needle was confirmed under arthroscopy after ablation of the rotator cuff by VAPR. (**c**) The needle was exposed and removed using curette forceps. (**d**) The suture punch and the broken needle are shown

6.16.3 Breakage of the Suture Passer Needle Tip

The tip of a Scorpion needle was broken during arthroscopic rotator cuff repair (Fig. 6.4b). The needle tip remained in the rotator cuff and could not be identified under arthroscopic view. We abandoned retrieving the needle tip from inside the rotator cuff because it was too small. The patient and family were informed of the situation, using the X-ray image that showed the needle tip after the operation (Fig. 6.4c): the needle tip was virtually nonremovable, and it was unlikely to become a problem because it was presumably embedded in the rotator cuff. Fortunately, the patient's postoperative course was favorable, without troubles.

6.16.4 Dropping of the Lid Portion of a Suture Passer

The lid portion of a BiPass tip was dropped during arthroscopic rotator cuff repair (Fig. 6.5a). Fortunately, it was immediately identified under arthroscopic view (Fig. 6.5b), and this lid portion was removed using curette forceps. It was presumed that repeated opening and closing of the lid had caused metal fatigue at the root portion of the lid (Fig. 6.5c), resulting in a breakage.

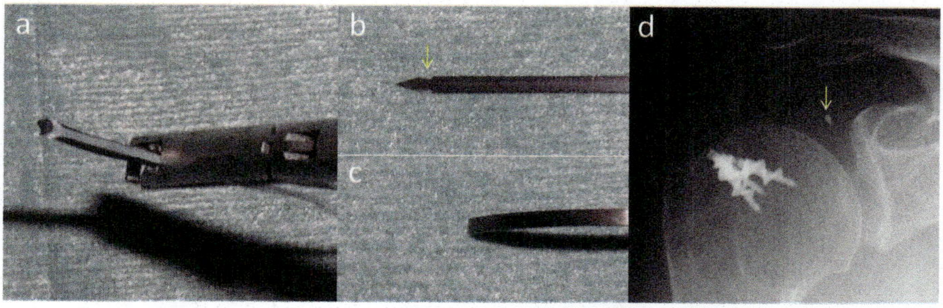

Fig. 6.4 Breakage of suture passer needle tip. (**a**) Suture passer (Scorpion) is an implement for passing the thread through the rotator cuff. (**b**) The Scorpion needle before use. Breakage may occur at the constricted portion indicated by the *arrow*. (**c**) A needle lacking its tip, which was broken at the constricted portion of the needle. (**d**) X-ray image after arthroscopic rotator cuff repair. The broken needle tip was still in the rotator cuff

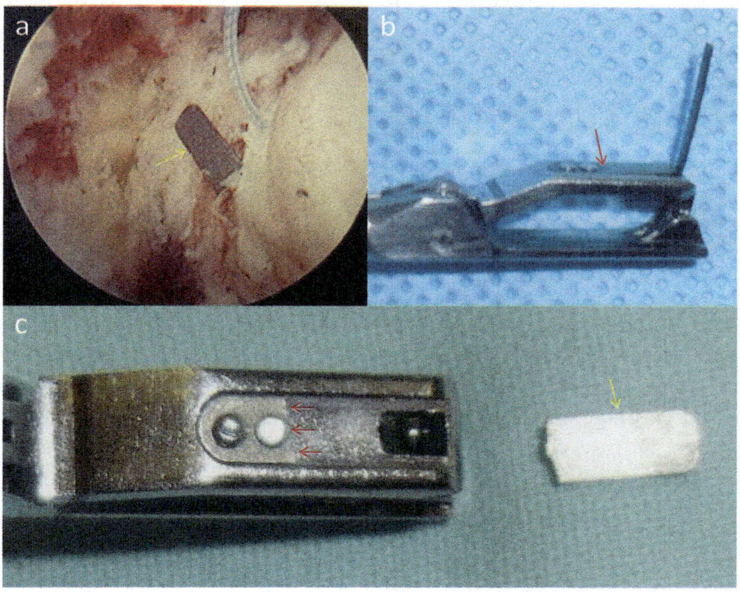

Fig. 6.5 Breakage of the lid portion of a suture passer tip. (**a**) The lid portion of the BiPass was found in surface of the rotator cuff. (**b**) The root of the lid portion of the BiPass has an opening and closing function (*arrow*). (**c**) The breakage root of the lid portion (*arrow*)

6.17 Burn Caused by Heated Irrigation Fluid from VAPR

We formerly used irrigation fluid heated in a warmer box to prevent the patient's body from cooling excessively (Fig. 6.6a, b). However, the subacromial irrigation fluid was heated employing VAPR to a high temperature, and hot irrigation fluid

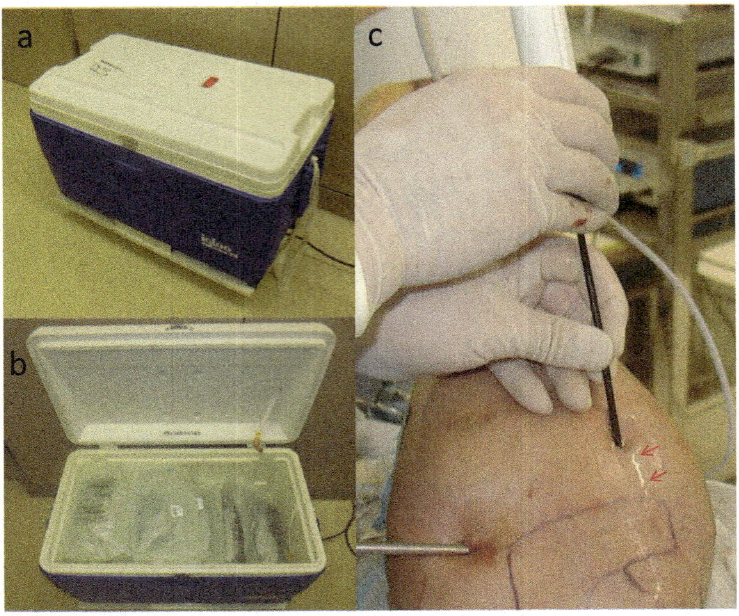

Fig. 6.6 Burn from heated irrigation fluid from VAPR. (**a**, **b**) We formerly used irrigation fluid warmed in a warmer box to avoid lowering the patient's body temperature. (**c**) The irrigation fluid in the subacromial region was heated employing VAPR to a high temperature. The hot irrigation fluid exiting the portal caused the skin burn pictured (*arrows*)

exiting the portal (Fig. 6.6c) occasionally caused skin burns. Fortunately, such burns were mild and restricted to a small area, but such burns can be very dangerous. The synovial membrane and rotator cuff in the subacromial space and the articular cartilage and articular capsule in the shoulder are at risk of sustaining burn injuries. Diffuse chondrolysis reportedly occurred as a result of arthroscopic thermal capsulorrhaphy [7, 8].

6.18 Bone Absorption and Osteolysis in Areas Surrounding the Absorbable Anchor

It has been reported that bone absorption and osteolysis may occur in the anchor hole when an absorbable anchor is used employing the arthroscopic Bankart repair [9–11]. We also experienced a case with enlargement of the anchor hole and formation of a concavity in the anteroinferior part of the glenoid. Case 4 was a 45-year-old man in whom four absorbable anchors (Panalok Loop) were used. Two threads were passed through each loop, and the capsular ligament and labrum were repaired using a total of eight threads (Fig. 6.7a). The postoperative course was

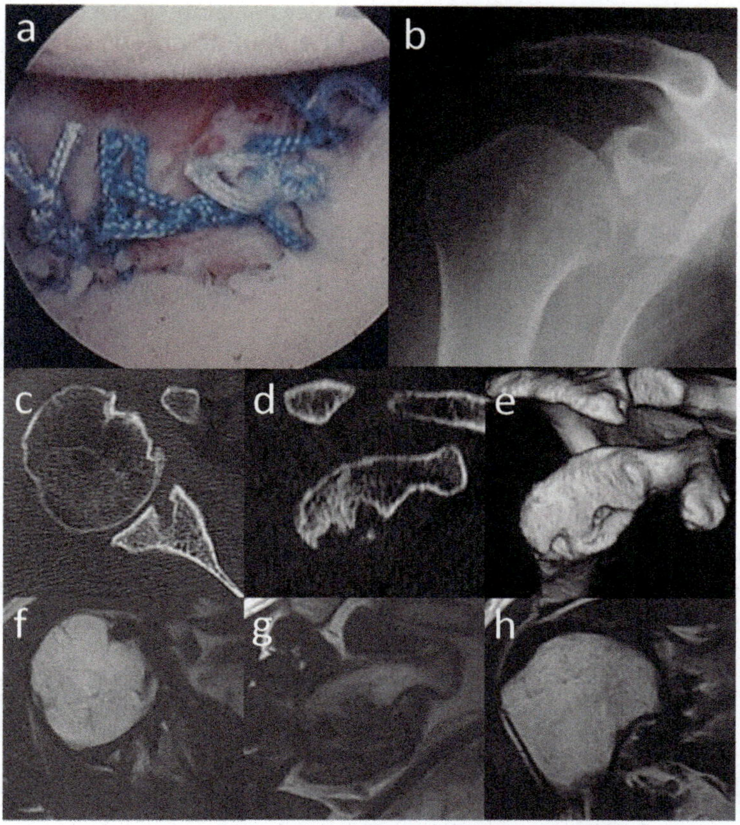

Fig. 6.7 Bone absorption and osteolysis in areas surrounding the absorbable anchor (**b–h** are images obtained 1 year and 3 months after surgery). (**a**) Case 4. A 46-year-old man. Arthroscopic Bankart repair was performed for the treatment of recurrent dislocation of the shoulder joint. Four absorbable anchors (Panalok Loop) were used. Two threads were passed through each loop, and the capsular ligament and labrum were repaired using a total of eight threads. (**b**) At 1 year and 3 months after surgery, the X-ray image showed concavity in the anteroinferior part of the glenoid. (**c**) Enlarged anchor holes can be seen in the CT image. (**d**, **e**) CT and 3D CT images demonstrated osteolysis in the anteroinferior part of the glenoid. (**f–h**) T_2-weighted MRI showed low signal intensity in the osteolytic area, without accompanying edema fluid

temporarily favorable, with no further dislocation and favorable conversion to a negative anterior apprehension test. However, 1 year and 3 months after surgery, the patient suffered pain and rotational motion disorder of the shoulder. The X-ray image obtained at the time showed concavity in the anteroinferior part of the glenoid (Fig. 6.7b), and enlarged anchor holes were observed on a CT image (Fig. 6.7c). The sagittal section of the CT image and the three-dimensional (3D) CT image demonstrated osteolysis in the anteroinferior part of the glenoid

(Fig. 6.7d, e). T_2-weighted MRI showed low signal intensity in the osteolytic area without accompanying edema fluid (Fig. 6.7f–h). Thereafter, the pain resolved after about 6 months of follow-up, achieving restoration of the range of rotational motion.

6.19 Osteolysis of the Undersurface of the Acromion from Knot Impingement

It has been reported that osteolysis may occur in the undersurface of the acromion, causing pain, several months after arthroscopic rotator cuff repair [12]. Case 5 was a 39-year-old man who underwent arthroscopic repair surgery for a bursal side tear of the rotator cuff, employing the single-row technique using two Ethibond threads and two FiberWire threads with two absorbable anchors (Panalok loop RC) (Fig. 6.8a). Acute pain in the shoulder occurred 5 months after surgery. X-ray, CT, and 3D CT images taken at the time showed concavity of the bone in the undersurface of the acromion and thinning of the acromion (Fig. 6.8b–d). MRI T_2-weighted images showed retention of edema fluid in the concave portion of the acromion (Fig. 6.8e). Because pain and swelling persisted, another arthroscopic

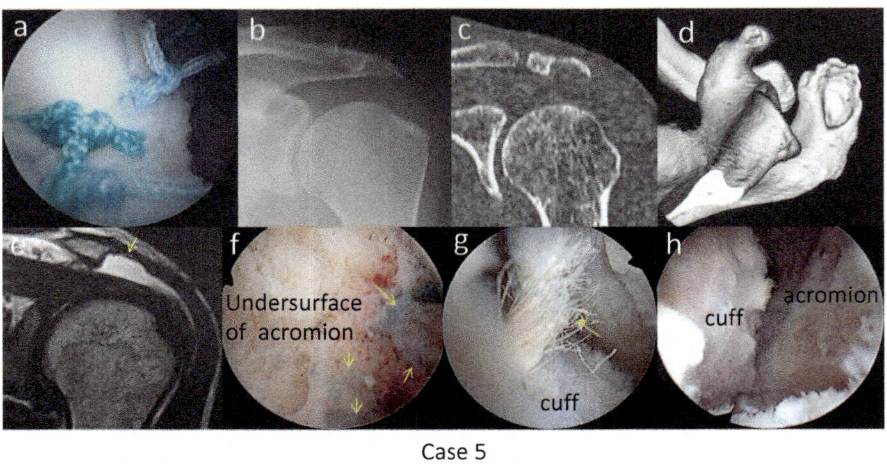

Fig. 6.8 Osteolysis of the undersurface of the acromion caused by knot impingement. (**a**) Case 5. A 39-year-old man underwent arthroscopic repair surgery for the bursal side tear of the rotator cuff, employing the single-row technique using two Ethibond threads and two FiberWire threads with two absorbable anchors (Panalok loop RC). (**b–d**) X-ray, CT, and 3D CT images showed concavity of the bone in the undersurface of the acromion and thinning of the acromion. (**e**) T_2-weighted MRI showed retention of edema fluid in the concave portion of the acromion. (**f**) Broken Ethibond thread was found to be adherent to the concave part of the undersurface of the acromion. (**g**) The FiberWire thread impinged at the undersurface of the acromion. (**h**) The thread was removed, and the absence of impingement was then confirmed

surgery was conducted. Broken Ethibond thread was found in the concave portion of the undersurface of the acromion (Fig. 6.8f). Although the rotator cuff had been repaired favorably, there was a hard protrusion in the rotator cuff surface. It was presumed that the tip of the hard protrusion and the undersurface of the acromion caused impingement. When this protrusion was shaved, a FiberWire thread emerged from inside (Fig. 6.8g). This thread was then entirely removed (Fig. 6.8h). Immediate pain alleviation was obtained with arthroscopic removal of the thread.

It was presumed that physical abrasion of the knot had caused scraping of the undersurface of the acromion, resulting in osteolysis. However, we recently experienced a case with osteolysis of the undersurface of the acromion occurring after rotator cuff repair employing the bridging suture technique without knot tying, and came to suspect that knot impingement might not be the only cause of osteolysis. Because there are reports raising doubts about knot impingement, further investigations are required to elucidate the cause of osteolysis [13].

6.20 Postoperative Infection

Although infection associated with arthroscopic shoulder surgery is rare, it may induce osteomyelitis or secondary osteoarthritis if not treated in an early phase. If there are signs of infection such as fever, pain, and redness, hematological examinations including C-reactive protein (CRP), sedimentation, and leukocytes should be carried out. X-ray examination should also be conducted to look for indications of bone absorption and downward shift of the humeral head. The presence/absence and extent of edema in the shoulder joint and the undersurface of the acromion should be examined by MRI. Shoulder joint puncture under X-ray fluoroscopy is necessary to conduct culture of joint fluid and antibiotic sensitivity studies. Culture of joint fluid is indispensable before the initiation of antibiotic therapy.

If pain, redness, and swelling are mild, intravenous drip infusion of an antibiotic chosen based on the results of sensitivity studies should be conducted for consecutive days. Oral antibiotic therapy employing a series with different sensitivity may also be given concomitantly.

If redness or swelling is severe, and antibiotic therapy alone is judged to be inadequate to treat the infection, irrigation and debridement under arthroscopy should be performed in an early phase. Whether to remove the anchor should be decided on a case-by-case basis. If there is evidence of bone absorption around the anchor, the anchor and thread should be removed. An antibiotic to which the pathogen is sensitive should also be drip infused postoperatively.

Case 6 was a 73-year-old woman who underwent arthroscopic rotator cuff repair. Three months after this surgery, there was redness at the wound site in the lateral portal, which gradually resulted in the formation of a subcutaneous abscess (Fig. 6.9a). Horizontal T_2-weighted MRI revealed continuity from the subacromial space to the subcutaneous abscess (Fig. 6.9b). Sagittal T_2-weighted MRI showed

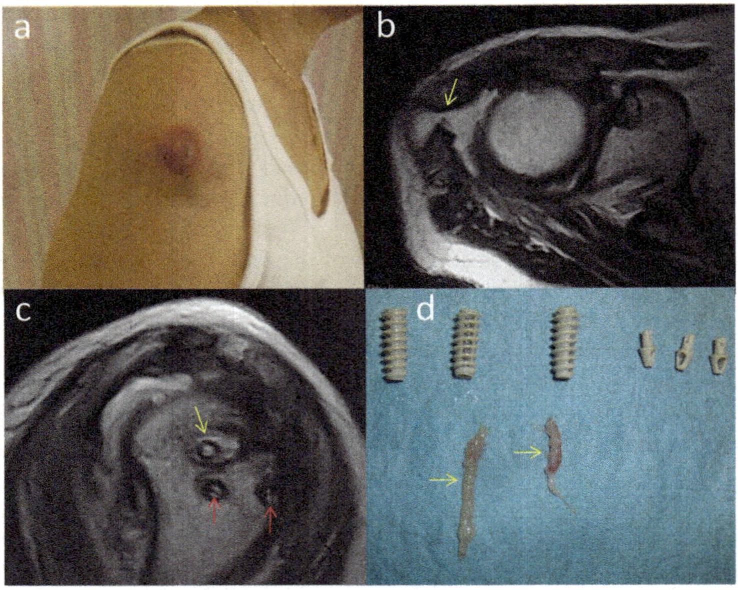

Case 6

Fig. 6.9 Postoperative infection. (**a**) Case 6. A 73-year-old woman. Subcutaneous abscess developed at the wound site in the lateral portal after arthroscopic rotator cuff repair. (**b**) Horizontal T_2-weighted MRI revealed continuity from the subacromial space to the subcutaneous abscess. (**c**) Sagittal T_2-weighted MRI showed edema around the anchors. (**d**) After removal of the anchors, granulation tissue (*arrows*) was found in the lumen of the SwiveLock

edema around the anchors (Fig. 6.9c). *Pseudomonas aeruginosa* was detected by culture. The subacromial space and shoulder joint were irrigated under arthroscopy, and the anchors were removed under direct vision after slightly augmenting the skin incision at the site of abscess resection. Granulation tissue was found in the lumen of the SwiveLock (Fig. 6.9d). Intravenous antibiotic therapy to which the pathogen was sensitive was continued for 2 weeks postoperatively, leading to subsidence of the infection.

6.21 Pneumothorax and Subcutaneous Emphysema

It has been reported that pneumothorax and/or subcutaneous emphysema may occur in arthroscopic shoulder surgery [14–16]. We experienced 15 patients with pneumothorax or subcutaneous emphysema after arthroscopic rotator cuff repair.

We have consistently conducted arthroscopic surgery of the shoulder with patients in the lateral decubitus position under general anesthesia. Until 2009, no cases developed pneumothorax or subcutaneous emphysema after arthroscopic surgery of the shoulder. However, there was one pneumothorax after arthroscopic rotator cuff repair in 2010 and 15 cases with pneumothorax or subcutaneous emphysema during the 6 years between 2010 and 2015. Among these cases, there were 11 with pneumothorax alone, 3 with pneumothorax accompanied by subcutaneous emphysema, and 1 with subcutaneous emphysema alone. In all 15 cases, pneumothorax or subcutaneous emphysema occurred on the side of arthroscopic rotator cuff repair, whereas neither occurred in cases undergoing surgery other than arthroscopic rotator cuff repair. As shown in Table 6.1, pneumothorax and subcutaneous emphysema occurred rather frequently, that is, in 4 patients in 2012 and 6 in 2013. Arthroscopic rotator cuff surgery was conducted in 646 patients during the 6 years between 2010 and 2015, and the incidence of pneumothorax or subcutaneous emphysema after arthroscopic rotator cuff repair was 2.3 %. During the same period of time, arthroscopic Bankart repair was performed in 177 shoulders, but neither pneumothorax nor subcutaneous emphysema was noted.

The 15 patients who suffered pneumothorax or subcutaneous emphysema were 69.6 years old (range, 54–84 years), with 8 men and 7 women. The affected site was the right shoulder in 11 cases and the left shoulder in 4. The size of the rotator cuff tear was medium in 2 cases, large in 9, and massive in 4, whereas neither pneumothorax nor subcutaneous emphysema occurred after surgery for small or incomplete rotator cuff tear. The mean surgical time was 138 min (range, 93–185 min). Interscalene block was conducted concomitantly in 3 cases.

We obtain X-ray images in every patient immediately after surgery before awakening from general anesthesia. If pneumothorax is confirmed in the X-ray image taken immediately after surgery, chest X-ray images are promptly ordered to confirm the size and site of pneumothorax. A surgeon is called into the operating room to decide whether to conduct chest tube drainage.

In 11 of our 15 patients, pneumothorax was confirmed in X-ray images of the shoulder immediately after surgery, and chest X-ray examination was performed (Fig. 6.10a, b). A chest drainage tube was inserted by a surgeon in the operating room before awakening the patient from general anesthesia, and the drainage tube was connected to a negative pressure pump. After confirming amelioration of the

Table 6.1 Number of cases undergoing arthroscopic shoulder surgery and the number and frequency of cases developing pneumothorax and subcutaneous emphysema by year

	2010	2011	2012	2013	2014	2015	Total
Arthroscopic shoulder surgery	160	168	167	156	150	150	**951**
Arthroscopic rotator cuff repair	93	110	110	112	116	105	**646**
Arthroscopic Bankart repair	30	42	34	29	21	21	**177**
Others	37	16	23	15	13	24	**128**
Pneumothorax and/or subcutaneous emphysema	1	2	4	6	1	1	**15**
Incidence of pneumothorax and/or subcutaneous emphysema in arthroscopic rotator cuff repair	1.1 %	1.8 %	3.6 %	5.4 %	0.9 %	1.0 %	**2.3 %**

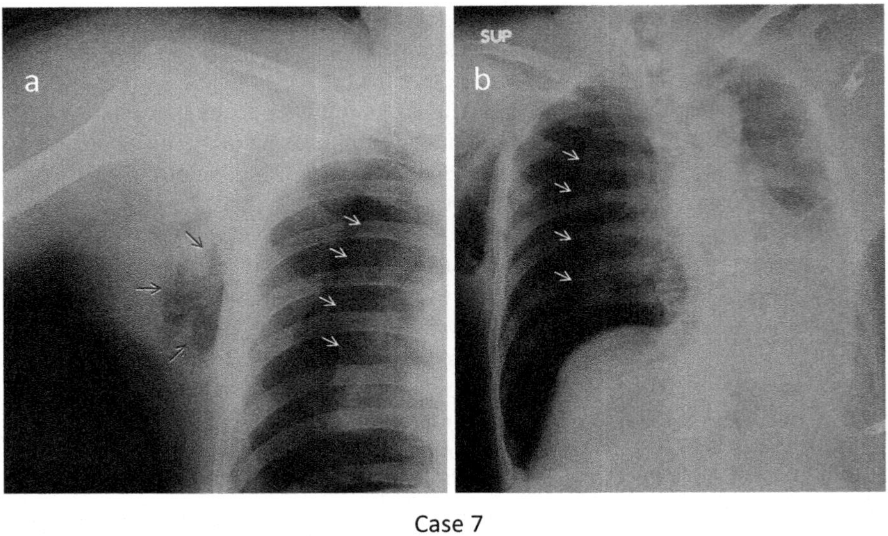

Fig. 6.10 Pneumothorax and subcutaneous emphysema after arthroscopic rotator cuff repair. (**a**) Case 7. A 84-year-old man. Arthroscopic rotator cuff repair was performed for the medium-sized rotator cuff tear. The surgical time was 93 min. Pneumothorax (*yellow arrow*) and subcutaneous emphysema (*red arrow*) were present based on the X-ray image of the shoulder taken immediately after surgery. (**b**) Chest X-ray examination showed marked pneumothorax (*arrow*). A trocar was inserted into the pleural space by a surgeon before awakening from general anesthesia

pneumothorax in the chest X-ray image, the patients were roused from anesthesia. Subcutaneous emphysema was present concomitantly in 2 of these 11 patients.

Pneumothorax was overlooked in the X-ray image of the shoulder immediately after surgery in 3 of our 15 patients. Oxygen saturation was as low as 95 in all 3 patients on the day after surgery. Therefore, chest X-ray examination was performed in 2 patients, and chest X-ray examination and CT of the lung in another patient, to confirm pneumothorax (Fig. 6.11a, b). Then, a chest drainage tube was inserted in each patient by a surgeon. In the 1 remaining patient, chest X-ray examination performed on the day after surgery revealed pneumothorax and subcutaneous emphysema. Because a surgeon judged there to be no space to insert a trocar, the patient was followed up without chest drainage until full resolution. No clinical symptoms associated with pneumothorax, such as chest pain and difficulty breathing, were present in the 2 patients in whom the chest drainage tube was inserted, whereas the other patient complained of mild chest pain.

In one of our 15 patients, subcutaneous emphysema alone was identified by X-ray examination of the shoulder immediately after surgery, and the patient was followed up under conservative treatment.

In these 15 patients, pneumothorax and/or subcutaneous emphysema resolved without causing residual disability. There were 2 smokers: 1 was a 54-year-old man and the other was a 74-year-old woman. No patient had a respiratory disease such as

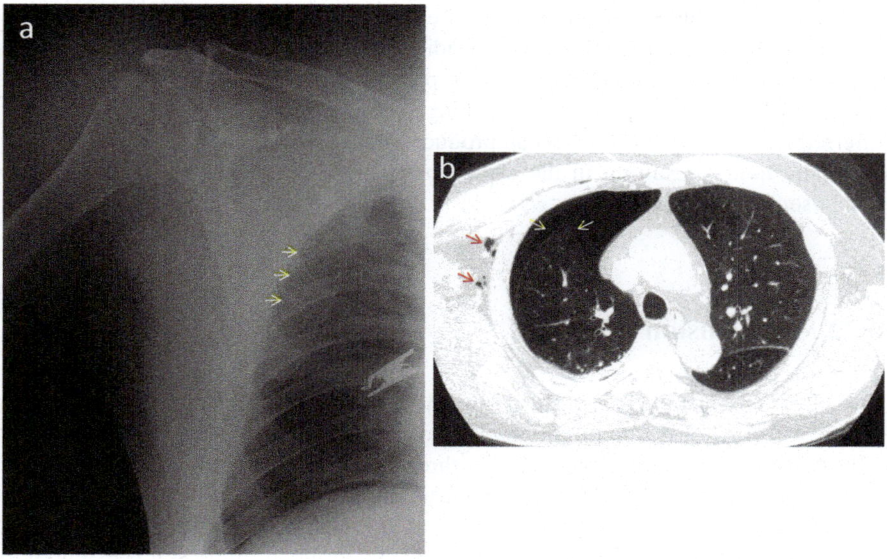

Case 8

Fig. 6.11 Pneumothorax after arthroscopic rotator cuff repair. (**a**) Case 8. A 70-year-old man. Arthroscopic rotator cuff repair was performed for the large-sized rotator cuff tear. Operating time was 134 min. Pneumothorax was missed in the X-ray image of the shoulder obtained immediately after surgery. Careful retrospective study of the X-ray image led to the identification of a *subtle line* indicating pneumothorax (*arrows*). (**b**) Because oxygen saturation was as low as 95 on the day after surgery, chest X-ray and CT images were obtained, which confirmed obvious pneumothorax (*yellow arrows*) and emphysema outside the chest wall (*red arrows*). A trocar was inserted into the pleural space

asthma. No bullae were found by chest X-ray examination in any of our patients before surgery.

In three patients, interscalene block was combined with general anesthesia. However, because the needle was inserted under ultrasonic guidance, it is unlikely that interscalene block causes pneumothorax.

A needle is inserted from the lateral acromion to position the anchor portal, but there is virtually no possibility based on the anatomic positional relationship that the needle tip damages the pleural membrane.

Possible causes of pneumothorax and subcutaneous emphysema include the following: (1) positive pressure on the lung from the respirator under endotracheal intubation; (2) extensive infiltration of irrigation fluid into not only the area around the shoulder on the affected side but also subcutaneous tissue in the thoracic wall and the neck, which would cause edema, thereby diminishing movement of the thorax, resulting in insufficient extension of the thorax under positive pressure on the lung; (3) load imposition on the thoracic region because of water pressure of the perfusion pump; and (4) low-temperature burn in the thoracic region by heated irrigation fluid because of the use of a radiofrequency device.

Pneumothorax occurred frequently in patients who had large or massive tears, and the surgical time was relatively long, 138 min on average. Therefore, it is inferred that a variety of factors can produce a load on the lung on the affected side for many hours, resulting in the occurrence of pneumothorax and subcutaneous emphysema.

6.22 Conclusion

Complications include those caused by anesthesia, surgical position, and the perfusate. The risk of developing complications rises as the surgical time increases. Efforts should be made to complete arthroscopic shoulder surgery within 2 h. If surgery is prolonged, edema of soft tissue caused by the perfusate impairs the operative view and leads to a longer surgical time with ever-increasing edema, that is, causing a vicious circle. In regard to nerve and vascular injuries, it is essential to fully understand the anatomic courses and variations of the nerves and blood vessels. Unreasonable manipulation should be avoided to prevent breakage of surgical instruments. When a part of a broken metal instrument remains in the body, every effort must be made to remove the fragment, using an image intensifier without hesitation. X-ray examination of the shoulder should be performed immediately after surgery to assess whether pneumothorax is present.

We hope that this chapter will help arthroscopic surgeons in obtaining informed consent and in other relevant situations.

References

1. Warner JJP, Krushell RJ et al (1992) Anatomy and relationship of the suprascapular nerve: anatomical constraints to mobilization of the supraspinatus and infraspinatus muscle in the treatment of massive rotator-cuff tears. J Bone Joint Surg 74-A:36–45
2. Huberty DP, Schoolfield JD et al (2009) Incidence and treatment of postoperative stiffness following arthroscopic rotator cuff repair. Arthroscopy 25:880–890
3. Kuremsky M, Cain EL et al (2011) Thromboembolic phenomena after arthroscopic shoulder surgery. Arthroscopy 27:1614–1619
4. Koh JL, Levin SD et al (2013) Cerebral oxygenation in the beach chair position: a prospective study on the effect of general anesthesia compared with regional anesthesia and sedation. J Shoulder Elbow Surg 22:1325–1331
5. Moerman AT, De Hert SG, Jacobs TF et al (2012) Cerebral oxygen desaturation during beach chair position. Eur J Anaesthesiol 29:82–87
6. Orebaugh SL (2003) Life-threatening airway edema resulting from prolonged shoulder arthroscopy. Anesthesiology 99:1456–1458

7. Levine WN, Clark AM Jr et al (2005) Chondrolysis following arthroscopic thermal capsulorrhaphy to treat shoulder instability. A report of two cases. J Bone Joint Surg 87-A:616–621
8. Petty DH, Jazrawi LM et al (2004) Glenohumeral chondrolysis after shoulder arthroscopy: case reports and review of literature. Am J Sports Med 32:509–515
9. Athwal GS, Shridharani SM et al (2006) Osteolysis and arthropathy of the shoulder after use of bioabsorbable knotless suture anchors. J Bone Joint Surg 88-A:1840–1845
10. Take Y, Yoneda M et al (2008) Enlargement of drill holes after use of a biodegradable suture anchor: quantitative study on consecutive postoperative radiographs. J Arthrosc Relat Surg 24:251–257
11. Takubo Y, Morihara T et al (2008) Anchor hole enlargement after arthroscopic Bankart repair using absorbable suture anchors: a report of three cases. J Shoulder Elbow Surg 17:e16–e18
12. Hotta T, Yamashita T (2010) Osteolysis of the inferior surface of the acromion caused by knots of the suture thread after rotator cuff repair: knot impingement after rotator cuff repair. J Shoulder Elbow Surg 19:e17–e23
13. Park YE, Shon MS et al (2014) Knot impingement after rotator cuff repair: is it real? J Arthrosc Relat Surg 30:1055–1060
14. Lee HC, Dawan N et al (1992) Subcutaneous emphysema, pneumomediastinum, and potentially life-threatening tension pneumothorax. Pulmonary complications from arthroscopic shoulder decompression. Chest 101:1265–1267
15. Dietzel DP, Ciullo JV (1996) Spontaneous pneumothorax after shoulder arthroscopy: a case report of four cases. J Arthrosc Relat Surg 12:99–102
16. Calvisi V, Lupparelli S et al (2009) Subcutaneous emphysema and pneumomediastinum, following shoulder arthroscopy with brachial plexus block: a case report and review of literature. Arch Orthop Trauma Surg 129:349–352

Chapter 7
Instability

Keisuke Matsuki and Hiroyuki Sugaya

Abstract Outcomes after surgical treatment for shoulder instability have been improving with the innovations in surgical techniques and devices, especially arthroscopic surgeries. However, there still remain several concerns, and various attempts have been made to further improve the outcomes. One of the remaining issues is the high recurrence rate in collision/contact athletes with shoulder instability. Although open procedures such as the Latarjet procedure are often indicated for such patients, the arthroscopic remplissage technique as an augmentation can be another treatment option to reduce the recurrence rate. Another issue is management of bone loss in the glenoid and humeral head. Precise evaluation of the bone defect is important for choosing treatment options, and CT is the current gold standard of imaging. If the bony fragment in the Bankart lesion is well preserved, arthroscopic bony Bankart repair can work well even with a small fragment because restoration of the glenoid shape can be expected after reduction and fixation of the fragment in the longer term. If the fragment is nonexistent or too small, bone grafting should be considered. For large Hill–Sachs lesions, the arthroscopic remplissage has demonstrated lower recurrence rates without severe restriction of external rotation.

Keywords Shoulder instability • Glenoid bone loss • Arthroscopic bony Bankart repair • Arthroscopic iliac bone grafting • Arthroscopic Hill–Sachs remplissage

7.1 Introduction

7.1.1 Advances in Treatment for Shoulder Instability

Shoulder dislocation and recurrent glenohumeral instability are a common shoulder problem, especially in active young patients. Traumatic anterior instability is the most common, and surgical stabilization is often required when conservative

K. Matsuki • H. Sugaya (✉)
Sports Medicine and Joint Center, Funabashi Orthopaedic Hospital, 1-833 Hazama, Funabashi, Chiba 274-0822, Japan
e-mail: hsugaya@nifty.com

K. Tamai et al. (eds.), *Advances in Shoulder Surgery*,
DOI 10.1007/978-4-431-55988-7_7

treatment has failed [1]. Historically, open stabilization has been considered the gold standard treatment. Since Wolf et al. [2] introduced an arthroscopic technique using suture anchors in 1991, arthroscopic stabilization techniques have become more popular with advances in the techniques and devices. Surgeons may prefer arthroscopic surgeries because of the advantages over open surgeries: better diagnostic ability and repair of all accompanying intraarticular lesions, less risk of postoperative shoulder stiffness, and avoidance of tenotomy or splitting of the subscapularis [3]. In the United States, 71.2 % of Bankart repairs were arthroscopic from 2003 to 2005, whereas 87.7 % were arthroscopic from 2006 to 2008 [4].

Results of arthroscopic stabilization in the early era were not satisfactory in terms of the high recurrence rates. The recurrence rate in open procedures is approximately 8 %, according to systematic reviews [3, 5, 6]. Harris et al. [5] conducted a systematic review on long-term outcomes of arthroscopic Bankart repairs performed mostly in the 1990s and reported that the recurrence rate was 24 %. However, Petrera et al. [6] reported in their systematic review that the recurrence rate of arthroscopic stabilization in the studies after 2002 was 2.9 % and that there was a significant difference in the rate with open procedures (9.2 %). Thus, the outcomes of arthroscopic surgeries have overtaken those of open procedures with the innovation of the surgical techniques and devices. However, several issues still remain, and various attempts have been made to further improve the outcomes. In this chapter, we describe the current issues in treatments for shoulder instability and recent advances in management of such problems.

7.1.2 Current Issues in Treatment for Shoulder Instability

7.1.2.1 Issues in Soft Tissue Bankart Repair

Although it has been believed that arthroscopic soft tissue stabilization can achieve an excellent outcome [6], extremely poor longer-term outcomes after soft tissue Bankart repair by European surgeons have recently been published [7, 8]. Castagna et al. [7] reported long-term outcome after arthroscopic soft tissue stabilization and revealed their failure rate as high as 22.5 % in 31 patients with 71 % of follow-up rate. In addition, van der Linde et al. [8] reported a 35 % failure rate in their long-term follow-up study with 97 % of follow-up rate in 65 patients. They stated that the use of fewer than three suture anchors might increase the risk of postoperative failure, as described by other authors [3, 9]. Seroyer and colleagues [10] proposed the four-quadrant approach for capsulolabral repair in glenohumeral instability and insist upon the importance of reinforcing the anteroinferior and posteroinferior capsule, in addition to the anterior capsule, by inserting inferior suture anchors using the anteroinferior and posterolateral portals in lateral decubitus position [9–12]; thus, at least four suture anchors are required to stabilize the anterior and inferior quadrant for standard Bankart repair. Their concept is exactly the same as the one that we have in terms of restoring proper tension to the entire entire inferior

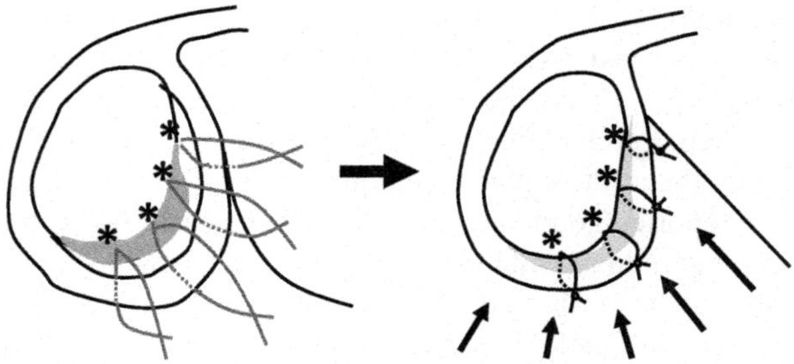

Fig. 7.1 Schematic drawing of entire inferior glenohumeral ligament (IGHL) retensioning. En face view, right shoulder. *Dark grey area* indicates inferior glenoid surface where cartilage is removed. *Light grey area* indicates the same area but covered by labrum by repair

glenohumeral ligament (IGHL) [13–16]. Soft tissue Bankart repair is the procedure of not simply reattaching the disrupted anterior labrum but also providing proper tension to the entire IGHL (Fig. 7.1) [14–16]. Seroyer and colleagues [10] also stated the lateral decubitus position is advantageous to reinforce the anteroinferior and posteroinferior quadrant; however, we do not find any disadvantage in reinforcing the entire IGHL using the beach-chair position after the introduction of the arm holder. In addition, in the beach-chair position, we can obviate the use of cannulas, which in return provides freedom to the joint for instruments; therefore, we can access the anteroinferior and posteroinferior quadrant without the use of additional portals such as trans-subscapularis or posterolateral portals [17].

7.1.2.2 Management of Bone Loss

It is well accepted that shoulder dislocation can cause bony defects in the humerus and the glenoid. Itoi et al. [18] conducted a cadaveric study and concluded that a bony defect of the glenoid that is more than 21 % of the glenoid width may cause instability and limitation of the range of motion after Bankart repair. Burkhart and De Beer [19] named the glenoid with significant bony defect as "inverted-pear" glenoid, and Lo et al. [20] reported 11 of 53 shoulders with inverted-pear glenoid through arthroscopic observation. They also investigated amount of bone loss to produce an inverted-pear glenoid and found that bone loss with at least 25 % of the glenoid width is required. Thus, we have recognized the importance of restoring the glenoid bone loss, and various procedures have been reported regardless of open or arthroscopic procedures.

A bone defect in the posterior aspect of the humerus is well known as the Hill–Sachs lesion, which was first described by Hill and Sachs in 1940 [21]. Burkhart and De Beer [19] pointed out a potential risk that a large, "engaging" Hill-Sachs lesion could cause recurrence after surgical stabilization and recommended open procedures such as the Latarjet procedure for shoulders with large bone loss. A recent major innovation in arthroscopic treatment for large Hill–Sachs lesions may be the remplissage technique. This technique aims to fill the Hill–Sachs lesions with the posterior aspect of the capsule and rotator cuff tendon to prevent engaging the bony defects and glenoid rim. Originally, Connolly [22] proposed this technique as an open procedure. Then, Purchase and Wolf [23] first described, as a modification of the open procedure, the arthroscopic technique of Hill–Sachs "remplissage." Many authors have been reported good outcomes of combined arthroscopic Bankart repair and remplissage for shoulder instability with a large Hill–Sachs lesion. We assume that this technique can be used not only for shoulders with a large Hill–Sachs lesion but also for high-risk shoulders such as young collision/contact athletes as an augmentation.

7.1.2.3 Management of Collision/Contact Athletes

Management of collision/contact athletes with shoulder instability remains controversial. Generally, collision/contact athletes tend to have a higher recurrence rate than other athletes [24, 25]. Lower recurrence rates of open stabilization for collision/contact athletes have been reported, and open surgery is considered the gold standard treatment for recurrent shoulder instability in collision/contact athletes [26]. Recently, combined arthroscopic Bankart repair and open coracoid transfer has been also proposed, and good outcomes in rugby athletes were reported with no recurrence in the short term [27].

However, better outcomes of arthroscopic stabilization have been reported recently [28, 29]. Mazzocca et al. [28] reviewed 18 collision/contact athletes who underwent arthroscopic anterior stabilization and found 2 shoulders with recurrent dislocation (11 %). Petrera et al. [29] studied 43 patients, including 22 collision and 21 non-collision athletes, and the recurrence rates were not significantly different between collision and non-collision athletes (9 % versus 0 %). We also investigated the outcomes of arthroscopic stabilizations that were performed in 702 athletes between 2004 and 2010, and the recurrence rate in collision athletes was 8.7 % whereas the overall recurrence rate was 4 % [30]. We believe that arthroscopic surgeries can be comparable to or superior to open procedures even for collision/contact athletes. With the results of our study, we have recently performed arthroscopic Bankart repairs with additional procedures for such high-risk athletes to improve the outcomes. This issue is described later in this chapter.

7.2 Management of Bone Loss

7.2.1 Evaluation of Glenoid Bone Loss

7.2.1.1 Radiography

X-ray images are helpful in detecting bony lesions of the glenoid, but its capability to detect the lesions is limited with conventional anteroposterior images [31]. However, Bernageau et al. [32] proposed an effective method for detecting anterior glenoid lesions with patients in the standing position. Edwards et al. [31] reported that 79 % of shoulders with chronic anterior instability demonstrated anterior glenoid rim lesions using the Bernageau view. We have developed a modified Bernageau method with patients lying on their axilla in their most relaxed position, which we called the "TV-watching position" (Fig. 7.2) [33]. This method enables us to acquire clear images to detect the anterior glenoid rim lesions with a high probability (Fig. 7.3). This X-ray method may be useful as a screening at a patient's first visit to the clinic.

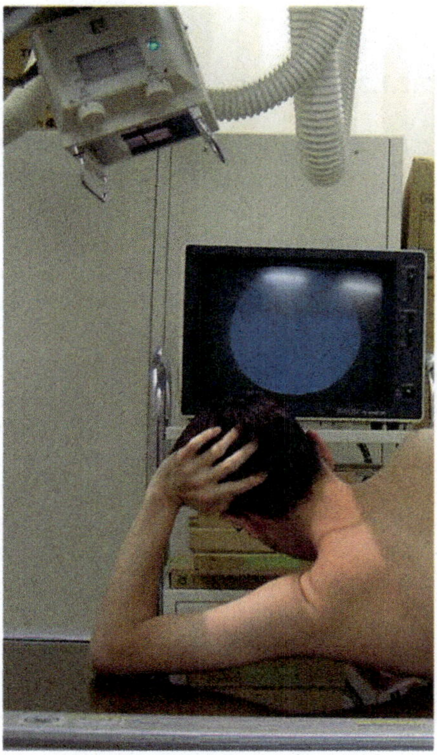

Fig. 7.2 Modified Bernageau method. Patients lie on their axilla in their most relaxed position. In this position, the scapula needs to incline 5° to the *vertical line*. Then, the incident X-ray needs to be aimed craniocaudally with 15°–20° of inclination to the *vertical line*

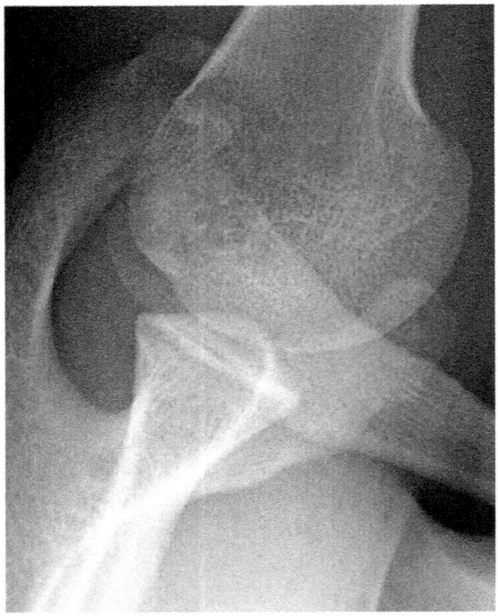

Fig. 7.3 X-ray image of normal glenoid obtained by the modified Bernageau methods. We call this image the "TV-watching view"

7.2.1.2 Computed Tomography (CT)

CT should be the gold standard for evaluation of the glenoid bone loss at present (Fig. 7.4). Especially, three-dimensional (3D) CT has several benefits in preoperative evaluation of the bony lesion: first, surgeons can recognize glenoid shape and the degree of bone loss intuitively at a glance; second, accurate quantification of bone loss can be possible by using an estimated inferior circle on the en face view of 3D CT; and last, surgeons can easily assess the size and shape of the bony fragment in shoulders with a bony Bankart lesion [33].

Several methods have been proposed to quantify bone loss and bony fragment of the glenoid using CT images. Most studies utilized assumed inferior circle of the glenoid on en face view of 3D CT images, and the bone loss was measured as width or area [13, 16, 34–36]. Some authors described the bone loss as a ratio of the width of missing bone to the anteroposterior diameter of the assumed circle [13, 16, 34, 35, 37]. The width measurement is easy and reproducible but may be insufficient in terms of accuracy. Recently, several authors reported area measurement of the defect [36, 38]. The area measurement will be more ideal to quantify bone loss because the defect is two dimensional. However, our recent study indicated that bone loss measured with width and area was highly correlated [16].

Several notable CT studies on the glenoid morphology in shoulders with anterior instability have been published. Sugaya et al. [34] revealed through a 3D CT study with the humeral head digitally subtracted that the prevalence of glenoid rim lesions in chronic anterior shoulder instability was as high as 90 %, including 50 % of bony Bankart lesion and 40 % of erosion. This study demonstrated a higher prevalence of

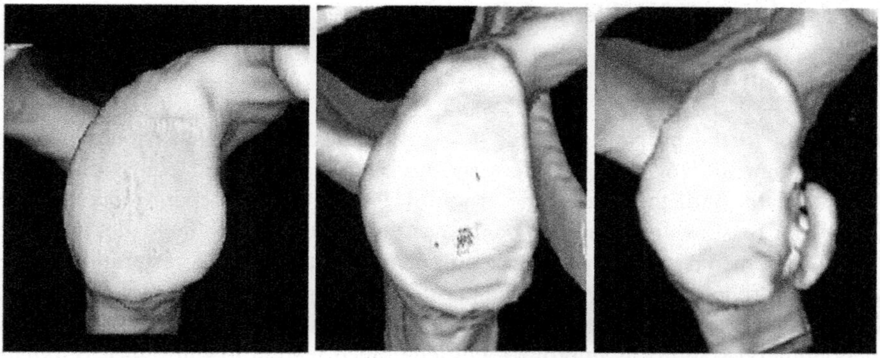

Fig. 7.4 Typical three subtypes of the glenoid morphology in recurrent shoulder instability by three-dimensional computed tomography (3D CT): normal (**a**), erosion (**b**), bony Bankart (**c**)

the glenoid rim lesions than it had been thought and indicated the importance of preoperative evaluation of the glenoid morphology. Saito et al. [39] investigated the location of the glenoid bone defect in shoulders with anterior instability and found that the mean orientation of the defect was pointing toward 3 o'clock on the clock face of the glenoid. This study demonstrated that bony defects of the glenoid were located more anterosuperiorly than had been thought. Sugaya et al. [13] assessed short-term outcomes of arthroscopic osseous Bankart repairs including pre- and postoperative CT evaluation and indicated the possibility to achieve good union of the bony fragment if reduction and fixation of the fragment were performed properly. This study suggested the importance to repair bony Bankart lesions without removing bone fragments. Thus, CT is important in evaluation of the glenoid bone loss.

7.2.1.3 Magnetic Resonance Imaging (MRI)

Although CT is the gold standard for evaluation of the glenoid bone loss, it requires radiation exposure. To avoid radiation exposure, several studies have attempted to utilize MRI for quantification of the bone loss and demonstrated that ability of MRI to quantify the bone loss was equally accurate with that of CT [40–42]. With the advances in MRI systems and techniques, MRI might take the place of CT in evaluation of the glenoid bone loss in the near future.

7.2.2 Surgery for Glenoid Bone Loss

7.2.2.1 Open Surgeries

According to the previous studies, it is generally accepted that shoulders with greater than 20°–25 % loss of the anteroinferior glenoid need bone grafting to achieve stability of the glenohumeral joint [19–21]. Open procedures such as the Latarjet or Bristow are thought to be the best for shoulders with large glenoid bone loss. The coracoid transfer is theorized to increase stability with restoration of the glenoid morphology and dynamic support of the repositioned conjoined tendon, which is called a "sling effect" [43]. A biomechanical study has proved that glenohumeral stability is improved with conjoined tendon loading [44]. Burkhart et al. [45] investigated results of the Latarjet procedure in shoulders with significant bone loss and reported that none of 47 patients showed recurrence except 1 patient with a positive apprehension test. Recently, excellent long-term results of the Latarjet procedure have been reported in several published articles [46–48]; however, these studies did not evaluate the glenoid bone loss in detail, such as the size of the defect.

Free bone grafting can be another treatment option for shoulders with a large glenoid bone loss or for high-risk patients, and good clinical results have been reported [49–51]. Warner et al. [39] performed glenoid reconstruction in 11 shoulders with severe glenoid bone loss using the autogenous iliac crest bone, and there was no recurrence at a mean follow-up of 33 months. Weng et al. [50] used allografts from the femoral head for glenoid reconstruction in nine shoulders with large glenoid erosion. Although one subluxation and one dislocation occurred after seizure, the remaining patients did not report recurrent instability. Mascarenhas et al. [51] reconstructed the glenoids with large bone defect with the iliac crest allograft in ten patients, and none of the patients experienced recurrent instability at mean follow-up of 16 months.

One of the major concerns in bone grafting may be resorption of the graft. The high incidence of graft resorption has been reported in recently published articles [52, 53]. Balestro et al. [52] reported that 8 of 12 shoulders exhibited a severe osteolysis or almost complete disappearance of the graft after the Latarjet procedure using bioabsorbable screws with 4 shoulders experienced recurrent instability. Zhu et al. [53] examined 57 patients who underwent the Latarjet procedure and found the graft resorption in 90.5 % of patients; however, there were no recurrent dislocations during the 2-year follow-up. Although the graft resorption may not be always associated with recurrence, surgeons should be cautious about this issue.

7.2.2.2 Arthroscopic Surgeries

Some surgeons may be suspicious about the efficacy of arthroscopic surgeries for shoulders with large glenoid bone loss, but many surgeons continue performing arthroscopic treatment with efforts to improve the outcomes because of the superiority in visualization of the intraarticular pathologies, less risk of shoulder stiffness, and less invasiveness.

One breakthrough in arthroscopic management of the glenoid bone loss may be the osseous Bankart repair. In the early arthroscopic era, bony fragments in the Bankart lesion frequently ignored or removed when mobilizing and repairing the lesion [19, 54], although half of shoulders with the anterior glenoid rim lesion retain an osseous fragment [34]. As mentioned earlier, Sugaya et al. [13] introduced an arthroscopic technique to repair chronic bony Bankart lesions using suture anchors and reported successful short-term outcomes and the possibility of achieving good union of the bony fragment if the fragment was properly reduced and fixed. Recently, Kitayama, Sugaya, and colleagues [16] reported the mid- to long-term outcomes of arthroscopic chronic bony Bankart repair. Although one patient experienced recurrent dislocation from a major trauma in a traffic accident, the remaining 37 patients were rated excellent or good. Postoperative 3DCT of the glenoid demonstrated that the shape of the glenoid was restored to nearly normal or slightly hypertrophic at the 5- to 8-year follow up. Thus, they proved that chronic bony fragments of the Bankart lesion could heal after proper reduction and fixation of the fragment. They insisted that proper ligament tensioning based on extensive labrum release was the key to perform successful arthroscopic bony Bankart repair. Extensive labrum release enables excellent fragment reduction and proper retensioning of the entire IGHL, and this eventually prevents bone fragment absorption and, instead, promotes new bone formation. In addition, they also insisted that proper ligament tensioning based on the extensive labrum release was a key to successful soft tissue Bankart repair [16].

Another effort in arthroscopic management of the glenoid bone loss will be development of arthroscopic techniques for bone grafting. Open bone grafting procedures have provided satisfactory results, but it may be a big problem that the open procedures do not treat the damaged capsulolabral complex and that they tend to develop postoperative loss of external rotation [55]. Thus, several surgeons have made efforts to develop arthroscopic techniques for bone grafting [56–58]. Lafosse et al. [56] first introduced the arthroscopic Latarjet procedure in 2007. At a minimum of 5-year follow-up, there was no recurrent dislocation except one subluxation after this arthroscopic procedure [59]. Boileau et al. [55, 58] also developed an all-arthroscopic technique combining the Bristow-Latarjet procedure with the Bankart repair. They reported excellent outcomes of this technique in 70 shoulders at a mean of 35-month follow-up with stable shoulders in 69 shoulders and 9° loss of external rotation at side compared to the contralateral side [55]. Several authors have reported various arthroscopic techniques for free bone grafting [60–65]. Although most of these articles were a technical note or a case report, Zhao et al. [63] reported outcomes in 52 patients with 2- to 5-year follow-up. They used a technique to tether allogeneic iliac graft to the glenoid by sutures, and 3 of 52 patients exhibited recurrent instability. Skendzel and Sekiya [61] introduced a technique to fix a glenoid allograft with cannulated screws, and we also prefer rigid fixation of the graft with screws [64, 65].

7.2.3 Our Strategy for Management of Glenoid Bone Loss

7.2.3.1 Choice of Surgical Option

First, evaluation of glenoid morphology with 3D CT is very important. We choose surgical procedures based on these morphological data combining additional patient information for the risk of recurrence such as age, gender, sports activity, and size of the Hill–Sachs lesion [16].

If the bony defect is less than 20 %, we perform the arthroscopic Bankart repair with or without soft tissue augmentation, such as the rotator interval closure or the Hill–Sachs remplissage, according to the patient's risk of recurrence. If the defect is 20 % or larger and the bony fragment is large enough, we choose the arthroscopic osseous Bankart repair with or without soft tissue augmentation because restoration of the glenoid shape can be expected after reduction and fixation of the fragment (Fig. 7.5) [16]. If the fragment is small or none in active patients, or if the Hill–Sachs lesion is large, bone grafting should be considered. In most of such cases, especially in young, active athletes, we usually perform arthroscopic autologous iliac bone grafting. We have used this technique since 2003, and the technique has

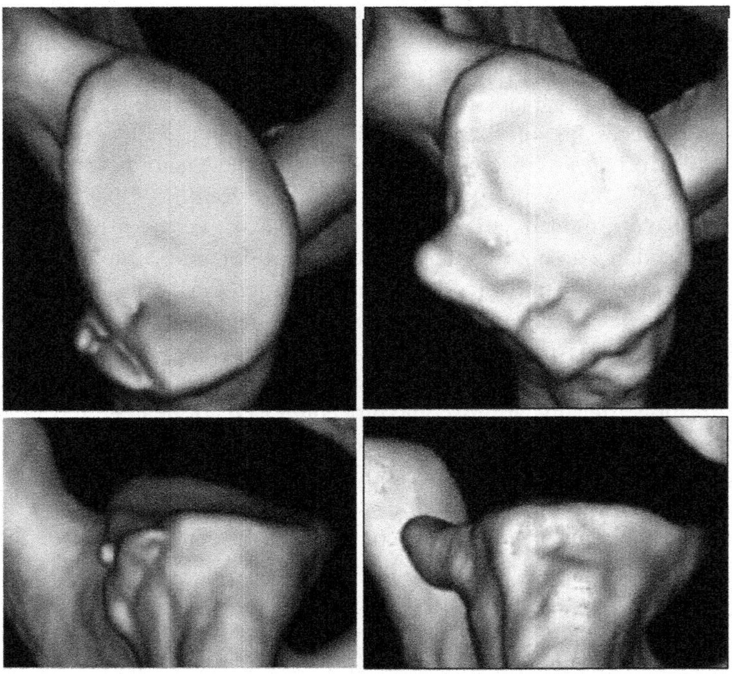

Fig. 7.5 Glenoid morphology before and after arthroscopic bony Bankart repair in 24-year-old judo athlete. *Left*: before surgery. *Right*: 7 years after surgery. Not only is bony union confirmed, but glenoid bone volume was obviously increased

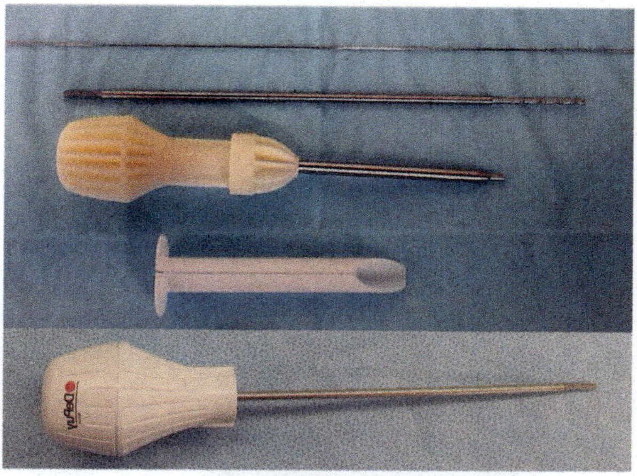

Fig. 7.6 Free bone grafting kit. Guidewire, drill, cannulated screw-guide and obturator, cannulated sheath for graft introduction, screwdriver (*top* to *bottom*)

been refined with developing original instruments (Fig. 7.6). We reviewed 20 patients (18 males and 2 females) with a mean age of 28 (range, 16–41) years old who underwent arthroscopic iliac bone grafting. There was no recurrent instability at a mean 21-month follow-up (range, 16–41 months) without significant loss of external rotation at side [64]. Three shoulders exhibited significant absorption of the graft with postoperative 3D CT, but the other cases demonstrated good restoration of the glenoid shape (Fig. 7.7).

7.2.3.2 Our Techniques for the Arthroscopic Osseous Bankart Repair

The patient is placed in the beach-chair position under general anesthesia. A routine diagnostic arthroscopy is carried out through a standard posterior portal, and an anterior portal is then established just superior to the subscapularis and lateral to the conjoined tendon. Surgeries are performed using the posterior portal as a viewing portal and the anterior and the anterosuperior portal as working portals.

The displaced osseous fragment with the labroligamentous complex is separated from the glenoid neck using a rasp introduced through the anterior portal (Fig. 7.8a). Mobilization of the labroligamentous complex together with the fragment is performed up to the 7 o'clock position (right shoulder). This extensive labrum release enables excellent fragment reduction. In addition, a small amount of articular cartilage at the face of the inferior glenoid from 3 to 7 o'clock is removed to promote tissue healing after repair. Two suture anchors loaded with #2 high-strength suture are inserted at the face of the anteroinferior glenoid (6:00, 4:40) through the anterior portal. One limb of a suture from both anchors is placed through the labrum adjacent to the inferior side of the fragment using a Caspari punch (Conmed Linvatec, Largo, FL, USA). Knot-tying is then performed (Fig. 7.8b).

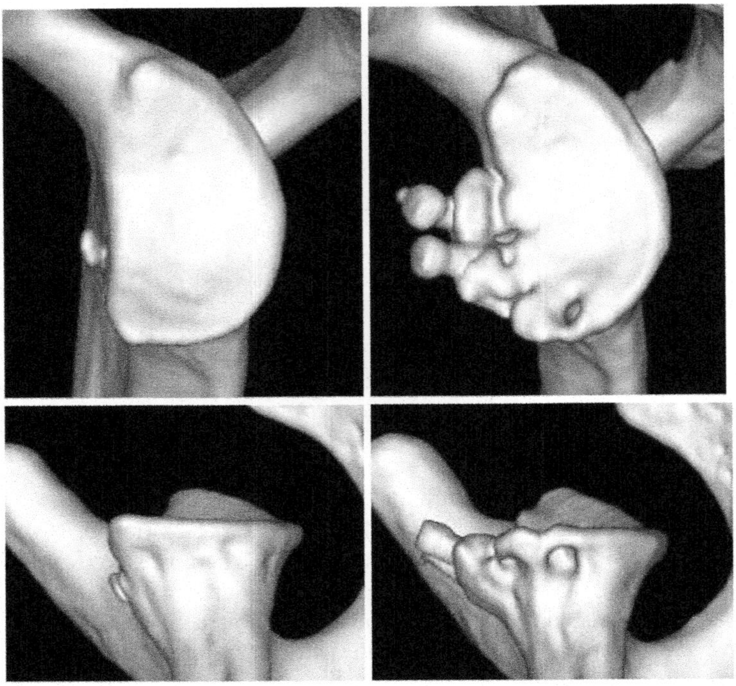

Fig. 7.7 Glenoid morphology before and after successful iliac crest grafting. *Left*: before surgery. *Right*: 2 years after surgery

The next step is the fixation of the osseous fragment, either by passing the suture through the fragment or around the fragment with use of a bone penetrator or Bone Stitcher (Smith & Nephew, Norwood, MA, USA). Two more suture anchors are used for the fragment and anterior labrum fixation. In this step, the labrum together with the fragment are held and stabilized by a robust grasper introduced from the anterosuperior portal to facilitate the fragment management by the bone penetrator introduced from the anterior portal. The fragment is usually reattached to a higher position than the anatomic position as a result of retensioning of the entire inferior glenohumeral ligament (Fig. 7.8c). After completing the repair, the arm is freed, and it is confirmed that there is no limitation of external rotation. In most shoulders, especially in collision/contact athletes, rotator interval closure is performed with the arm in more than 60° of external rotation as an augmentation of the bony Bankart repair.

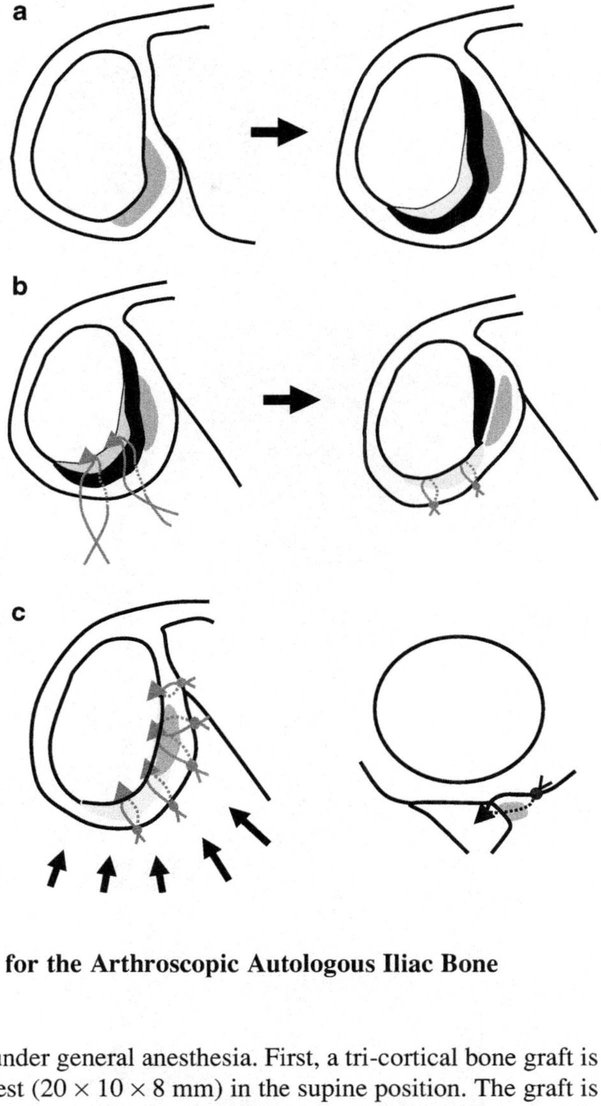

Fig. 7.8 Arthroscopic bony Bankart repair. (**a**) Complex release and mobilization. Fragment together with the adjacent labrum needed to be completely release from the glenoid neck, and cartilage at the face of inferior glenoid also removed. *Dark grey* area indicates bony fragment. *Light grey* area indicates inferior glenoid face where cartilage was removed. (**b**) Inferior labrum repair. Two anchors were used for repairing labrum inferior to the fragment. (**c**) Repair completed. *Left*, en face view. *Right*, inferior view

7.2.3.3 Our Techniques for the Arthroscopic Autologous Iliac Bone Grafting

The surgery is performed under general anesthesia. First, a tri-cortical bone graft is harvested from the iliac crest (20 × 10 × 8 mm) in the supine position. The graft is trimmed to fit the glenoid, and one hole for a superior 3.2-mm cannulated screw is created. In addition, two small holes are created at the center of the graft for temporary fixation of the graft using a suture anchor (Fig. 7.9a).

Then, the patient is placed in the beach-chair position, and a routine diagnostic arthroscopy is carried out. An anterior portal is established, and the labroligamentus complex is mobilized using a rasp through the anterior portal. The mobilized complex is retracted anteriorly with a nylon suture for visualization of the anterior glenoid. An anchor is inserted at the glenoid rim around 3:00 (right shoulder) for temporary fixation of the graft. Originally a developed cannula was introduced from

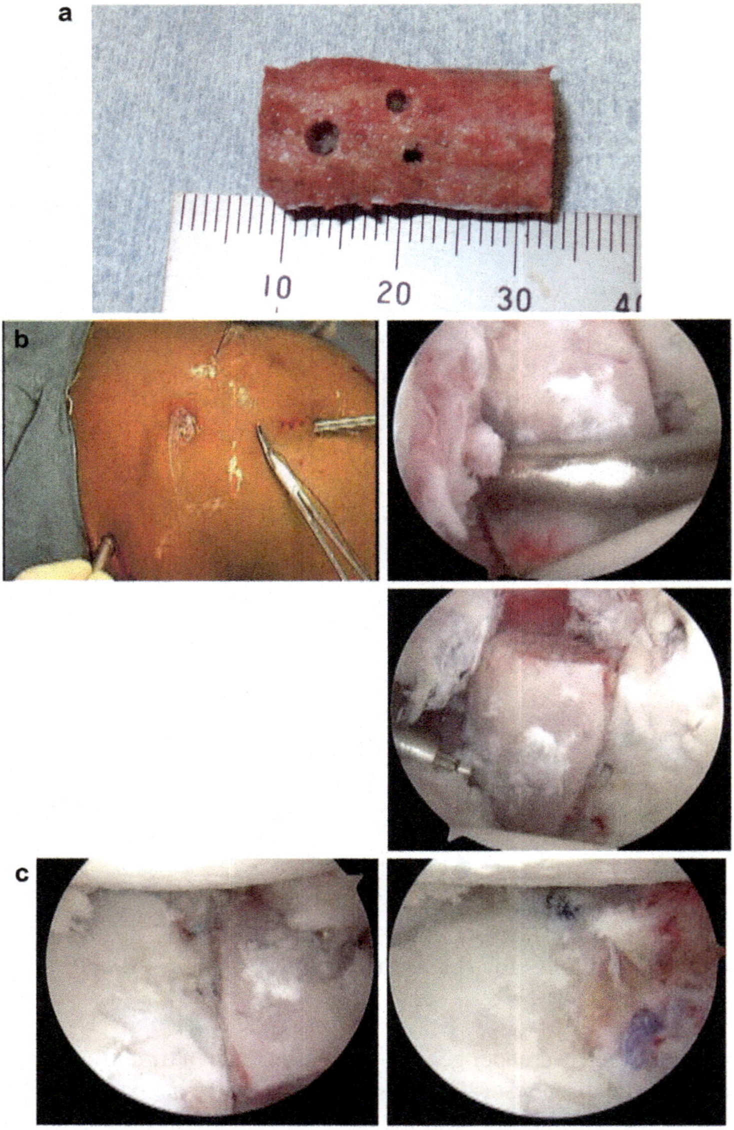

Fig. 7.9 Arthroscopic iliac crest grafting. (**a**) Harvested tri-cortical iliac bone graft ($20 \times 10 \times 8$ mm). The graft is trimmed to fit the glenoid, and one drill hole for 3.2-mm cannulated screw and two small holes for sutures for temporal graft fixation are created before introduction to the joint. (**b**) After temporal graft fixation, a switching rod introduced from the posterior portal is pushed and penetrated through the subscapularis muscle using inside-out technique to the skin (*top right*). Then, a "suicide portal" is created at the anteromedial side of the chest (*left*). The screws are then inserted through this portal and screw-guide (*bottom*, *right*). (**c**) Anterior view after graft fixation (*left*), and after capsulolabrum reconstruction (*right*)

the anterior portal, and the sutures of the anchor are pulled out through this cannula. The sutures are passed through the holes of the graft, and the graft is introduced into the joint through the cannula with the sutures used like a "zipline." The graft is inserted between the glenoid neck and the labroligamentus complex and temporarily fixed with the sutures (Fig. 7.9b).

At this point, the arthroscope is introduced to the bursa from the posterior portal. Then, posterolateral and anterolateral portals are established and bursal tissue cleaned up. The scope is then introduced to the anterolateral portal and the glenohumeral joint can be seen looking down from this portal. This view provides excellent visualization for the graft and glenoid. Then, a switching stick introduced from the posterior portal is pushed and penetrated through the subscapularis muscle using an inside-out technique to the skin. Then, a "suicide portal" is created at the anteromedial side of the chest, using this prominent skin as a landmark, then having the switching stick going through the skin incision. An original screw-guide is inserted over the switching stick, and screws are inserted through this portal and screw-guide (Fig. 7.9b). Last, the labroligamentus complex is repaired with anchors inserted at the glenoid so that the graft is located outside the glenohumeral joint (Fig. 7.9c) [65].

7.3 Management of High-Risk Athletes

7.3.1 Evaluation of Hill–Sachs Lesion

Preoperative evaluation of the Hill–Sachs lesion may be challenging compared to the evaluation of the glenoid rim lesion because of its three-dimensional nature. Area, depth, and location can be all related to instability of the glenohumeral joint. Several studies have attempted to measure the Hill–Sachs lesion and to define the critical size and location of the lesion [66–69], but no consensus has been reached because of differences in the measuring methods. Kralinger et al. [66] measured the size of the Hill–Sachs lesion with X-ray and reported that the Hill–Sachs lesions greater than 2.5 cm^3 in volume yielded four times higher recurrence rate than those smaller than 2.5 cm^3 in volume. Cho et al. [67] measured width, depth, orientation, and location of the Hill–Sachs lesion with CT images and reported that engaging Hill–Sachs lesions were significantly larger in size and more horizontally oriented to the humeral shaft than nonengaging lesions. Yamamoto et al. [70] advocated a novel concept of glenoid track and emphasized the importance of the location of the lesion in terms of interaction of the Hill–Sachs lesion and the anterior glenoid rim lesion. Although there is no gold standard method to evaluate the Hill–Sachs lesion, it will be essential to preoperatively assess the size and location of the lesion to minimize the risk of postoperative recurrences. CT may be the best imaging study to evaluate the lesion because we can measure the lesion three dimensionally and grasp the location at a glance using multiplanar reconstruction or 3D reconstruction images.

7.3.2 Arthroscopic Remplissage Procedure

Since Purchase, Wolf, and colleagues [23] introduced the arthroscopic Hill–Sachs remplissage technique in 2008, this technique has rapidly become widespread among shoulder surgeons because of its effectiveness to prevent recurrence in shoulders with large Hill–Sachs lesion without severe loss of motion. This technique aims to fill bony defects of the Hill–Sachs lesions with the posterior aspect of the capsule and rotator cuff tendon to prevent engaging the bony defects and glenoid rim. There have been many articles to report the outcomes of the arthroscopic remplissage procedure performed in combination with the arthroscopic Bankart repair [71–74]. Boileau et al. [71] performed this procedure in 47 of 459 shoulders, and only 1 shoulder (2.1 %) experienced recurrent instability at the mean 24-month follow-up. Wolf et al. [72] reported 2- to 10-year follow-up results of the Hill–Sachs remplissage, and noted that postoperative recurrence occurred in 2 of 45 patients (4.4 %). Brilakis et al. [73] reported recurrences in 3 of 48 patients (6.3 %) after the remplissage procedure. Zhu et al. [74] retrospectively investigated the outcomes of the Hill–Sachs remplissage, and found 4 recurrences in 49 patients (8.2 %). Recent systemic reviews have described the overall recurrence rate after the Hill–Sachs remplissage to be 3.4–5.4 %, without significant range-of-motion (ROM) restrictions [75, 76].

The major problem in the remplissage technique will be uncertainty in suture passage. The original remplissage procedure employed a technique in which sutures were put through the posterior capsule and cuff tendon with a penetrating grasper in a blind manner with the scope being maintained in the glenohumeral joint [23]. Lädermann et al. [77] conducted a cadaveric study to evaluate the anatomic relationship between the position of anchors and sutures placed for the remplissage and the infraspinatus and teres minor using ten cadaveric shoulders. The sutures of the superior anchor penetrated the infraspinatus muscle in six cases, the musculotendinous junction in three cases, and the infraspinatus tendon in one case. The sutures of the inferior anchor were located in the muscle of the musculotendinous junction in all cases. They concluded that the arthroscopic remplissage of a Hill–Sachs lesion as currently performed was a capsulomyodesis of both the infraspinatus and teres minor and not a capsulotenodesis of the infraspinatus as previously believed. Considering this study and a recent anatomic study on the shoulder capsule and rotator cuff [78], we have modified the technique to pass sutures securely through the infraspinatus and teres minor tendons.

7.3.3 Our Technique of Hill–Sachs Remplissage

7.3.3.1 Indications

The commonly accepted indications are shoulders with an engaging, large Hill–Sachs lesion. We also performed the remplissage for shoulders with a large Hill–Sachs lesion or revision cases, especially for young cases, until 2010. Based on our study on the outcomes of 702 arthroscopic stabilization between 2004 and 2010, which indicated that the recurrence rates were higher in young contact and collision athletes [30], we have expanded the indications of the remplissage and have performed the remplissage as an augmentation for high-risk patients. The current indications of the remplissage include young contact/collision athletes who are thought to have high risk of recurrence in addition to the conventional indications. We performed the remplissage as an augmentation for 90 high-risk shoulders between 2011 and 2014, and no shoulders have reported recurrence with minimum ROM limitation (unpublished data).

7.3.3.2 Surgical Technique

The surgery is performed in the beach-chair position under general anesthesia. Our basic concept for the remplissage is (1) to avoid inserting anchors too medial to minimize loss of external rotation, (2) to manage sutures with direct visualization, and (3) to securely pass sutures through the infraspinatus tendon, the teres minor tendon, and the thick capsule between the two tendons, based on the recent anatomic study [78].

First, we create a standard posterior portal and carry on diagnostic arthroscopy through this portal. Next, we perform the remplissage using three portals: the posterior portal, a portal at the posterolateral corner of the acromion, and a portal in the posterolateral aspect created so that the three portals form an equilateral triangle (Fig. 7.10a). Viewing in the glenohumeral joint through the posterior portal, two or three anchors are inserted through the portal at the posterolateral corner of the acromion into the middle of the medial edge and the valley of the bone defect (Fig. 7.10b). Viewing in the subdeltoid bursa through the posterior portal, the infraspinatus tendon is penetrated with a suture grasper from the posterolateral portal, and then, viewing in the glenohumeral joint, one or two sutures are caught and pulled out. Repeating these procedures, we pass sutures through the infraspinatus tendon, the teres minor tendon, and the thick capsule between the two tendons using the posterolateral portal or the third portal (Fig. 7.10c). Then, we move back to the glenohumeral view and perform Bankart repair and rotator interval closure, if necessary. Last, the sutures for the remplissage are tied, viewing in the bursa (Fig. 7.10d). Postoperative MR arthrography shows good union of the posterior cuff tendon to the bone defect (Fig. 7.10e).

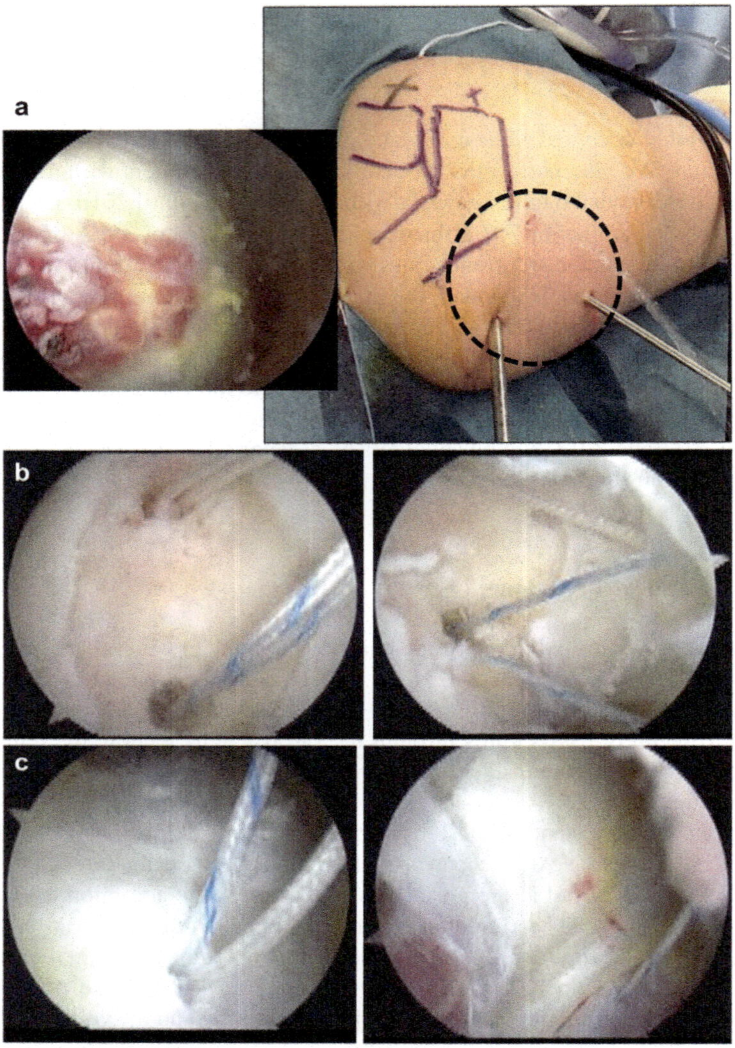

Fig. 7.10 Our new Hill–Sachs remplissage. (**a**) Portals (*right*) and bursal view of the infraspinatus and teres minor (*left*). (**b**) After anchor insertion (*left*), and after suture placement viewing from the joint (*right*). (**c**) After suture placement viewing from the bursa. Infraspinatus (*left*) and teres minor (*right*). (**d**) After knot-tying. Infraspinatus (*left*) and teres minor (*right*). (**e**) Magnetic resonance angiogram (MRA) at 1 year after surgery. *White circle* indicates the site of fixation

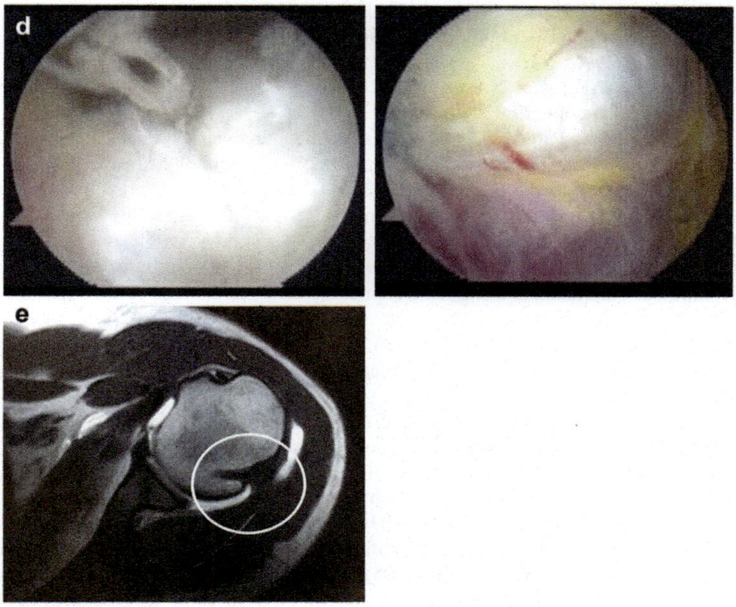

Fig. 7.10 (continued)

7.4 Conclusions

The surgical outcomes for shoulder instability have been improving with the innovations in surgical techniques and devices. To achieve better results, it is important to precisely comprehend the pathology in each patient, including the glenoid rim lesion and Hill–Sachs lesion. The current gold standard study for evaluation of the lesions is the CT scan. Based on the morphology of the glenoid and humerus and other factors such as age, gender, and sports activity, we should choose the appropriate treatment to minimize the recurrence rate as well as maximize the sports performance level.

References

1. Brophy RH, Marx RG (2009) The treatment of traumatic anterior instability of the shoulder: nonoperative and surgical treatment. Arthroscopy 25:298–304
2. Wolf EM, Wilk RM, Richmond JC (1991) Arthroscopic Bankart repair using suture anchors. Oper Tech Orthop 1:184–191
3. Randelli P, Ragone V, Carminati S et al (2012) Risk factors for recurrence after Bankart repair: a systematic review. Knee Surg Sports Traumatol Arthrosc 20:2129–2138

4. Owens BD, Harrast JJ, Hurwitz SR et al (2011) Surgical trends in Bankart repair: an analysis of data from the American Board of Orthopaedic Surgery certification examination. Am J Sports Med 39:1865–1869
5. Harris JD, Gupta AK, Mall NA et al (2013) Long-term outcomes after Bankart shoulder stabilization. Arthroscopy 29:920–933
6. Petrera M, Patella V, Patella S et al (2010) A meta-analysis of open versus arthroscopic Bankart repair using suture anchors. Knee Surg Sports Traumatol Arthrosc 18:1742–1747
7. Castagna A, Markopoulos N, Conti M et al (2010) Arthroscopic Bankart suture-anchor repair: radiological and clinical outcome at minimum 10 years of follow-up. Am J Sports Med 38:2012–2016
8. van der Linde JA, van Kampen DA, Terwee CB et al (2011) Long-term results after arthroscopic shoulder stabilization using suture anchors: an 8- to 10-year follow-up. Am J Sports Med 39:2396–2403
9. Frank RM, Mall NA, Gupta D et al (2014) Inferior suture anchor placement during arthroscopic Bankart repair: influence of portal placement and curved drill guide. Am J Sports Med 42:1182–1189
10. Seroyer ST, Nho SJ, Provencher MT et al (2010) Four-quadrant approach to capsulolabral repair: an arthroscopic road map to the glenoid. Arthroscopy 26:555–562
11. Gupta AK, McCormick FM, Abrams GD et al (2013) Arthroscopic bony Bankart fixation using a modified Sugaya technique. Arthrosc Tech 2(3):e251–e255
12. Cvetanovich GL, McCormick F, Erickson BJ et al (2013) The posterolateral portal: optimizing anchor placement and labral repair at the inferior glenoid. Arthrosc Tech 2(3):e201–e204
13. Sugaya H, Moriishi J, Kanisawa I et al (2005) Arthroscopic osseous Bankart repair for chronic recurrent traumatic anterior glenohumeral instability. J Bone Joint Surg 87-A:1752–1760
14. Sugaya H (2011) Arthroscopic treatment of glenoid bone loss: surgical technique. In: Provencher M, Romeo A (eds) Shoulder instability. A comprehensive approach. Elsevier, Philadelphia, pp 186–196
15. Sugaya H (2010) Instability with bone loss. In: Angelo RL, Esch JC, Ryu RKN (eds) AANA advanced arthroscopy: the shoulder. Elsevier, Philadelphia, pp 136–146
16. Kitayama S, Sugaya H, Takahashi N et al (2015) Clinical outcome and glenoid morphology after arthroscopic chronic bony Bankart repair: a 5- to 8-year follow-up. J Bone Joint Surg 97-A:1833–1843
17. Sugaya H, Kon Y, Tsuchiya A (2004) Arthroscopic Bankart repair in the beachchair position: a cannulaless method using an intra-articular suture relay technique. Arthroscopy 20 (suppl 2):116–120
18. Itoi E, Lee SB, Burglund LJ et al (2000) The effect of a glenoid defect on anteroinferior stability of the shoulder after Bankart repair: a cadaveric study. J Bone Joint Surg 82-A:35–46
19. Burkhurt SS, De Beer JF (2000) Traumatic glenohumeral bone defects and their relationship to failure of arthroscopic Bankart repairs: significance of the inverted-pear glenoid and the humeral engaging Hill–Sachs lesion. Arthroscopy 16:677–694
20. Lo IKY, Parten PM, Burkhurt SS (2004) The inverted pear glenoid: an indicator of significant glenoid bone loss. Arthroscopy 20:169–174
21. Hill HA, Sachs MD (1940) The grooved defect of the humeral head. Radiology 35:690–700
22. Connolly J (1972) Humeral head defects associated with shoulder dislocations. AAOS Instr Course Lect 21:42–54
23. Purchase RJ, Wolf EM, Hobgood ER et al (2008) Hill–Sachs "remplissage": an arthroscopic solution for the engaging Hill–Sachs lesion. Arthroscopy 24:723–726
24. Cole BJ, L'Insalata J, Irrgang J et al (2000) Comparison of arthroscopic and open anterior shoulder stabilization: a two to six-year follow-up study. J Bone Joint Surg 82-A:1108–1114
25. Cho NS, Hwang JC, Rhee YG (2006) Arthroscopic stabilization in anterior shoulder instability: collision athletes versus noncollision athletes. Arthroscopy 22:947–953
26. Pagnani M, Dome DC (2002) Surgical treatment of traumatic anterior shoulder instability in American football players. J Bone Joint Surg 84-A:711–715

27. Tasaki A, Morita W, Yamakawa A et al (2015) Combined arthroscopic Bankart repair and coracoid process transfer to anterior glenoid for shoulder dislocation in rugby players: evaluation based on ability to perform sport-specific movements effectively. Arthroscopy 31:1693–1701
28. Mazzocca AD, Brown FM Jr, Carreira DS et al (2005) Arthroscopic anterior shoulder stabilization of collision and contact athletes. Am J Sports Med 33:52–60
29. Petrera M, Dwyer T, Tsuji MRS et al (2013) Outcomes of arthroscopic Bankart repair in collision versus noncollision athletes. Orthopedics 36:621–626
30. Sugaya H (2014) Arthroscopic stabilization for collision athletes with anterior shoulder instability. MB Orthop 27:14–20 (in Japanese)
31. Edwards TB, Boulahia A, Walch G (2003) Radiographic analysis of bone defects in chronic anterior shoulder instability. Arthroscopy 19:732–739
32. Bernageau J, Patte D, Bebeyre D et al (1976) Intérêt du profil glénoïdien dans les luxations récidivantes de l'épaule. Rev Chir Orthop 62(Suppl 2):142–147
33. Sugaya H (2014) Techniques to evaluate glenoid bone loss. Curr Rev Musculoskelet Med 7:1–5
34. Sugaya H, Moriishi J, Dohi M et al (2003) Glenoid rim morphology in recurrent anterior glenohumeral instability. J Bone Joint Surg 85-A:878–884
35. Chuang TY, Adams CR, Burkhurt SS (2008) Use of preoperative three-dimensional computed tomography to quantify glenoid bone loss in shoulder instability. Arthroscopy 24:376–382
36. Dumont GD, Russell RD, Browne MG et al (2012) Area-based determination of bone loss using the glenoid arc angle. Arthroscopy 28:1030–1025
37. Griffith JF, Antonio GE, Tong CWC et al (2003) Anterior shoulder dislocation: quantification of glenoid bone loss with CT. AJR 180:1423–1430
38. de Filippo M, Castagna A, Steinbach LS et al (2013) Reproducible noninvasive method for evaluation of glenoid bone loss by multiplanar reconstruction curved computed tomographic imaging using a cadaveric model. Arthroscopy 29:471–477
39. Saito H, Itoi E, Sugaya H et al (2005) Location of the glenoid defect in shoulders with recurrent anterior dislocation. Am J Sports Med 33:889–893
40. Hujismans PE, Haen PS, Kidd M et al (2007) Quantification of a glenoid defect with three-dimensional computed tomography and magnetic resonance imaging: a cadaveric study. J Shoulder Elbow Surg 16:803–809
41. Gyftopoulos S, Hasan S, Bencardino J et al (2012) Diagnostic accuracy of MRI in the measurement of glenoid bone loss. AJR 199:873–878
42. Lee RK, Griffith JF, Tong MMP et al (2013) Glenoid bone loss: assessment with MR imaging. Radiology 267:496–502
43. May VR (1970) A modified Bristow operation for anterior recurrent dislocation of the shoulder. J Bone Joint Surg 52-A:1010–1016
44. Giles JW, Boons HW, Elkinson I et al (2013) Does the dynamic sling effect of the Latarjet procedure improve shoulder stability? A biomechanical evaluation. J Shoulder Elbow Surg 22:821–827
45. Burkhurt SS, De Beer JF, Barth JR et al (2007) Results of modified Latarjet reconstruction in patients with anteroinferior instability and significant bone loss. Arthroscopy 23:1033–1041
46. Bessière C, Trojani C, Carles M et al (2014) The open Latarjet procedure in more reliable in terms of shoulder stability than arthroscopic Bankart repair. Clin Orthop Relat Res 472:2345–2351
47. Bouju Y, Gadéa F, Stanovici J et al (2014) Shoulder stabilization by modified Latarjet-Patte procedure: results at a minimum 10 years' follow-up, and role in the prevention of osteoarthritis. Orthop Traumatol Surg Res 100:S213–S218
48. Mizuno N, Denard PJ, Raiss P et al (2014) Long-term results of the Latarjet procedure for anterior instability of the shoulder. J Shoulder Elbow Surg 23:1691–1699

49. Warner JJP, Gill TJ, O'Hollerhan JD et al (2006) Anatomical glenoid reconstruction for recurrent anterior glenohumeral instability with glenoid deficiency using an autogenous tricortical iliac crest bone graft. Am J Sports Med 34:205–212
50. Weng PW, Shen HC, Lee HH, et al (2009) Open reconstruction of large bony glenoid erosion with allogeneic bone graft for recurrent anterior shoulder dislocation. Am J Sports Med 37:1792–1797
51. Mascarenhas R, Raleigh E, McRae S et al (2014) Iliac crest allograft glenoid reconstruction for recurrent anterior shoulder instability in athletes: surgical technique and results. Int J Shoulder Surg 8:127–132
52. Balestro JC, Young A, Maccioni C et al (2015) Graft osteolysis and recurrent instability after the Latarjet procedure performed with bioabsorbable screw fixation. J Shoulder Elbow Surg 24:711–718
53. Zhu YM, Jiang CY, Lu Y, et al (2015) Coracoid bone graft resorption after Latarjet procedure is underestimated: a new classification system and a clinical review with computed tomography evaluation. J Shoulder Elbow Surg 24:1782–1788
54. Bigliani LU, Newton PM, Steinmann SP et al (1998) Glenoid rim lesions associated with recurrent anterior dislocation of the shoulder. Am J Sports Med 26:41–45
55. Boileau P, Thélu CE, Mercier N et al (2014) Arthroscopic Bristow-Latarjet combined with Bankart repair restores shoulder stability in patients with glenoid bone loss. Clin Orthop Relat Res 472:2413–2424
56. Lafosse L, Lejeune E, Bouchard A et al (2007) The arthroscopic Latarjet procedure for the treatment of anterior shoulder instability. Arthroscopy 23:1242.e1–1242.e5
57. Lafosse L, Boyle S (2010) Arthroscopic Latarjet procedure. J Shoulder Elbow Surg 19:2–12
58. Boileau P, Mercier N, Roussanne Y et al (2010) Arthroscopic Bankart-Bristow-Latarjet procedure: the development and early results of a safe and reproducible technique. Arthroscopy 26:1434–1450
59. Dumont GD, Fogerty S, Rosso C et al (2014) The arthroscopic Latarjet procedure for anterior shoulder instability. Am J Sports Med 42:2560–2566
60. Mochizuki Y, Hachisuka H, Kashiwagi K et al (2007) Arthroscopic autologous bone graft with arthroscopic Bankart repair for a large bony defect lesion caused by recurrent shoulder dislocation. Arthroscopy 23:677.e1–667.e4
61. Skendzel JG, Sekiya JK (2011) Arthroscopic glenoid osteochondral allograft reconstruction without subscapularis takedown: technique and literature review. Arthroscopy 27:129–135
62. Anderl W, Kriegleder B, Heuberer PR (2012) All-arthroscopic implant-free iliac crest bone grafting: new technique and case report. Arthroscopy 28:131–137
63. Zhao J, Huangfu X, Yang X et al (2014) Arthroscopic glenoid bone grafting with nonrigid fixation for anterior shoulder instability. Am J Sports Med 42:831–839
64. Sugaya H, Takahashi N, Kawai N et al (2012) Arthroscopic iliac bone grafting for large glenoid defect in shoulders with recurrent anterior instability. Katakansetsu 36:383–387 (in Japanese)
65. Sugaya H (2015) Arthroscopic anterior glenoid bone block stabilization. In: Ryu RKN, Angelo RL, Abrams JS (eds) The shoulder: AANA advanced arthroscopic surgical techniques, 1st edn. SLACK Books, Thorofare
66. Kralinger FS, Gloser K, Wischatta R et al (2002) Predicting recurrence after primary anterior shoulder dislocation. Am J Sports Med 30:116–120
67. Cho SH, Cho NS, Rhee YG (2011) Preoperative analysis of the Hill–Sachs lesion in anterior shoulder instability. Am J Sports Med 39:2389–2395
68. Saito H, Itoi E, Minagawa H et al (2009) Location of the Hill–Sachs lesion in shoulder with recurrent anterior dislocation. Arch Orthop Trauma Surg 129:1327–1334
69. Ozaki R, Nakagawa S, Mizuno N et al (2014) Hill–Sachs lesions in shoulders with traumatic anterior instability: evaluation using computed tomography with 3-dimensional reconstruction. Am J Sports Med 42:2597–2605

70. Yamamoto N, Itoi E, Abe H et al (2007) Contact between the glenoid and the humeral head in abduction, external rotation, and horizontal extension: a new concept of glenoid track. J Shoulder Elbow Surg 16:649–656
71. Boileau P, O'Shea K, Vargas P et al (2012) Anatomical and functional results after arthroscopic Hill–Sachs remplissage. J Bone Joint Surg 94-A:618–626
72. Wolf EM, Arianjam A (2014) Hill–Sachs remplissage, an arthroscopic solution for the engaging Hill–Sachs lesion: 2- to 10-year follow-up and incidence of recurrence. J Shoulder Elbow Surg 23:814–820
73. Brilakis E, Mataragas E, Deligeorgis A, et al (2016) Midterm outcomes of arthroscopic remplissage for the management of recurrence anterior shoulder instability. Knee Surg Sports Traumatol Arthrosc 24:593–600
74. Zhu YM, Lu Y, Zhang J et al (2011) Arthroscopic Bankart repair combined with remplissage technique for the treatment of anterior shoulder instability with engaging Hill–Sachs lesion: a report of 49 cases with a minimum 2-year follow-up. Am J Sports Med 39:1640–1647
75. Leroux T, Bhatti A, Khoshbin A et al (2013) Combined arthroscopic Bankart repair and remplissage for recurrent shoulder instability. Arthroscopy 29:1693–1701
76. Buza JA III, Iyengar JJ, Anakwenze OA et al (2014) Arthroscopic Hill–Sachs remplissage: a systematic review. J Bone Joint Surg 96-A:549–555
77. Lädermann A, Arrigoni P, Barth J, et al (2016) Is arthroscopic remplissage a tenodesis or capsulomyodesis? An anatomic study. Knee Surg Sports Traumatol Arthrosc 24:573–577
78. Nimura A, Kato A, Yamaguchi K et al (2012) The superior capsule of the shoulder joint complements the insertion of the rotator cuff. J Shoulder Elbow Surg 21:867–872

Chapter 8
Arthroscopic Rotator Cuff Repair

Yozo Shibata

Abstract In recent years, an increasing number of rotator cuff repairs have been performed arthroscopically because advances have been made in arthroscopic devices, suture anchors, and various techniques. Arthroscopic rotator cuff repair (ARCR) is of greater benefit than open rotator cuff repair (ORCR) in several aspects. By using various arthroscopic portals, arthroscopy enables the pathological examination of all sites in both the subacromial bursa and the shoulder joint, which allows evaluation of rotator cuff tear morphology as well as planning for its mobilization and repair. Compared to ORCR, ARCR facilitates the introduction of rehabilitation to allow for early return of range of motion, because there are smaller surgical scars, minimal invasion to the deltoid muscle, and less postoperative pain.

In the early 1990s, the availability of suture anchors dramatically increased the numbers of ARCR. However, surgeons must perform it while using various instruments inserted into a very narrow space and looking at a magnified arthroscopic image on a TV monitor. The narrow space involved, the difficult in recognizing the three-dimensional structures, and the inaccessibility of shoulder joint structures without the use of instruments all add to the difficulty of the procedure, which requires a great deal of time for surgeons to master ARCR.

In this section, basic procedures of ARCR for partial and small- and medium-sized cuff tears are described.

Keywords Arthroscopic rotator cuff repair • Cuff tear • Partial rotator cuff tear

8.1 Trends in Arthroscopic Rotator Cuff Repair (ARCR)

In recent years, an increasing number of ARCR have been performed because of the advances in arthroscopic instruments, suture anchors, and various techniques. In particular, the invention of the suture anchor during the first half of 1990 led to a

---

Y. Shibata (✉)
Department of Orthopaedic Surgery, Fukuoka University Chikushi Hospital, 1-1-1 Zokumyoin, Chikushino, Fukuoka 818-8502, Japan
e-mail: yshibata.01@me.com

K. Tamai et al. (eds.), *Advances in Shoulder Surgery*,
DOI 10.1007/978-4-431-55988-7_8

switch in surgical methodology, from detaching the anterior fibers of the deltoid muscle to repair the rotator cuff tear from above the shoulder, to the arthroscopic procedure of mobilization, and suturing of the cuff stump while leaving the deltoid muscle intact. As for ARCR, Snyder reported a preliminary study in 1993 [1] that the supraspinatus tendon was sutured on the footprint with anchors inserted in a single row.

In contrast to cuff repair using this single-row technique, a double-row technique [2] was developed in an attempt to enlarge footprint coverage, which was further followed by the development of a transosseous-equivalent technique [3] to improve not only footprint coverage but also footprint contact. Although no difference in postoperative shoulder functions exists between the single-row and double-row techniques except for large, massive tears, the double-row technique is reported to provide better structural healing. However, Sano et al. reported that the double-row technique caused stress concentration in the medial row at the knot-tying site on the bursal side, and that, in the transosseous suture fixation, the stress extended proximally into the tendon substance. No significant stress concentration was observed inside the tendon [4]. In addition, Yamakado reported four cases of medial-row failure after double-row ARCR, in which there was pullout of mattress sutures of the medial row and knots were caught between the cuff and the greater tuberosity [5]. Because of these certain shortcomings remain, including difficulty with reoperation in cases of repeat tear, anchor dislodgement, knot impingement, and financial cost, Kuroda et al. developed an anchorless technique for arthroscopic transosseous suture rotator cuff repair [6]. Moreover, although those are anchor techniques, surface-holding repair [7] to improve the contact of the cuff stump to the footprint, and a bone marrow stimulation technique [8] to improved cuff repair integrity have been reported.

Furthermore, Colvin et al. reported a 1.4-fold increase in the number of rotator cuff repairs in the United States in 2006 compared to 1996. Of these, open rotator cuff repairs (ORCR) increased 1.3 fold while ARCR increased 6 fold, with a dramatic increase seen in the latter. Although the number of ORCR performed in 1996 was four times greater than that of ARCR, by 2006, the number of ARCR had increased to about the same level as that of ORCR [9]. In Japan, the Japan Shoulder Society reported the results of a questionnaire survey on shoulder surgeries performed by its members in 2009 [10]. The number of shoulder-related surgeries performed during the year was 18,153, 44 % of which were for rotator cuff injury and 10 % each for proximal humeral fracture, clavicle fracture, and instability surgeries. The number of ARCR performed was 2.5 times greater than ORCR. These survey results show that rotator cuff surgery is the most commonly performed shoulder surgery in Japan, suggesting that ARCR is a technique that shoulder surgeons must be able to perform.

8.2 Indication of Arthroscopic Rotator Cuff Repair

The clinical symptoms of rotator cuff tear include shoulder joint pain, limited range of motion, and muscle weakness. Because asymptomatic rotator cuff tears occasionally occur without such symptoms [11], however, it is meaningful to treat symptomatic rotator cuff tears conservatively to achieve an asymptomatic state. Therefore, rotator cuff repair is indicated for nonresponders to conservative therapy. The roles of rotator cuff repair include regaining the source of force, improving concentricity of the humeral head by restoring dynamic stability, and a spacer between the acromion and the humeral head. Therefore, middle-aged males or manual laborers are good candidates for rotator cuff repair.

8.3 Advantages and Disadvantages of Arthroscopic Rotator Cuff Repair

ARCR is more beneficial than open repair in several aspects: small skin incision, less postoperative pain, and minimal deltoid muscle weakness because it is not necessary to detach the anterior fibers of the deltoid. From these aspects, ARCR is thought to be less invasive than open repair. Interleukin-6 is produced by monocytes, macrophages, fibroblasts, and T_2 lymphocytes during tissue traumatization. Therefore, measurement of this marker is used as an indicator of the degree of surgical invasion [12, 13]. Shinoda et al. performed ARCR and ORCR in a prospective, randomized fashion, and measured preoperative and postoperative serum interleukin-6 levels as an indicator of surgical invasion. The mean preoperative serum interleukin-6 level was 1.12 pg/ml for ARCR and 1.20 pg/ml for ORCR ($P > 0.05$). The mean postoperative serum interleukin-6 level at 24 h was 24.3 pg/ml for ARCR and 77.0 pg/ml for open repair. Postoperative serum interleukin-6 levels differed significantly between the two groups ($P < 0.01$). They concluded that ARCR is less invasive than ORCR based on serum interleukin-6 levels [14]. ARCR also allows detailed assessment of the tear pattern by enabling observation of the cuff stump from both the joint side and bursal side, as well as by facilitating the pathological evaluation within the glenohumeral joint, which is impossible to examine by open repair. Such detailed pathological information helps the surgeon to determine appropriate methods of release, mobilization, and suturing of the cuff stump.

On the other hand, arthroscopic repair can also be disadvantageous for reasons of technical challenges, including disappearance of the perspective within the surgical field via a two-dimensional TV monitor; all surgical procedures are performed with instruments inserted via portals, which deprives the surgeon of direct contact with the anatomic structures; difficulty in controlling the instruments in the narrow surgical space; and further narrowing of the surgical space over time from edema of the soft tissue covering the subacromial bursa, which can lead to a missing suture.

Gartsman et al., based on their clinical experience, reported significant shortening of operation time with ARCR in a second set of 10 cases compared to the first 10 cases [15]. In addition, Takeda reviewed his 180 cases of ARCR, finding rapid shortening of operation time up to the first 100 cases, and reporting a necessity for experiencing at least 60 cases of ARCR before stabilization of operation time to around 80 min occurred [16]. Although ARCR is a very attractive and sophisticated procedure, the aforementioned points suggest that surgeons wanting to learn it should receive appropriate cadaver training, start out with a mini-open repair method on patients, and gradually switch to all procedures arthroscopically.

8.4 Patient Position

ARCR can be performed in a beach-chair or lateral decubitus position (Fig. 8.1). Although cuff repair can be performed in either position, the author prefers the beach-chair position because of the following two advantages: the beach-chair position allows the surgeon to easily move to a position anterior or posterior to the patient, constantly keeping his or her eyes in the direction of the arthroscopy (Fig. 8.2); this position allows easy switching to open surgery. The arm holder enabling the sterilization (Ohta, Japan) is used to hold the affected limb.

8.5 Portals

To make detailed observations of an intraarticular or intrabursal lesion and accurately carry out the procedure, creation of an appropriate portal is essential. Representative portals are described next (Fig. 8.3).

Posterior standard portal: This portal is made two fingerbreadths inferior to and two fingerbreadths medial to the posterior angle of the acromion and is used for the evaluation of glenohumeral joint pathology and the joint side of the cuff. It is used as a viewing portal for suturing a joint side tear of the subscapularis tendon or to change bursal or joint side tears of the supraspinatus tendon to a complete tear. When viewing from the lateral standard portal, the suture passing from the cuff can be pulled out of the posterior standard portal.

Lateral standard portal: This portal is made two fingerbreadths inferior to the lateral margin of the acromion on the line extending from the posterior margin of the distal end of the clavicle and is suitable for observation of the inside of the subacromial bursa or the bursal side of the cuff. It is used as a viewing portal for suturing most supraspinatus, infraspinatus, or subscapularis tendon tears.

Rotator interval portal: In posterior standard portal viewing, this portal is used for synovectomy within the glenohumeral joint, or to insert an anchor into the anterior humeral head for subscapular tendon suture. In lateral standard portal viewing, this portal is used to pull out the suture passing through the cuff.

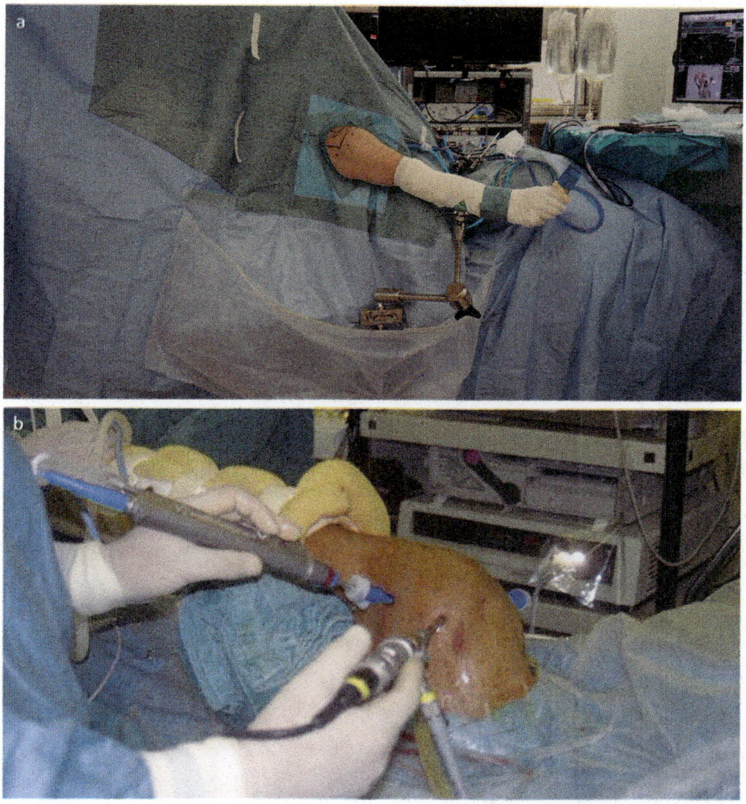

Fig. 8.1 Patient position. (**a**) Beach-chair position and arm controller. Upper extremity is held by an autoclavable arm controller (Oota, Okayama, Japan). (**b**) Lateral decubitus position. Although no dedicated operating table is needed as with the beach-chair position, it is difficult for the surgeon to carry out the observation or surgery with a scope inserted to the glenohumeral joint or subacromial bursae from the anterior portal as the surgeon cannot stand between the arthroscopic tower and the patient

Anterolateral portal: This portal is used to insert the ExpressSew (DePuy-Mitek) or Scorpion (Arthrex), which enables both the holding of the cuff stump and the penetration of the suture, to antegradely pass the suture through the cuff. It is also used as a portal for insertion of a lateral row anchor.

Posterolateral portal: This portal allows the surgeon to insert a suture grasper into the posterior cuff stump to retrogradely pull out the suture.

Medial row anchor insertion portal: This portal is used to insert a medial row anchor from the lateral margin of the acromion.

Neviaser portal: This portal is made in a position corresponding to the superior margin of the glenoid between the clavicle and the scapular spine. A suture grasper can be inserted via this portal to retrogradely pull out the suture.

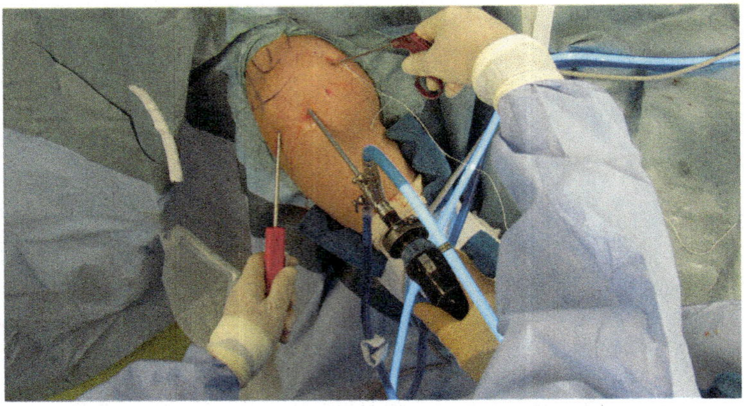

Fig. 8.2 Advantage of the beach-chair position. With an assistant holding a camera between the surgeon's hands, the surgeon can use both hands to operate in the same manner as during open surgery, which is likely to shorten the learning curve compared to the lateral decubitus position

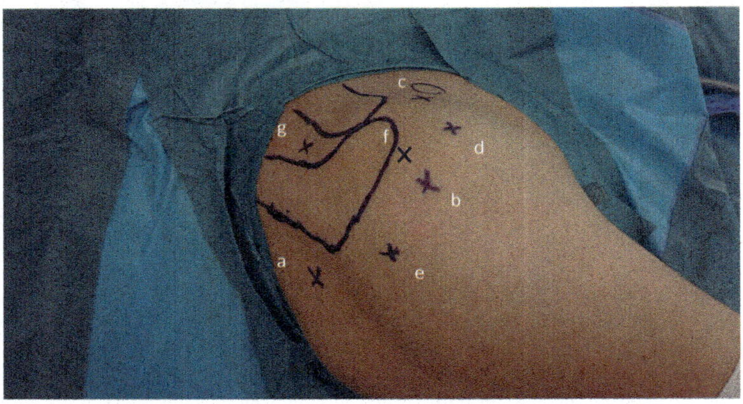

Fig. 8.3 Portals. (**a**) Posterior standard portal; (**b**) lateral standard portal; (**c**) rotator interval portal; (**d**) anterolateral portal; (**e**) posterolateral portal; (**f**) medial row anchor insertion portal; (**g**) Neviaser portal

8.6 Small- and Medium-Sized Full-Thickness Tendon Tears

Cofield et al. classified the size of rotator cuff tears into small (<1 cm), medium (1 to <3 cm), large (3 to <5 cm), and massive (>5 cm) tears [17]. Small and medium tears are generally the most suitable for rotator cuff repairs because they are associated with mild fatty degeneration in the rotator cuff muscles, with excellent footprint coverage of the cuff stump and a low incidence (5–20 %) of retear after the surgery [18–20]. First, the inside of the glenohumeral joint is observed from the posterior standard portal to determine the size and shape of the cuff tear and to evaluate damage of the long head of the biceps tendon.

Next, observation is carried out through the lateral standard portal, the inflammatory synovial tissue is removed and the cuff stump is minimally trimmed, and the cuff stump is then pulled with an instrument to confirm its mobility (Fig. 8.4a, b). If the footprint coverage of the cuff stump is insufficient, a radiofrequency device is inserted from the anterolateral portal, and the subacromial bursa and the coracohumeral ligament are released (Fig. 8.4c, d). If the mobility of the cuff stump is still poor (not frequent for small and medium tears), intraarticular observation is carried out again from the posterior standard portal, a radiofrequency device is inserted from the rotator interval portal, and the joint capsule around the glenoid is then released. Bearing in mind the possibility of suprascapular nerve injury in the outside of the capsule, care should be taken to ensure that only the capsule is separated by the tip of the radiofrequency device (Fig. 8.5). Once

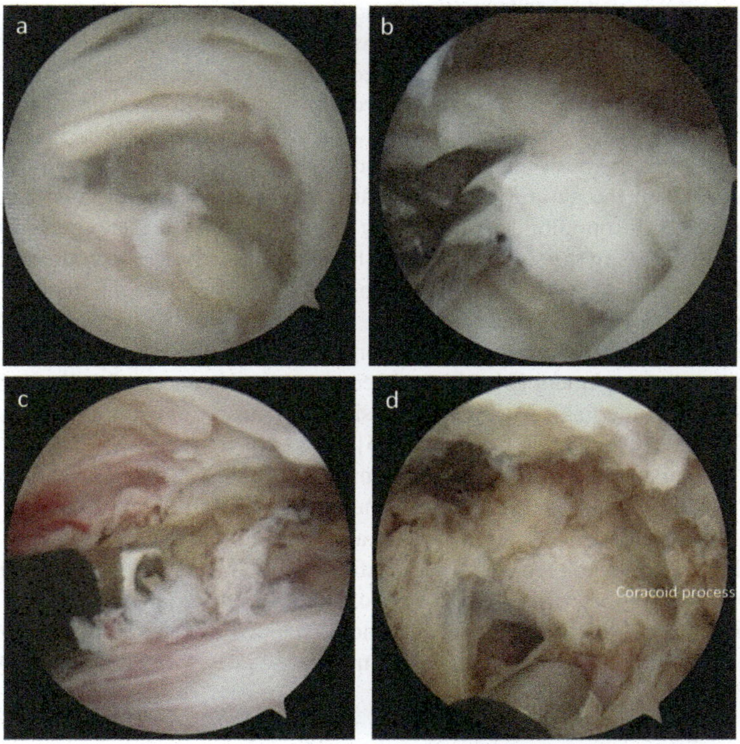

Fig. 8.4 Treatment for the bursal side. (**a**) Medium-size tear (left shoulder). (**b**) Pull the cuff stump with a grasper to see whether it can cover the footprint of the greater tuberosity. (**c**) Release the margin of the subacromial bursa. (**d**) The position of the coracoid process can be confirmed by probing its base surrounded by soft tissue with the tip of a radiofrequency device. Dissociate the coracohumeral ligament attaching to the external wall of the base of the coracoid process

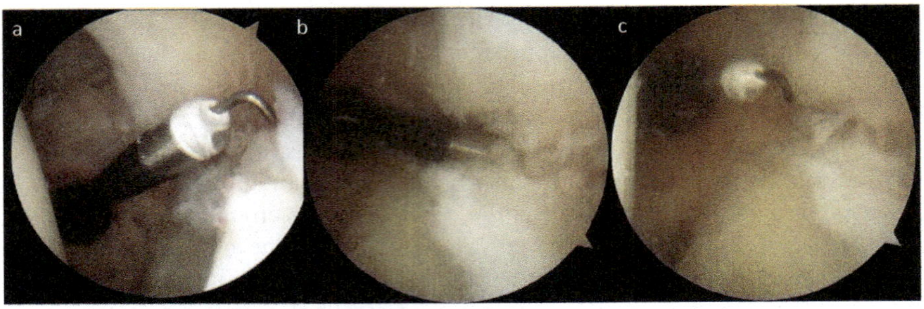

Fig. 8.5 Treatment for the joint side. Employing an arthroscopic view from the posterior standard portal, release the joint capsule using the radiofrequency device inserted from the anterior rotator interval

adequate mobility of the cuff stump is obtained, a triple-loaded suture anchor as a medial row anchor is inserted into medial side of the abraded footprint (Fig. 8.6a). The suture from a medial row anchor is antegradely passed through using ExpressSew (DePuy-Mitek), Scorpion (Arthrex), etc. (Fig. 8.6b). Suture passing is relatively easy, when the suture is passed through the anterior margin of the cuff stump, the suture is passed retrogradely from the anterior portal using a 60° suture grasper (DePuy-Mitek). Similarly, when it is passed through the posterior margin of the stump, it is done from the posterior portal using the suture grasper. If the suture is followed with the suture grasper to catch it, the grasper hook has the risk of lodging in the surrounding soft tissue. By grasping the suture using an additional grasper and dropping the suture inside the hook of the suture grasper, the suture can be easily placed (Fig. 8.6c, d). After passing all sutures from the medial row anchor through the cuff stump, a bridging suture is applied using the transosseous equivalent technique to exert uniform contact pressure on the footprint (Fig. 8.7a, b). To prevent knot impingement [21, 22], and because there is concern that ligation of the sutures from the medial row on the bursal side can cause stress concentration, which in turn can increase the risk of retear [4, 5], we avoided to knot-tying in the medial row on the bursal side (Fig. 8.7c). This caution is because no problems arise even if ligation of the medial row is not performed because of the high tendinous fusion rate in rotator cuff tear repair for small and medium tears. Such knotless suture methods have been developed and successfully applied with good results by Kuroda et al., who developed arthroscopic transosseous suture repair without the use of anchors [23], and by Taniguchi et al., who developed surface-holding repair with anchors used only for the medial row and not for the lateral row, without knot-tying on the bursal side [7].

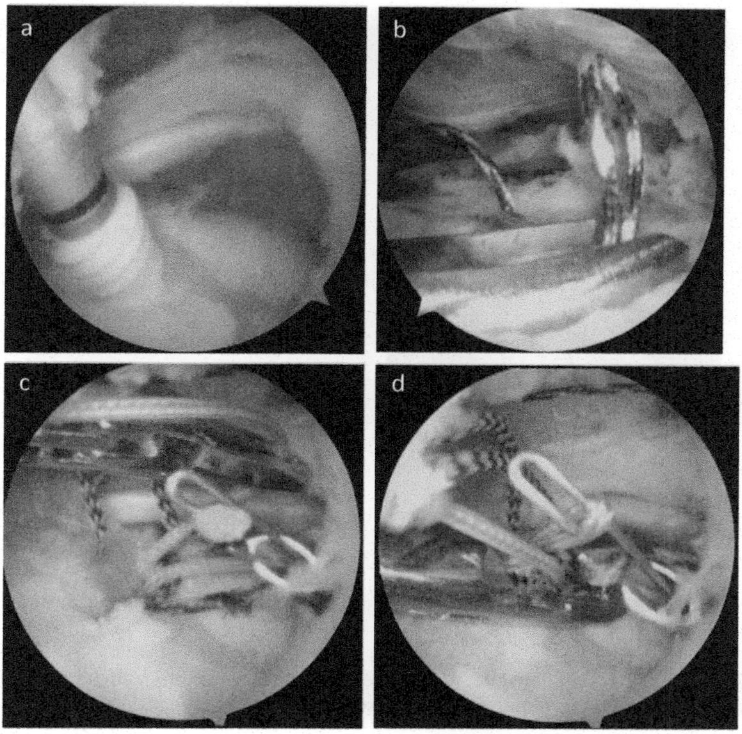

Fig. 8.6 Medial row anchor insertion (**a**), suture penetration using the ExpressSew (**b**); insert a suture grasper in the direction from the bursal side of the cuff to the joint side (**c**); and wind a suture held with an additional grasper around the tip of the suture grasper (**d**). If the suture grasper (Depuy-Mitec) follows the suture, the hook will lodge in the soft tissue and the grasper will become damaged

8.7 Subscapular Tendon Repair

In the case of a complete subscapularis tendon tear, the working space anterior to the subscapularis tendon is narrow. Therefore, suturing can be facilitated by simultaneous escape of the shuttle relay suture passing through the cuff and the suture from the anchor inserted into the footprint posteriorly to the shoulder joint before relaying [24] (Fig. 8.8).

In this case, the author first checks the mobility of the subscapular tendon by observing from the posterior standard portal (Fig. 8.9a, b). If mobility is insufficient, release of the coracohumeral ligament and anterior and posterior side of the subscapularis tendon is performed. After confirming the reach of the cuff stump to the footprint, an anchor is inserted from the anterior portal. The suture from the anchor is released to the anterolateral portal, and then a suture grasper is inserted from the anterior portal with the anchor inserted therein to suture the cuff (Fig. 8.9c-e).

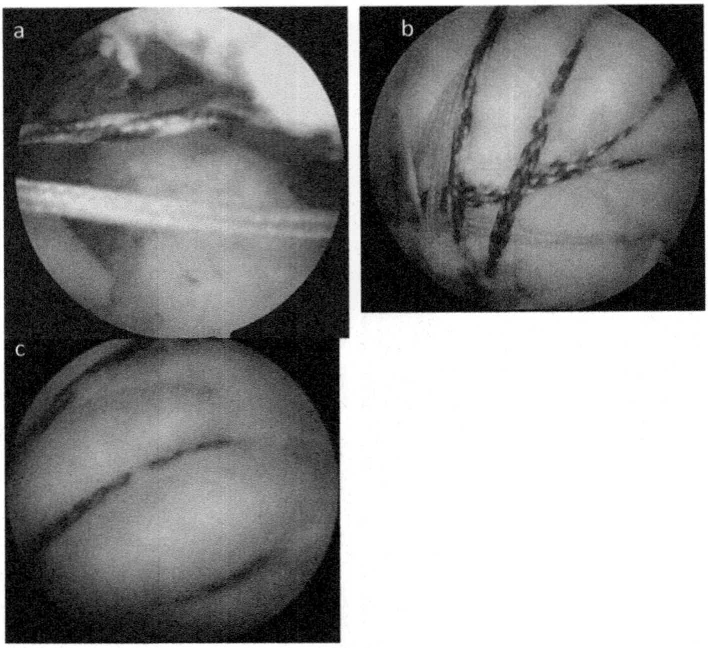

Fig. 8.7 (**a**) Insertion of an anchor to the lateral row; (**b**) completion of bridging using the transosseous-equivalent technique; (**c**) knotless suture bridge on the bursal side

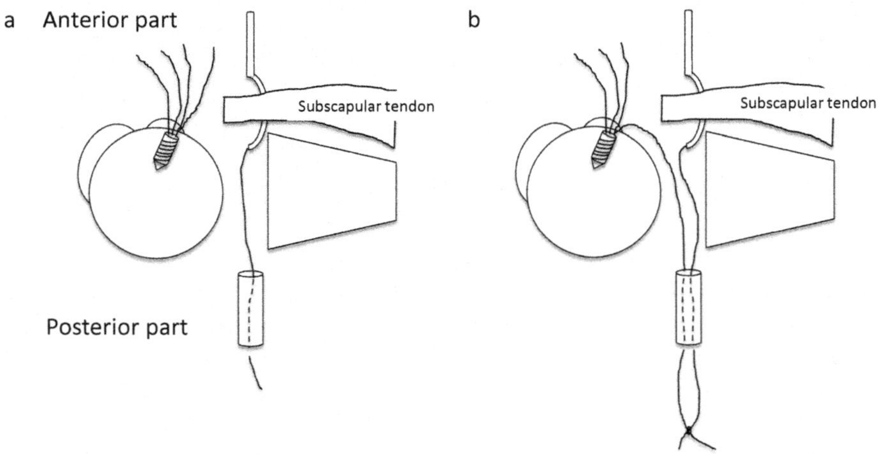

Fig. 8.8 Suture of subscapular tendon tear by Ide (left shoulder). (**a**) Pass a nylon suture for shuttle relay through the subscapular tendon stump from the anterior portal and pull out the suture from the back of the glenohumeral joint. (**b**) Pull out the anchor suture from the posterior portal and suture the subscapularis tendon using the shuttle-relay method

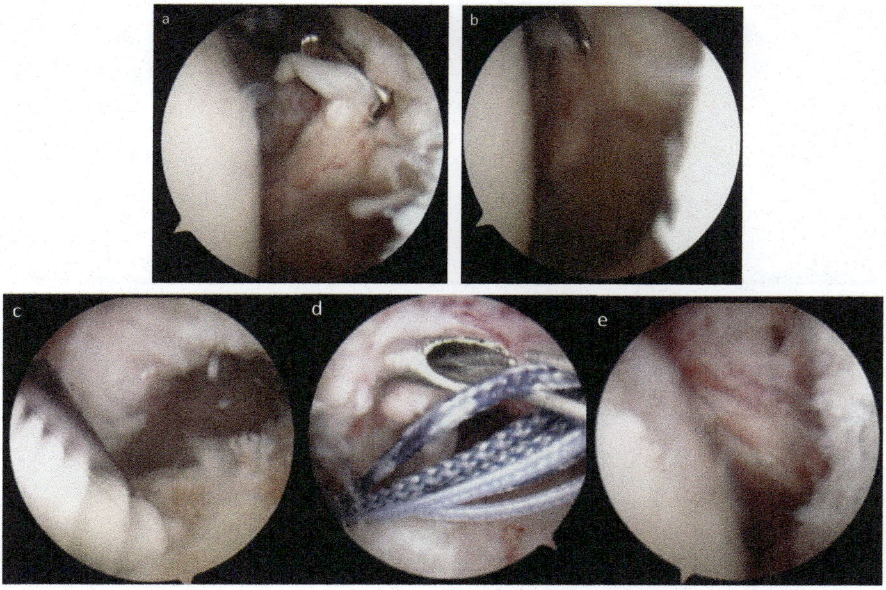

Fig. 8.9 Suture of the subscapular tendon tear (left shoulder). (**a**, **b**) Hold the subscapular tendon stump and check its mobility. (**c**) Insert an anchor from the anterior portal. (**d**) Escape the anchor suture to the superior working portal. Catch the suture using the suture grasper, which penetrates into the cuff from the anterior portal. (**e**) The sutured subscapularis tendon

8.8 Partial-Thickness Rotator Cuff Tear

Partial-thickness rotator cuff tears include joint side tears, bursal side tears, and intratendinous tears. Ellman classified these partial tears by depth as follows: grade I, less than 3 mm; grade II, 3–6 mm; and grade III, greater than 6 mm or greater than 50 % of total tendon thickness [25]. For grade I or II tears, the partial tear stump is debrided, and then arthroscopic subacromial decompression is performed if impingement is observed on the anteroinferior acromion. For grade III partial tears, there are two types of repair—repair after converting the tear to a complete tear (a full-thickness tear) and trans-tendon repair. The former is performed for both joint side and bursal side tears, and the latter is done for joint side incomplete tears.

When a joint side tear is converted to a full-thickness tear, a needle is inserted to the joint side tear via the bursal side while observing the inside of the joint from the posterior standard portal (Fig. 8.10a, b). Once the needle reaches the partial tear, an arthroscope is inserted from the lateral standard portal while observing the site of needle insertion on the bursal side, through which the needle is intraarticularly penetrated with a radiofrequency device or a shaver (Fig. 8.10c, d). After confirming the preparation of a small hole and entry of the tip of a radiofrequency (RF) device into the joint from the hole, arthroscopic observation is carried out once

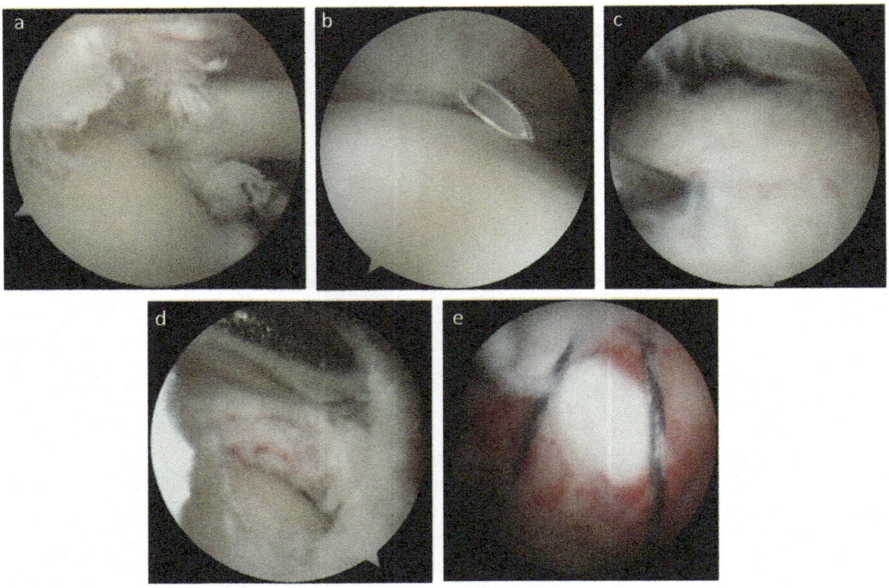

Fig. 8.10 Repair of a joint side tear of the supraspinatus tendon (left shoulder). (**a**) Joint side tear of the supraspinatus tendon; (**b**) needle insertion from the bursal side; (**c**) needle insertion point on the bursal side; (**d**) converted to a full-thickness tear; (**e**) completed rotator cuff repair

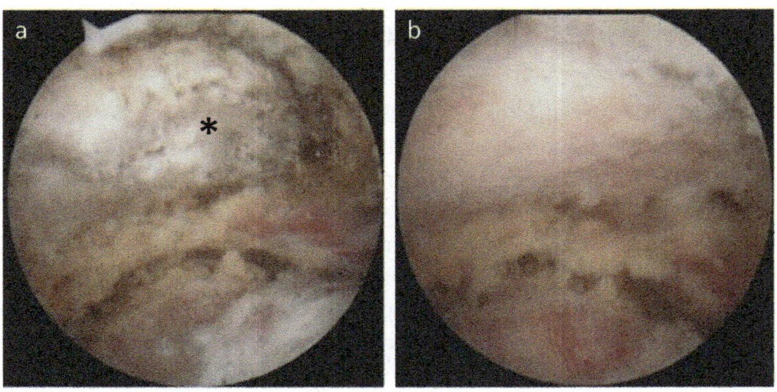

Fig. 8.11 Arthroscopic subacromial decompression (*right shoulder*). (**a**) The acromial undersurface where soft tissue is removed. A distinct bony protrusion (*) is observed. (**b**) The acromial undersurface after bone resection

again from the posterior standard portal, and the RF device is carefully manipulated to enlarge the tear size without damaging the long head of the biceps tendon. Once conversion to a full-thickness tear has been completed, standard arthroscopic repair is performed (Figs. 8.10e and 8.11). Similarly, for a bursal side tear, repair is performed after converting the tear to a complete tear.

Although the repair can easily be performed by converting a partial-thickness tear to a complete tear, disruption of the continuous tendon leads to disturbed intratendinous blood flow, which is disadvantageous for tendon healing. Attempts by Ide et al. [26] and Seo et al. [27] to prevent such an outcome in trans-tendon repair have shown favorable results, although increased technical difficulty was noted.

8.9 Arthroscopic Subacromial Decompression

In the case of ORCR, subacromial decompression is performed not only to treat subacromial impingement but also to enlarge the surgical field. Gartsman randomly performed ARCR with or without arthroscopic subacromial decompression (ASD) in patients with a single supraspinatus tendon tear with type 2 acromion. Patients were kept unaware as to which group they had been assigned. Results showed no difference between the two groups in the American Shoulder and Elbow Surgeons (ASES) score at 1 year after the surgery [28]. Milano et al. randomly assigned patients with type 2 or 3 acromion to either an ASD or non-ASD group and reported that there was no difference between the two groups in the Constant score and responses to the Disabilities of the Arm, Shoulder and Hand (DASH) questionnaire at 2 years after ARCR [29]. Additionally, in a double-blind multicenter study, MacDonald et al. performed ARCR with or without ASD and found no difference between the two groups in the ASES score at 2 years after ARCR [30].

Because ARCR is accomplished within the subacromial space, subacromial decompression is not essential. Having ASD-associated concerns with regard to increased soft tissue swelling, damage to the anterior deltoid fiber, and anterosuperior instability of the humeral head at occurrence of cuff retear [31], we perform ASD when type III acromion or inferior acromion erosions are observed.

ARCR for partial tears and small- or medium-sized rotator cuff tears is not only less invasive but also brings excellent clinical results. The procedure will continue to be the most commonly performed by shoulder surgeons. However, this surgical procedure is continuously evolving, and further advancement in anchors, sutures, instruments, and surgical techniques is expected.

References

1. Randelli P, Cucchi D, Ragone V et al (2015) History of rotator cuff surgery. Knee Surg Sports Traumatol Arthrosc 23:344–362
2. Lo IK, Burkhart SS (2003) Double-row arthroscopic rotator cuff repair; re-establishing the footprint of the rotator cuff. Arthroscopy 19:1035–1042
3. Park MC, Elattrache NS, Ahmad CS et al (2006) "Transosseous-equivalent" rotator cuff repair technique. Arthroscopy 22:1360.e1361–1360.e1365
4. Sano H, Yamashita T, Wakabayashi I et al (2007) Stress distribution in the supraspinatus tendon after tendon repair: suture anchors versus transosseous suture fixation. Am J Sports Med 35:542–546

5. Yamakado K, Katsuo S, Mizuno K et al (2010) Medial-row failure after arthroscopic double-row rotator cuff repair. Arthroscopy 26:430–435
6. Kuroda S, Ishige N, Mikasa M (2013) Advantages of arthroscopic transosseous suture repair of the rotator cuff without the use of anchors. Clin Orthop Relat Res 471:3514–3522
7. Taniguchi N, Suenaga N, Oizumi N et al (2014) Surface-holding repair: an original arthroscopic rotator cuff repair technique. J Shoulder Elbow Surg 23:620–627
8. Taniguchi N, Suenaga N, Oizumi N et al (2015) Bone marrow stimulation at the footprint of arthroscopic surface-holding repair advances cuff repair integrity. J Shoulder Elbow Surg 24:860–866
9. Colvin AC, Egorova N, Harrison AK et al (2012) National trends in rotator cuff repair. J Bone J Surg Am 94:227–233
10. Yoneda M (2011) Questionnaire survey report of shoulder surgery in 2009. Katakansetsu (Shoulder Joint) 35:697–705 (in Japanese)
11. Yamamoto A, Takagishi K, Kobayashi T et al (2010) Prevalence and risk factors of a rotator cuff tear in the general population. J Shoulder Elbow Surg 19:116–120
12. Wirtz DC, Heller KD, Miltner O et al (2000) Interleukin-6: a potential inflammatory marker after total joint replacement. Int Orthop 24:194–196
13. Bilgen O, Atici T, Durak K et al (2001) C-reactive protein and erythrocyte sedimentation rates after total hip and total knee arthroplasty. J Int Med Res 29:7–12
14. Shinoda T, Shibata Y, Izaki T et al (2009) Comparative study of surgical invasion in arthroscopic and open rotator cuff repair. J Shoulder Elbow Surg 18:596–599
15. Gartsman D, Graham RD, MacLennan MJ et al (2005) Arthroscopic rotator cuff repair: the learning curve. Arthroscopy 21:394–400
16. Takeda H (2007) The learning curve of an arthroscopic rotator cuff repair. Katakansetsu (Shoulder Joint) 31:385–387 (in Japanese)
17. Cofield RH, Parvizi J, Hoffmeyer PJ et al (2001) Surgical repair of chronic rotator cuff tears: a prospective long-term study. J Bone Joint Surg Am 83:71–77
18. Goutallier D, Postel JM, Gleyze P et al (2003) Influence of cuff muscle fatty degeneration on anatomic and functional outcomes after simple suture of full-thickness tears. J Shoulder Elbow Surg 12:550–554
19. Harryman DT 2nd, Mack LA, Wang KY et al (1991) Repairs of the rotator cuff. Correlation of functional results with integrity of the cuff. J Bone Joint Surg Am 73:982–989
20. Sugaya H, Maeda K, Matsuki K et al (2007) Repair integrity and functional outcome after arthroscopic double-row cuff repair: a prospective outcome study. J Bone Joint Surg Am 89:953–960
21. Hotta T, Yamashita T (2010) Osteolysis of the inferior surface of the acromion caused by knots of the suture thread after rotator cuff repair surgery: knot impingement after rotator cuff repair. J Shoulder Elbow Surg 19:e17–e23
22. Nagasawa R (2010) Knot impingement after rotator cuff repair. Katakansetsu (Shoulder Joint) 34:815–819 (in Japanese)
23. Kuroda S, Ishige N, Mikasa M (2013) Advantages of arthroscopic transosseous suture repair of the rotator cuff without the use of anchors. Clin Orthop Relat Res 71:3514–3522
24. Ide J, Tokiyoshi A, Hirose J et al (2007) Arthroscopic repair of traumatic combined rotator cuff tears involving the subscapularis tendon. J Bone Joint Surg Am 89:2378–2388
25. Ellman H (1990) Diagnosis and treatment of incomplete rotator cuff tears. Clin Orthop Relat Res 254:64–74
26. Ide J, Maeda S, Takagi K (2005) Arthroscopic transtendon repair of partial-thickness articular-side tears of the rotator cuff: anatomical and clinical study. Am J Sports Med 33:1672–1679
27. Seo YJ, Yoo YS, Kim DY et al (2011) Trans-tendon arthroscopic repair for partial-thickness articular side tears of the rotator cuff. Knee Surg Sports Traumatol Arthrosc 19:1755–1759
28. Gartsman GM, O'Connor DP (2004) Arthroscopic rotator cuff repair with and without arthroscopic subacromial decompression: a prospective, randomized study of one- year outcomes. J Shoulder Elbow Surg 13:424–426

29. Milano G, Grasso A, Salvatore M et al (2007) Arthroscopic rotator cuff repair with and without subacromial decompression: a prospective randomized study. Arthroscopy 23:81–88
30. MacDonald P, McRae S, Leiter J et al (2011) Arthroscopic rotator cuff repair with and without acromioplasty in the treatment of full-thickness rotator cuff tears: a multicenter, randomized controlled trial. J Bone Joint Surg Am 93:1953–1960
31. Chahal J, Mall N, MacDonald PB et al (2012) The role of subacromial decompression in patients undergoing arthroscopic repair of full-thickness tears of the rotator cuff: a systematic review and meta-analysis. Arthroscopy 28:720–727

Chapter 9
Mini-Open Rotator Cuff Repair

Yukihiko Hata, Norio Ishigaki, and Tomoyuki Matsuba

Abstract We report the techniques of mini-open rotator cuff repair for rotator cuff tears and the postoperative outcomes in patients followed up for 10 or more years after surgery. The surgical procedure aimed to repair the torn rotator cuff with transosseous suture through the mini-open deltoid splitting approach. We evaluated 41 shoulders in 39 patients followed up for 10 or more years after surgery, with a mean age of 58.2 years at the time of surgery and mean postoperative follow-up period of 10.8 years. The University of California Los Angeles shoulder scale score significantly improved at 10 years after surgery, and 93 % of the patients had excellent or good results. The repeat tear (retear) rate at 10 years after surgery on cuff integrity evaluation by magnetic resonance imaging was 17 %. Favorable shoulder joint function has been maintained over the long term after mini-open rotator cuff repair, and the outcome of the repaired rotator cuff was also favorable. The results suggest that mini-open rotator cuff repair is an effective treatment option for rotator cuff tears.

Keywords Mini-open rotator cuff repair • Rotator cuff tear • MRI (magnetic resonance imaging) • Transosseous suture

9.1 Introduction

Surgical treatment is usually selected for symptomatic full-thickness rotator cuff tears that are resistant to conservative treatment, and many good early or intermediate (2–9 years) clinical results have been reported [1–3]. However, only a few articles report on the clinical results of patients followed up for 10 or more years after surgery [4–8].

In our institution, mini-open rotator cuff repair [9] has been performed in patients with rotator cuff tears since 1997. We previously reported that these surgical procedures are less invasive to deltoid anterior fibers than the conventional

Y. Hata (✉) • N. Ishigaki • T. Matsuba
Shoulder Medical Center, North Alps Medical Center Azumi Hospital, 3207-1 Ikedamachi, Kitaazumigun, Nagano 399-8695, Japan
e-mail: y.hata@azumi-ghp.jp

K. Tamai et al. (eds.), *Advances in Shoulder Surgery*,
DOI 10.1007/978-4-431-55988-7_9

open surgery and allow early return to work and sports [10]. Herein, we report the procedure and postoperative outcomes of mini-open rotator cuff repair in patients followed up for 10 or more years after surgery.

9.2 Mini-Open Rotator Cuff Repair

9.2.1 Surgical Indication

This procedure is indicated in cases in which pain or muscular weakness has reduced activities of daily living (ADL) or quality of life. We consider it to not be indicated in the following cases: (1) those with irreparable rotator cuff tears (three or more tears and 5 cm or wider retraction), (2) those with conditions complicated by severe underlying diseases, and (3) those with low ADL levels (e.g., retired persons).

9.2.2 Surgical Method

9.2.2.1 Anesthesia and Surgical Position

Surgery is performed under general anesthesia. The surgical position of the patient is the beach-chair position, with the back against the surgical table and the head elevated to 40°. Then the affected shoulder is brought to the outside sufficiently so that the arm can elevate posteriorly without contacting the edge of the surgical table during surgery.

9.2.2.2 Surgical Techniques

A 3-cm-long skin incision was made starting from the middle of the anterior margin of the acromion toward the axilla (mini-open deltoid splitting approach; Fig. 9.1). The anterior deltoid fascia was cut along the skin incision, and the muscle was bluntly dissected and retracted (Fig. 9.2), The coracoacromial ligament was resected, and acromioplasty was then carried out under direct vision by scraping the undersurface of the acromion with a nasal rasp (Medicon eG, Tuttlingen, Germany) until it is flat, the insertion of the deltoid being protected with a retractor.

The degenerated portion of the rotator cuff tear is excised as quickly as possible, and one to three stay sutures (No. 2 braided nylon sutures) are applied to the stump of the rotator cuff. At this time, the use of a Mayo–Hegar needle holder (19 cm) makes it easy to apply the suture to the rotator cuff drawn into the back. It is important to fully separate the adhesion around the rotator cuff (particularly the subacromial space and around the base of the coracoid process) manually while the

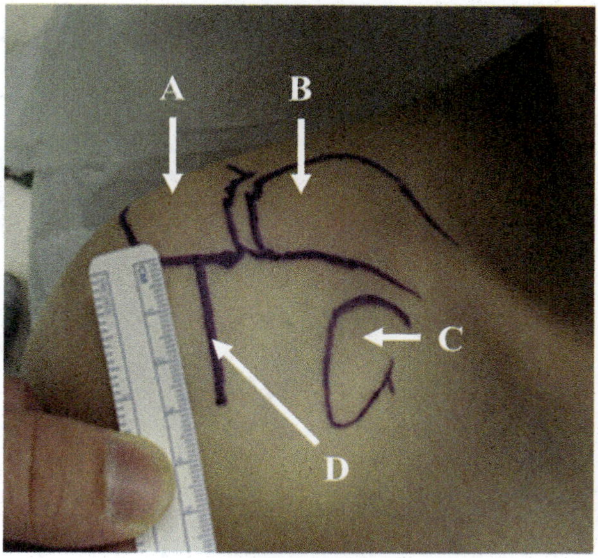

Fig. 9.1 Skin incision. A 3-cm-long skin incision was made starting from the middle of the anterior margin of the acromion toward the axilla. *A* Acromion; *B* clavicle; *C* coracoid process; *D* skin incision

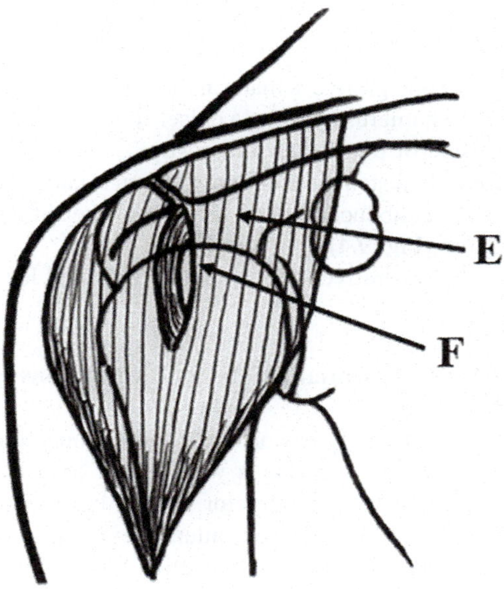

Fig. 9.2 Dissection and retraction of the deltoid anterior fibers. *E The deltoid anterior fibers; F* the deltoid muscle was bluntly dissected and retracted

stay suture is held and the rotator cuff is pulled out, by which the stump of the rotator cuff can be pulled out to the greater tuberosity of the humerus in most the patients. The rotator cuff should be pulled out along the direction of the rotator cuff muscle fibers when it is pulled out, and care should be taken not to make the surface of the repaired rotator cuff irregular at the time of suturing.

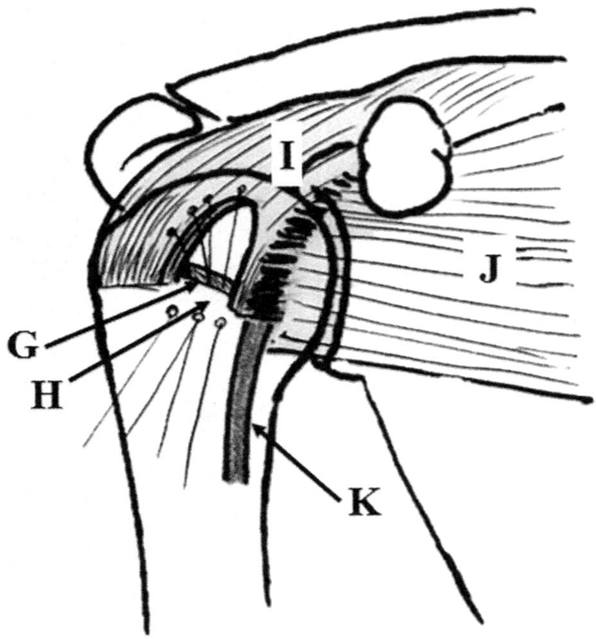

Fig. 9.3 Rotator cuff repair. Two-stitch mattress sutures to the posterior stump of the rotator cuff are passed from the groove to the outside of the greater tuberosity. *G* Groove; *H* greater tuberosity; *I* supraspinatus tendon; *J* subscapular tendon; *K* long head of the biceps tendon (*LHB*)

A bony groove is made at the insertion of the rotator cuff of the greater tuberosity of the humerus by using a chisel. Then, the sutures are passed from the groove to the outside of the greater tuberosity by using a gynecological no. 5 blunt needle and securely fasten the stump of the torn rotator cuff to the tuberosity with the arm in the shoulder abduction of 0° (Fig. 9.3). The slit left inside is sutured with a side-to-side suture (Fig. 9.4).

The operative time is about 1 h. Blood loss volume seldom exceeds 100 ml.

9.2.2.3 Essential Points and Precautions in Operative Techniques

1. Because the incision made for this operation is small, the visual field is narrow. However, securing a wide visual field by inappropriately pulling the deltoid muscle with a retractor should be avoided. The operative field needs to be secured by extension, internal/external rotation, or pulling down while the arm is held motionless. Posterior elevation or internal rotation of the shoulder facilitates bringing the posterior components of the rotator cuff (infraspinatus tendon or teres minor tendon) into the visual field. Arm depression facilitates bringing the superior components of the rotator cuff (supraspinatus tendon or infraspinatus tendon) into the visual field.
2. Treatment is often difficult in cases with subscapular tendon tears (Fig. 9.5). In such cases, repair is made possible by concomitant use of long head tendon anchoring [11]. First, the stump of the subscapular muscle is pulled out from the

Fig. 9.4 Side-to-side suture. After anchoring the posterior stump of the rotator cuff to the groove, the slit left inside is sutured with side-to-side suture. *L* Slit of the rotator cuff; *H* greater tuberosity

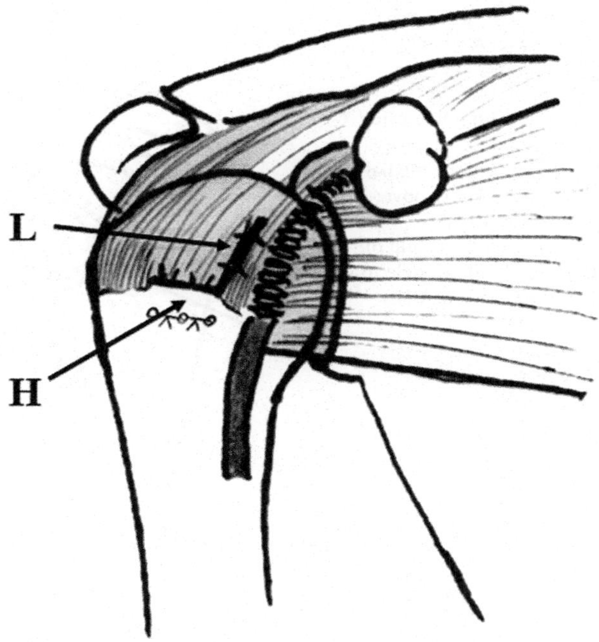

Fig. 9.5 Rotator cuff tears with subscapular tendon tears. *H* Greater tuberosity; *I* supraspinatus tendon; *J* subscapular tendon; *K* LHB

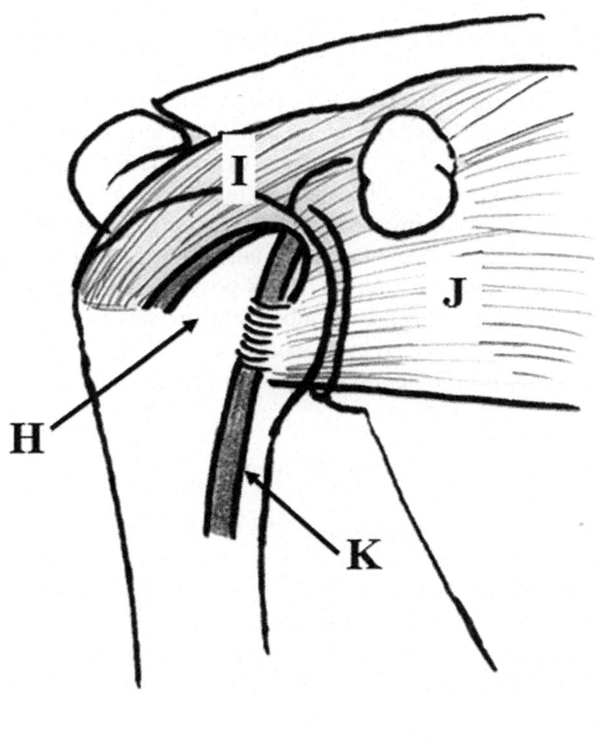

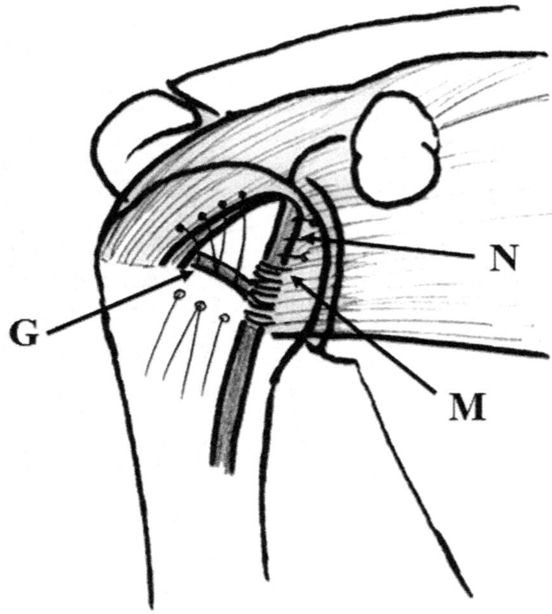

Fig. 9.6 Repair of subscapular tendon tear. The stump of the subscapular muscle is pulled out from the inside and sutured to the lesser tuberosity and the medial side of LHB. *G* Groove; *M* lesser tuberosity; *N* anchoring the stump of the subscapular muscle to the medial side of LHB

inside and sutured to the lesser tuberosity of the humerus and the medial side of the brachial biceps long head tendon (Fig. 9.6). Then, the posterior stump of the rotator cuff is pulled outward in an anteromedial direction and securely fastened to the bony groove created in the greater tuberosity with the arm in the shoulder abduction of 0° (Fig. 9.7). Finally, the slit left between the posterior stump of the rotator cuff and the lateral part of the long head tendon is sutured with a side-to-side suture (Fig. 9.8). What we emphasize during repair of a rotator cuff tear (involving the subscapularis tendon) is a well-balanced repair that can make tension uniform across the rotator cuff, rather than an anatomic repair.

3. In cases in which the rotator cuff stump cannot be pulled out sufficiently to reach the greater tubercle, repair is possible if a bony groove is created about 1 cm proximal to the greater tuberosity attachment point and the rotator cuff is sutured to it, as described by Nobuhara et al. [11]. Liu et al. reported that this technique poses no problem with postoperative functional recovery [12].

9.2.2.4 Postoperative Protocol

Passive elevation exercise of the shoulder joint is started with the patient wearing a shoulder abduction orthosis on the day after surgery. The orthosis is changed to a shoulder abduction pillow at 2 weeks after surgery, and the pillow is gradually changed to smaller ones while the patient is provided with a shoulder girdle-strengthening exercise and passive range-of-motion exercise. An active-assistive exercise is started at 3 weeks after surgery, and active exercise is gradually started

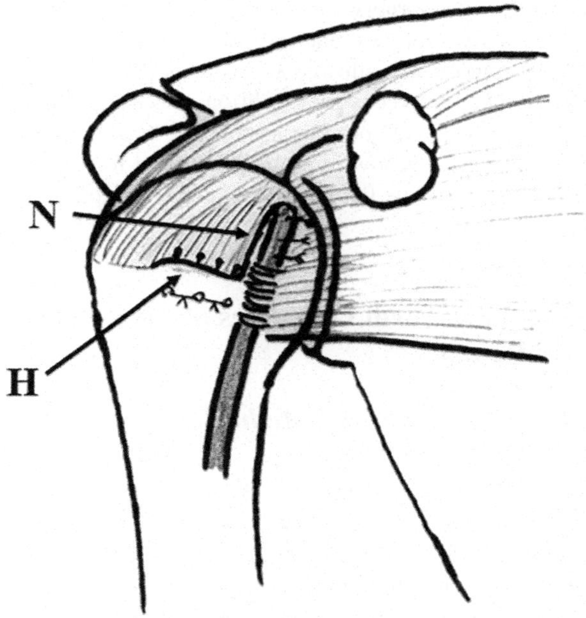

Fig. 9.7 Repair of posterior rotator cuff tears. Posterior stump of the rotator cuff is anchored to the bony groove created in the greater tuberosity. *H* Greater tuberosity; *N* slit left between the posterior stump of the rotator cuff and the lateral part of LHB

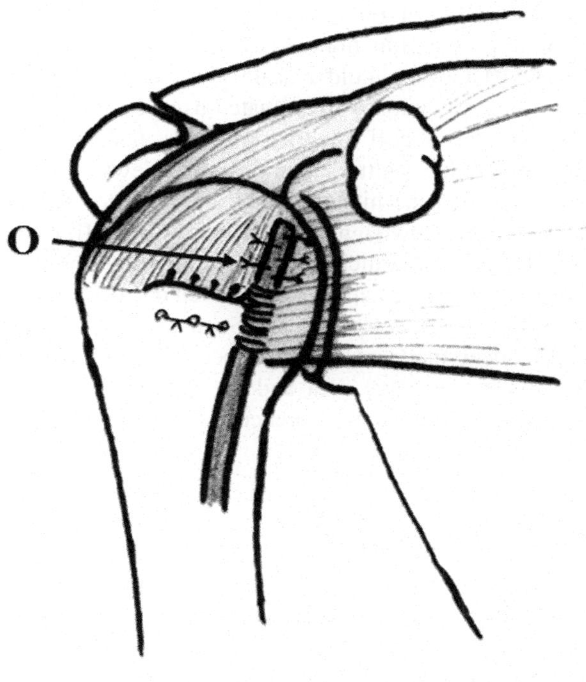

Fig. 9.8 Side-to-side suture. *O* The posterior stump of the rotator cuff is sutured to the lateral part of LHB

at 6 weeks after surgery. An outer muscle-strengthening exercise is started from 2 to 3 months after surgery, and the patient is gradually allowed to do light work. The patient is gradually allowed to do manual labor and sports from 6 months after surgery when the recovery condition is evaluated.

In cases with concomitant use of long head tendon anchoring, active flexion and extension of the elbow joint are prohibited for 3 weeks after surgery. During this period, only passive flexion and extension of the elbow joint are permitted.

9.3 Short-Term Outcomes of Mini-Open Rotator Cuff Repair

9.3.1 Materials and Methods

Four hundred ten patients who underwent mini-open rotator cuff repair for rotator cuff tears were evaluated at 2 years after surgery. Mean age at surgery was 60.8 years (range, 39–80 years). Surgery was performed on 231 male shoulders and 179 female shoulders. The tear size, according to the DeOrio and Cofield classification [13], was small in 48 shoulders, moderate sized in 231, large in 116, and massive in 15. The postoperative follow-up period was 42.6 months on average (range, 24–60 months).

Shoulder joint function was evaluated by using the University of California Los Angeles (UCLA) shoulder scale [14], and cuff integrity at the insertion of the supraspinatus tendon was evaluated using magnetic resonance imaging (MRI).

Postoperative cuff integrity was classified into three categories using oblique coronal, oblique sagittal, and transverse views of T_2-weighted images [15]: type I, cases in which the high-intensity area at the supraspinatus tendon insertion was visualized as a low signal on all images; type II, cases other than types I and III; type III, cases in which a full-thickness high-intensity area at the supraspinatus tendon insertion was visualized on even one of the images. Type III is equal to type IV or V with suspected retear in Sugaya's classification [16].

Statistical analysis was performed with the Wilcoxon signed-rank test to compare the preoperative data and the data at 2 years after surgery, with $p < 0.01$ indicating a significant difference.

9.3.2 Clinical Results

In the evaluation of clinical results according to the UCLA shoulder scale, the total score at 2 years after surgery was 33.6, indicating the outcome to be not inferior to that reported by Gartsman et al. (total score, 31.1) [17], Liu (32.7) [18], and Paulos et al. (30.2) [19] (Table 9.1).

Table 9.1 University of California Los Angeles (UCLA) shoulder scales 2 years after surgery

Items	Before surgery	2 years after surgery	p value
Pain	4.8 ± 2.2	9.3 ± 1.3	$p < 0.0001$
Function	7.2 ± 1.6	9.8 ± 0.7	$p < 0.0001$
Forward flexion	4.5 ± 0.7	4.9 ± 0.3	$p < 0.0001$
Muscle strength	4.1 ± 0.7	4.9 ± 0.4	$p < 0.0001$
Patient satisfaction	0.0	4.6 ± 0.6	$p < 0.0001$
Total score	20.7 ± 3.7	33.6 ± 2.2	$p < 0.0001$

Table 9.2 Cuff integrity evaluation on magnetic resonance imaging (MRI) at 2 years after surgery

Cuff integrity	Before surgery	2 years after surgery	p value
Type 1	0	235	
Type 2	0	114	
Type 3	410	61	$p < 0.0001$

Evaluation of supraspinatus tendon insertion by magnetic resonance imaging (MRI) revealed improvement over time, with 14.9 % of all cases rated as type 3 (retear) at 2 years after surgery (Table 9.2).

9.4 Long-Term Outcomes of Mini-Open Rotator Cuff Repair [20]

9.4.1 Materials and Methods

Forty one shoulders of 39 patients (follow-up rate, 85.4 %) which were followed up for 10 or more years after mini-open rotator cuff repair were evaluated. The mean age at the time of surgery was 58.2 years (range, 39–70 years), with were 23 men and 18 women, and 29 right and 12 left shoulders. This study had 4 small tears, 22 moderate-sized tears, 12 large tears, and 3 massive tears. The mean postoperative follow-up period was 10.8 years (range, 120–151 months).

Shoulder joint function was evaluated using the UCLA shoulder scale [14], and cuff integrity at the insertion of the supraspinatus tendon was evaluated using MRI [15].

Statistical analysis was performed by using the Wilcoxon signed-rank test to compare the preoperative data and the data at 10 or more years after surgery, with $p < 0.01$ indicating a significant difference.

9.4.2 Clinical Results

In the evaluation of the long-term clinical results according to the UCLA shoulder scale, a significant improvement was observed in all items, except for flexion muscle strength (Table 9.3). The results were excellent (34–35 points) in 24 shoulders (59 %), good (29–33 points) in 14 (34 %), and poor (28 points or less) in 3 (7 %).

On MRI, at the insertion of the supraspinatus tendon, a significant improvement was seen at 10 or more years after surgery compared with before surgery (Table 9.4). Of the shoulders, 17 % had type 3 cuff integrity.

9.4.3 Discussion

In the evaluation of the follow-up results at 10 or more years after rotator cuff repair, excellent or good results were reported in 80 % to 91 % [4, 5, 21], whereas Bell et al. [6] reported excellent or good results in 69 %. In our cases, the clinical results at 10 or more years after surgery were highly favorable, with 93 % excellent or good results based on the UCLA shoulder scale. Favorable shoulder joint function was maintained even at 10 or more years after surgery.

In the cuff integrity evaluation on MRI, the retear rate was 17 % at 10 or more years after rotator cuff repair. In previous reports, the retear rate ranged from 13 % to 94 % [8, 22, 23]. Clinical outcomes are thought to be better if cuff integrity is maintained.

Table 9.3 UCLA shoulder scales at 10 or more years after surgery

Items	Before surgery	10 years after surgery	*p* value
Pain	4.3 ± 2.3	9.1 ± 1.3	$p < 0.0001$
Function	8.3 ± 1.7	9.7 ± 0.7	$p < 0.01$
Forward flexion	4.5 ± 0.8	5.0 ± 0.2	$p < 0.01$
Muscle strength	4.6 ± 0.6	4.8 ± 0.5	NS
Patient satisfaction	0.0	4.4 ± 0.7	$p < 0.0001$
Total score	21.3 ± 4.0	33.1 ± 2.4	$p < 0.0001$

NS: not significant

Table 9.4 Cuff integrity evaluation on MRI at 10 or more years after surgery

Cuff integrity	Before surgery	10 years after surgery	*p* value
Type 1	0	27	
Type 2	0	7	
Type 3	41	7	$p < 0.0001$

9.5 Conclusion

Favorable shoulder joint function has been maintained over the long term after mini-open rotator cuff repair, and the retear rate was low at 10 or more years after surgery. The results suggest that mini-open rotator cuff repair is an effective treatment option for rotator cuff tears.

References

1. Goutallier D, Postel JM, Radier C et al (2009) Long-term functional and structural outcome in patients with intact repairs 1 year after open transosseous rotator cuff repair. J Shoulder Elbow Surg 18:521–528. doi:10.1016/j.jse.2008.11.006
2. Jost B, Zumstein M, Pfirrmann CW et al (2006) Long-term outcome after structural failure of rotator cuff repairs. J Bone Joint Surg Am 88:472–479
3. Lähteenmäki HE, Virolainen P, Hiltunen A et al (2006) Results of early operative treatment of rotator cuff tears with acute symptoms. J Shoulder Elbow Surg 15:148–153
4. Adamson G, Tibone JE (1993) Ten-year assessment of primary rotator cuff repairs. J Shoulder Elbow Surg 2:57–63. doi:10.1016/1058-2746(93)90001-W
5. Cofield RH, Parvizi J, Hoffmeyer PJ et al (2001) Surgical repair of chronic rotator cuff tears: a prospective long-term study. J Bone Joint Surg Am 83:71–77
6. Galatz LM, Griggs S, Cameron BD et al (2001) Prospective longitudinal analysis of postoperative shoulder function: a ten-year follow-up study of full-thickness rotator cuff tears. J Bone Joint Surg Am 83:1052–1056
7. Sperling JW, Cofield RH, Schleck C et al (2004) Rotator cuff repair in patients fifty years of age and younger. J Bone Joint Surg Am 86:2212–2215
8. Borgmästars N, Paavola M, Remes V et al (2010) Pain relief, motion, and function after rotator cuff repair or reconstruction may not persist after 16 years. Clin Orthop 468:2678–2689
9. Hata Y, Saitoh S, Murakami N et al (2005) A less invasive surgery for rotator cuff tear. Mini-open repair. J Shoulder Elbow Surg 10:11–16
10. Hata Y, Saitoh S, Murakami N et al (2004) Atrophy of the deltoid muscle following rotator cuff surgery. J Bone Joint Surg Am 86:1414–1419
11. Nobuhara K, Hata Y, Komai M (1994) Surgical procedure and results of repair of massive tears of the rotator cuff. Clin Orthop 304:54–59
12. Liu J, Hughes RE, O'Driscoll SW et al (1998) Biomechanical effect of medial advancement of the supraspinatus tendon. A study in cadavera. J Bone Joint Surg Am 80:853–859
13. Deorio JK, Cofield RH (1984) Results of a second attempt at surgical repair of a failed initial rotator-cuff repair. J Bone Joint Surg Am 66:563–567
14. Ellman H, Hanker G, Bayer M (1986) Repair of the rotator cuff. J Bone Joint Surg Am 68:1136–1144
15. Murakami N, Hata Y, Kobayashi H et al (2003) Examination of postoperative change in a repaired rotator cuff by MRI and sonography. Shoulder Joint 27:237–240
16. Sugaya H, Maeda K, Matsuki K et al (2007) Repair integrity and functional outcome after arthroscopic double-row rotator cuff repair. J Bone Joint Surg Am 89:953–960. doi:10.2106/JBJS.F.00512
17. Gartsman GM, Khan M, Hammerman SM (1998) Arthroscopic repair of full-thickness tears of the rotator cuff. J Bone Joint Surg Am 80:832–840
18. Li SH (1994) Arthroscopically-assisted rotator-cuff repair. J Bone Joint Surg (Br) 76:592–595
19. Paulos LE, Kody MH (1994) Arthroscopically enhanced "miniapproach" to rotator cuff repair. Am J Sports Med 22:19–25

20. Hata Y, Ishigaki N, Nakamura K et al (2011) Long-term outcomes of mini open repair for rotator cuff tears. Shoulder Joint 35:817–819
21. Bell S, Lim YJ, Coghlan J (2013) Long-term longitudinal follow-up of mini-open rotator cuff repair. J Bone Joint Surg Am 95:151–157. doi:10.2106/JBJS.K.00499
22. Vastamäki M, Lohman M, Borgmästars N (2013) Rotator cuff integrity correlates with clinical and functional results at a minimum 16 years after open repair. Clin Orthop Relat Res 471:554–561. doi:10.1007/s11999-012-2494-1
23. Zumstein M, Jost B, Hempel J et al (2008) The clinical and structural long-term results of open repair of massive tears of the rotator cuff. J Bone Joint Surg Am 90:2423–2431. doi:10.2106/JBJS.G.00677

Chapter 10
Massive and Irreparable Rotator Cuff Tears

Yu Mochizuki and Mitsuo Ochi

Abstract When primary repair of a massive rotator cuff tear is impossible, the lesion is called an irreparable rotator cuff tear. Treating irreparable rotator cuff tears is difficult as a result of the less satisfactory results and a higher retear rate. In addition, if massive rotator cuff rupture is left untreated, this complication frequently leads to cuff tear arthroplasty. Therefore, is would be helpful to change the concept of treatment from tissue repair and/or reconstruction to tissue regeneration. For tissue regeneration, the use of a scaffold is necessary. Based on the results of this experimental study, we concluded that the PGA sheet scaffold material allows for the regeneration of the tendon-to-tendon as well as tendon-to-bone interface in an animal model.

Based on the findings of the experimental study, we performed patch graft repair with a polyglycolic acid (PGA) sheet, an artificial biomaterial, for irreparable rotator cuff tear cases and successfully improved the results of repair for irreparable rotator cuff tears in terms of postoperative pain control and short-term outcomes. PGA sheets are a possible artificial scaffold material for promoting tendon regeneration in rotator cuff repair.

Keywords Rotator cuff • Massive and irreparable tear • Artificial material • Polyglycolic acid • Regeneration

10.1 Introduction

The management of massive rotator cuff tears is thought to be challenging because of the less satisfactory results and higher retear rate. In addition, if left untreated, massive rotator cuff rupture frequently leads to cuff tear arthroplasty [1]. Even when this complication is treated with total shoulder arthroplasty, shoulder pain and elevation disturbances frequently persist. In fact, there is a recent trend to

Y. Mochizuki (✉)
Hiroshima Prefectural Hospital, 1-5-54 Ujina-Kanda, Minami-ku, Hiroshima 734-8530, Japan
e-mail: yumochi@hph.pref.hiroshima.jp

M. Ochi
Hiroshima University, Hiroshima, Japan

K. Tamai et al. (eds.), *Advances in Shoulder Surgery*,
DOI 10.1007/978-4-431-55988-7_10

treat difficult cases using reverse total shoulder arthroplasty; however, this procedure is very invasive [2]. Therefore, various surgical techniques, including musculotendinous transfer [3–5] and patch grafts with autologous fascia lata [6] or artificial materials [7], have been used for the treatment of irreparable tears. However, the application of musculotendinous transfers necessitates the sacrifice of normal tissue and does not result in anatomic reconstruction unless rotator cuff repair is also performed. Furthermore, patch grafts made using fascia lata tend to degrade from normal wear and stretching [7], and those made using nonabsorbable artificial materials become mechanically weaker over time as a result of foreign-body reactions and/or infection. Hence, new strategies for the treatment of irreparable rotator cuff tears must be developed. The development of a tissue-engineering technique [8] offers a promising future for musculoskeletal tissue repair, and many studies have reported success in tendon engineering both in vitro [9, 10] and in vivo [11–13].

Based on the results of an experimental study, we performed a clinical study using a sophisticated artificial material. We hypothesized that it would be better to repair defects of the rotator cuff according to the patch graft technique using a polyglycolic acid (PGA) sheet without sacrificing the autologous tissues, such as the fascia lata, and employing a minimally invasive operative procedure using an arthroscopic patch graft. The purpose of this study was to investigate the short-term clinical results of arthroscopic PGA sheet patch graft repair for irreparable rotator cuff tears based on the concept of tissue regeneration.

10.2 Materials and Methods

We defined irreparable rotator cuff tears as those that, because of their size and retraction, cannot be repaired primarily to the site of insertion onto the tuberosity, despite conventional techniques of mobilization and soft tissue release. This study involved 75 patients selected from 436 patients who were evaluated in the shoulder surgery section of our department for shoulder pain in the years 2012–2013. The study was performed according to our hospital ethics committee guidelines and approved by our hospital ethics committee. All subjects [28 women and 47 men, with a mean age of 65.7 years (range, 57–77 years)] were diagnosed with irreparable rotator cuff tears. The patients were assigned to receive surgical treatment using repair with a PGA sheet (Neoveil, Gunze, Japan) patch graft (PGA group, 37 patients) or a fascia lata patch graft (PG group, 38 patients). Informed consent was obtained from all participants. The kind of patch to be used was selected randomly, and the patients were treated by the same surgical team. The exclusion criteria were as follows: (1) osteoarthritis of the glenohumeral joint; (2) inflammatory arthritis or any rheumatic condition; (3) labral lesions requiring additional procedures, such as type 2 superior labrum anterior posterior or Bankart lesions; (4) biceps lesions requiring tenodesis; and (5) injuries of the contralateral shoulder. The surgical procedure was performed arthroscopically in all patients. Partial

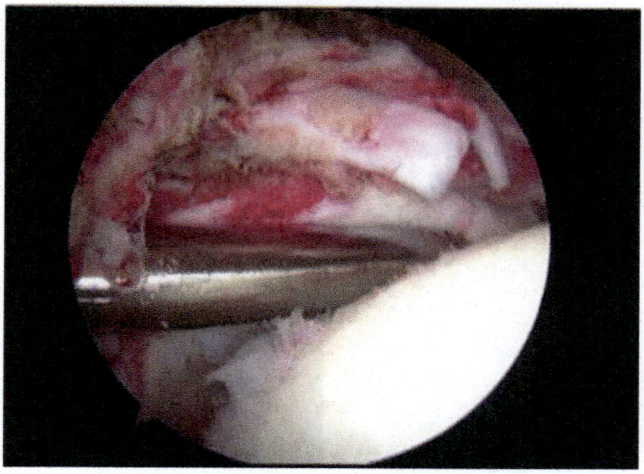

Fig. 10.1 Arthroscopic findings. The irreparable rotator cuff injury was found arthroscopically

bursectomy, minimal acromioplasty, and adhesion release were performed. The size of the defect was measured, and a graft of the same size as the defect was made using a PGA sheet (PGA group) or the fascia lata (PG group). The graft was placed underneath and overlapped with the edge of the torn tendon at a width of more than 5 mm to protect against superior migration of the humeral head. The sutures on the graft were passed through the tendon and tied up on the tendon surface. The fascia lata was harvested from the lateral side of the thigh just distal to the great trochanter. The footprint was prepared with a rasp, and two or three suture anchors were used in a single-row fashion (Figs. 10.1 and 10.2).

All patients followed the same rehabilitation regimen, which included the use of a rigid brace for 3 weeks and passive movement exercises under the supervision of a physical therapist for an additional 5 weeks. Active movement exercises were commenced at 3 weeks with limitation of the elevation angle. A strengthening exercise program was started at 12 weeks postoperatively.

The patients were clinically evaluated preoperatively and at 1, 3, 6, and 12 months postoperatively. The Japanese Orthopaedic Association (JOA) shoulder rating scale was used to evaluate the subjects preoperatively and at 12 months postoperatively. A magnetic resonance imaging (MRI) examination was performed at 1 year postoperatively in all patients. The intensity of the grafted patch was graded as high-, iso-, or low intensity, and the patients were classified into high-intensity, iso-intensity, and low-intensity groups.

Patients whose grafted patch contained a large amount of high-intensity areas were assigned to the high-intensity group, those with a large amount of iso-intensity areas in the grafted patch were assigned to the iso-intensity group, and those with a large amount of low-intensity areas in the grafted patch were assigned to the low-intensity group. High-intensity areas were thought to contain poorly matured tissues and low-intensity areas were considered to contain well-matured tissues. The rate obtained comparing the high-intensity group and the other groups was

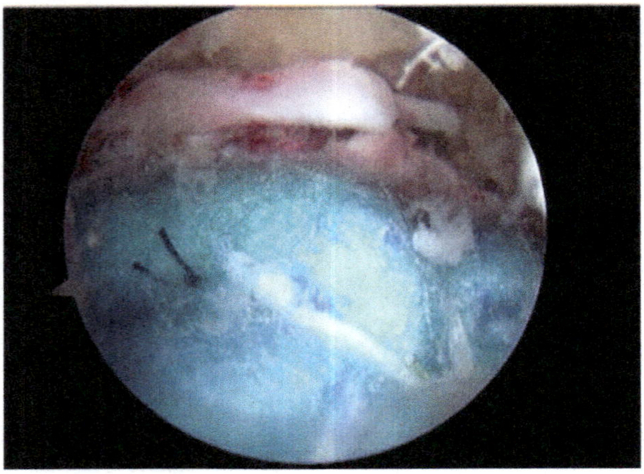

Fig. 10.2 Arthroscopic finding. Arthroscopic polyglycolic acid (PGSA) sheet patch graft was performed for an irreparable rotator cuff injury

defined as the high-intensity rate. No second-look arthroscopic surgeries or biopsies were performed.

Statistical analysis was conducted using the Mann–Whitney *U* test among the treatment groups. When comparing the pre–post treatments, the paired *t* test was performed. When comparing high-intensity rates, the Pearson chi-square test was used. A *p* value less than 0.05 was considered as being statistically significant.

10.3 Results

The follow-up analysis showed that each group benefited from the surgical treatment of irreparable rotator cuff tears. The mean JOA scores improved from 54.9 ± 1.1 points preoperatively to 90.7 ± 1.0 points at the 12-month follow-up ($p < 0.01$) in the PGA group and from 52.6 ± 1.5 points preoperatively to 91.7 ± 1.2 points at the 12-month follow-up ($p < 0.01$) in the PG group (Table 10.1). For the factor of pain, the mean scores improved from 15.8 ± 2.1 points preoperatively to 26.7 ± 1.1 points at the 12-month follow-up ($p < 0.01$) in the PGA group and from 14.7 ± 1.8 points preoperatively to 25.6 ± 1.4 points at the 12-month follow-up ($p < 0.01$) in the PG group. For the factor of function, the mean scores improved from 11.6 ± 2.2 points preoperatively to 17.6 ± 1.3 points at the 12-month follow-up ($p < 0.01$) in the PGA group and from 12.5 ± 1.4 points preoperatively to 16.8 ± 1.5 points at the 12-month follow-up ($p < 0.01$) in the PG group.

The MRI findings at 1 year showed a low-intensity rate of 51.4 % (19/37 patients), an iso-intensity rate of 35.1 % (13/37 patients), and a high-intensity rate of 13.5 % (5/37 patients) in the PGA group, and a low-intensity rate of 39.5 % (15/38 patients), iso-intensity rate of 28.9 % (11/38 patients), and high-intensity rate of 31.6 % (12/38 patients) in the PG group (Table 10.2). The MRI findings at 1 year

Table 10.1 The Japanese Orthopaedic Association (JOA) score of each group (points)

	Before surgery	12 months after surgery
PGA group	54.9 ± 1.1	90.7 ± 1.0*
PG group	52.6 ± 1.5	91.7 ± 1.2*

Mean JOA scores improved from 54.9 ± 1.1 points preoperatively to 90.7 ± 1.0 points at 12-month follow-up ($p < 0.01$) in the polyglycolic acid (PGA) group and from 52.6 ± 1.5 points preoperatively to 91.7 ± 1.2 points at 12-month follow-up ($p < 0.01$) in the patch graft (PG) group
*$p < 0.01$

Table 10.2 Magnetic resonance imaging (MRI) findings

	Low-intensity group	Iso-intensity group	High-intensity group
PGA group	51.4 % (19/37 patients)	35.1 % (13/37 patients)	13.5 % (5/37 patients)*
PG group	39.5 % (15/38 patients)	28.9 % (11/38 patients)	31.6 % (12/38 patients)*

MRI findings at 1 year showed a low-intensity group of 51.4 % (19/37 patients) and an iso-intensity group of 35.1 % (13/37 patients), a high-intensity group of 13.5 % (5/37 patients) in the PGA group, and a low-intensity group of 39.5 % (15/38 patients), an iso-intensity group of 28.9 % (11/38 patients), and a high-intensity group of 31.6 % (12/38 patients) in the patch graft (PG) group
The high-intensity rate was significantly lower for the PGA group ($p = 0.001$)
*$p = 0.001$

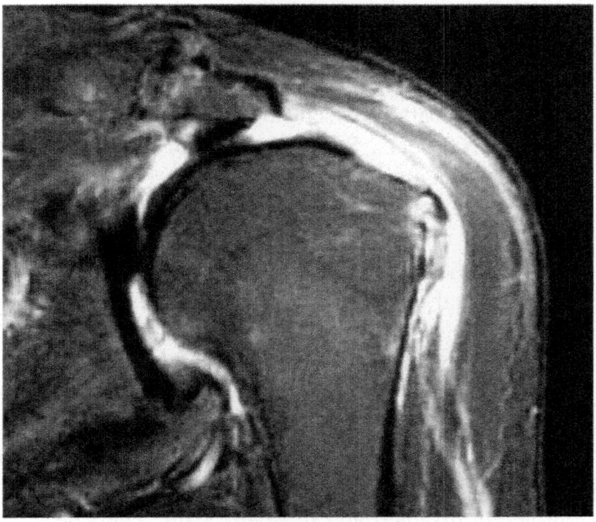

Fig. 10.3 Magnetic resonance imaging (MRI) finding before surgery

showed a high-intensity rate of 13.3 % (4/30 patients) in the PGA group and 31.2 % (10/32 patients) in the PG group (Figs. 10.3, 10.4). The high-intensity rate was significantly lower in the PGA group (p = 0.001). The type of implanted patch was the only factor affecting the retear rate. No major complications occurred, and no adverse events related to patch application were noted, including local inflammation, fibrosis, or subacromial adhesions affecting the joint function.

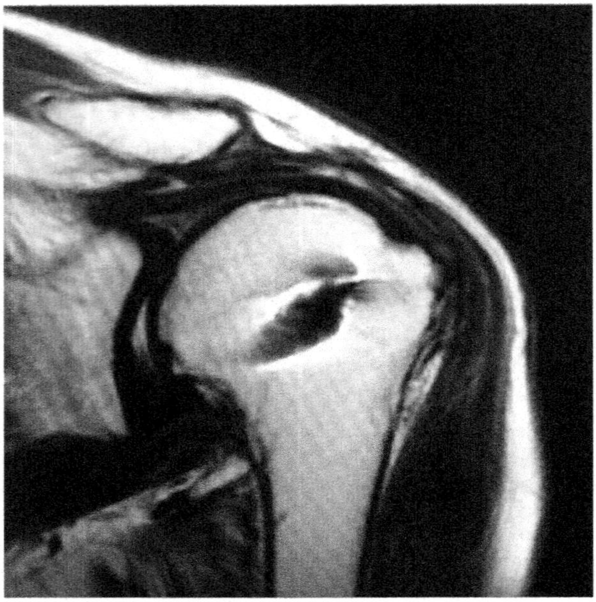

Fig. 10.4 Magnetic resonance imaging finding 1 year after surgery

10.4 Discussion

Rotator cuff tears represent the most common cause of shoulder pain in patients older than 60 years. Surgical repair of rotator cuff tears has become a common procedure with good clinical results [14–17]. However, failure of repair for massive rotator cuff tears occurs in 20 % to 68 % of patients, depending on tear size, patient age, degree of muscle atrophy, muscle fatty degeneration, and chronicity [18–24]. In addition, the high retear rates after surgery can be attributed to the quality of the residual tendon and healing capacity of the residual tendons. Native rotator cuff enthesis is characterized by complex morphological structures and involves direct insertion. The complex morphological structure of bone tendon insertion is difficult to repair. When primary repair of a massive rotator cuff tear is impossible, the lesion is called an irreparable rotator cuff tear. Treating irreparable rotator cuff tears is difficult for many reasons. Patients with irreparable rotator cuff tears may present with a variety of manifestations, such as no or mild symptoms, or may be completely disabled and in severe pain. The true incidence of irreparable rotator cuff tears is not known; however, anatomic studies of cadavers and imaging studies of asymptomatic patients have demonstrated rotator cuff tears in 30 % to 50 % of older patients, especially in those older than 70 years [25–27]. Tempelhof et al. [28] studied 411 asymptomatic individuals and found that 38 % of those older than 70 years had full-thickness rotator cuff tears. Rotator cuff tears with an increased degree of fatty infiltration and muscle atrophy, in association with a high-riding humeral head to the acromion, are at high risk of becoming irreparable. Goutallier et al. [22] used computed tomography (CT)scans to evaluate fatty infiltration, although magnetic resonance imaging (MRI) is probably more sensitive [17]. Irreparable rotator cuff tears occur in two physiologically distinct patient groups; however, they can be present in all age and activity groups. Most often, these tears occur in physiologically older, lower-demand patients (older than 70 years, and usually female) who are asymptomatic until a minor trauma creates symptoms. The second group consists of physiologically younger, more active patients, often in the sixth decade of life, who present with dramatic symptoms of pain and disability after an acute event or with a history of rotator cuff surgery or chronic rotator cuff injury. When the patient complains of symptoms of pain and disability, operative treatment should be considered. However, the development of a retear after surgical repair of a massive rotator cuff tear is an unsatisfactory result. Several factors, such as patient age, preoperative tear size, degree of muscular atrophy, degree of fatty infiltration of the cuff muscle, surgical technique, and inappropriate rehabilitation, have been demonstrated to be associated with tendon retears [29–32]. Generally, when massive rotator cuff tears are successfully repaired, excellent clinical results may be achieved and joint degeneration may be halted or at least markedly decelerated [33]. Trappey and Gartsman [34] insisted that a low-tension environment is critical for rotator cuff healing. Other biomechanical studies have demonstrated that the elements needed for the successful repair of rotator cuff tears are strong fixation [35], a high interface pressure, and a wide interface area between the tendon and bone [36], as well as minimizing the concentration of stress inside the tendon [37]. In cases of arthroscopic repair of massive rotator cuff tears, achieving effective anatomic repair is difficult because the repair construct is under inevitably undue tension even after adequate release. Therefore, the retear rate of massive rotator cuff tears is generally higher than that of smaller rotator cuff tears. Recent studies have demonstrated that the postoperative healing rate after arthroscopic repair of massive rotator cuff tears is 47 % to 94 % [23, 29, 38, 39].

Based on these reports, we considered that it would be better to change the concept of treatment from tissue repair and/or reconstruction to tissue regeneration. For tissue regeneration, a scaffold is necessary. We subsequently performed an experimental study for the purpose of selecting the optimal scaffold material to promote the regeneration of structures within the articular joint as a pilot study.

We selected three biomaterials for our pilot study—polytetrafluoroethylene (PTFE), poly-L-lactate-epsilon-caprolactone (PLC), and polyglycolic acid (PGA) sheets—that were used in clinical applications with different absorption speeds. We sutured these synthetic biomaterials to the surface of the medial joint capsules using 3-0 nylon sutures in the bilateral knee joints of 27 Japanese white rabbits weighing 3.0–3.4 kg (Japan SLC, Hamamatsu, Japan) and evaluated the histological findings. PTFE, a nonabsorbable synthetic material, is used in clinically vascular surgery for reconstruction of large vessels, including the heart and abdominal wall, and, indeed, for covering irreparable tears of the rotator cuff [3]. PLC, an absorbable material, is very flexible with a rubber-like elasticity to facilitate a complete recovery and is known to degrade very slowly depending on the hydrophilicity of each monomeric unit. This PLC sheet has been used for the dura mater [40] and blood vessels in experimental studies [41] and clinical applications [42]. PGA, which is known to degrade rapidly, is biocompatible and has been approved for human clinical applications [43]. PLC, PGA, and their copolymers have received great interest in the tissue-engineering field [44]. In our pilot studies, we confirmed that the PGA sheet hydrolyzes most rapidly, exhibiting a potential for producing abundant fibrous tissue with fewer foreign-body reactions. Subsequently, we examined which scaffold is adequate for regeneration of the rotator cuff between PGA and PLC and confirmed that the PGA sheet is more suitable. We did not consider the PTFE sheet to be suitable for tendon regeneration because it caused a substantial foreign-body reaction in the pilot study and fibrous cells did not infiltrate into the PTFE fibers. Moreover, polyglyconate is the strongest absorbable monofilament available [45]. Many experimental studies employing tissue engineering techniques have been performed using PGA [10, 46–50]. Polyglycolic acid sheets are used in thoracic surgery in various clinical applications and have been approved by the Ministry of Health and Welfare as a medical tool. We therefore considered it reasonable to use PGA sheets in clinical applications for tissue engineering (Fig. 10.5).

We subsequently performed an experimental study of patch grafts to compare the validity of the biomaterials, PGA and PLC sheets, using an irreparable rotator cuff injury model in rabbits.

As to the PLC group, on a gross examination, the remaining PLC scaffold sheets were covered with thin scar-like tissue at all time points. A histological examination of the tissues in the PLC group 4 weeks after surgery revealed the gross presence of PLC fibers. Randomly oriented fibroblasts and fibers with a small diameter exhibiting minimal wave formation surrounded by trabecular bone were found around the scaffolds at the tendon insertion sites. There was also infiltration of granulation tissue and blood vessels between the PLC fibers, and the interface was bridged by loose connective tissue. Some chondrocytes were seen, although they were not arranged along the long axis (Fig. 10.6). At 16 weeks after surgery, the PLC sheet grossly remained, and many multinuclear cells indicating a foreign-body

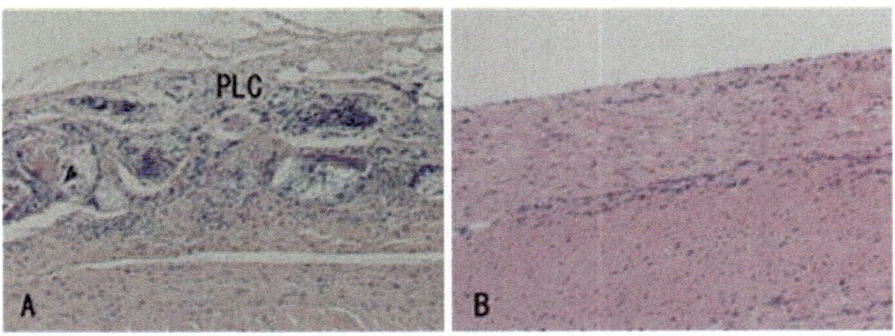

Fig. 10.5 Micrographs of specimens of the surface of the capsules of the knee joints 24 weeks after surgery with the poly-L-lactate-epsilon-caprolactone (PLC) sheet (**a**) and PGA sheet (**b**). Hematoxylin and eosin, ×100. (From Yokoya et al. [50])

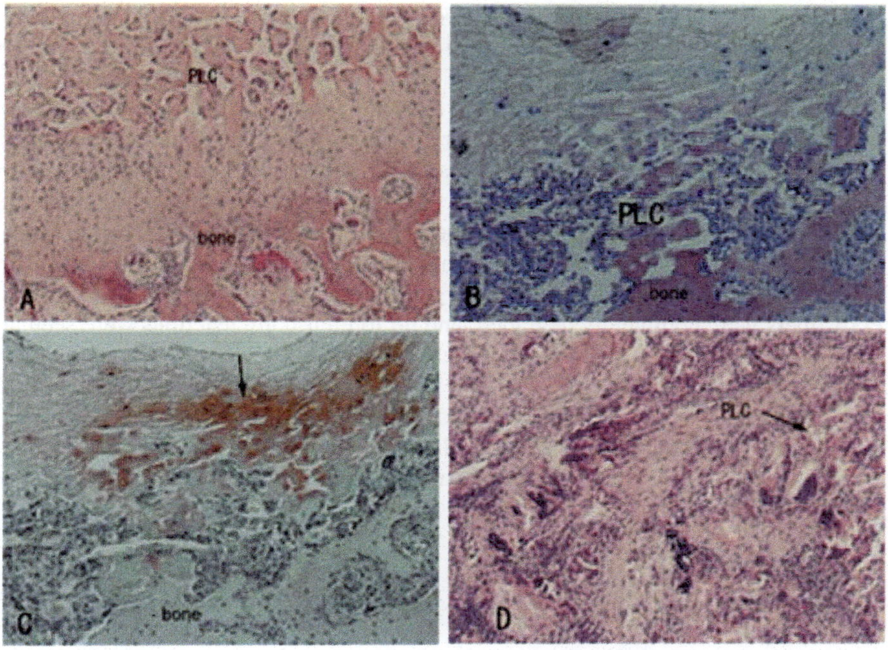

Fig. 10.6 Micrographs of specimens in PLC group. (**a**) At the PLC–bone interface at 4 weeks after the operation: *PLC* PLC scaffold, *bone* trabecular bone. Hematoxylin and eosin, ×100. (**b**) At the PLC–bone interface at 16 weeks: *PLC* PLC scaffold, *bone* trabecular bone. Hematoxylin and eosin, ×100. (**c**) At the PLC–bone interface at 16 weeks: *arrow* metachromasia indicating proteoglycan, *bone* trabecular bone. Safranin-O, ×100. (**d**) At the tendon proper at 16 weeks: *PLC* remaining PLC fibers. Hematoxylin and eosin, ×100. (From Yokoya et al. [50])

reaction were noted around the sheet. Although the conjunction area between the PLC fibers and trabecular bone was increased, the cell and fiber arrangement at the sites of tendon insertion was irregular. Some chondrocytes were scattered, and metachromasia was found around the chondrocytes on Safranin-O staining, thus indicating that the tissue contained proteoglycan. In the tendon proper, even at 4 and 16 weeks after surgery, the regenerated tendon-like tissue did not show good continuity between the PLC fibers and the proximal tendon edge, the border being quite clear, except for a small region. A few fibroblasts were found; however, they were highly scattered and many vessels were seen in the newly regenerated tendon at all time periods. Furthermore, significant foreign-body reactions were observed around the fiber areas at 8 and 16 weeks.

As to the PGA group, on a gross examination, the PGA sheets were covered with thick scar-like tissue on the implanted scaffold at 4 weeks after surgery. At 16 weeks, the PGA fibers were substituted with tendon-like scar tissue at the area of tendon insertion. A histological examination of the tissues in the PGA group 4 weeks after surgery revealed that the PGA fibers were partially degraded into small fragments, and extensive foreign-body reactions were detectable around the fragments of the PGA fibers. The tendon insertion site consisted of predominantly immature fibrous tissue aligned along the load axis (Fig. 10.7). At 8 weeks, most of the fibrous tissue was parallel to the long axis, although some direct collagen fibers were observed. At 16 weeks after surgery, tendon-to-bone healing was seen with the formation of continuous tissues, indicating the creation of parallel collagen fiber continuity between the tendon and bone with collagen fibers noted along the long axis. Fibrocartilage interface tissue stained with Safranin-O metachromasia, indicating the proteoglycan content, was partially found in smaller amounts than normal, although these amounts were larger than that seen in the PLC group. The PGA fibers were completely degraded, and no foreign-body reactions were seen at any sites at this time point. A histological examination of the tendon proper site 4 weeks after surgery revealed that the PGA-repaired areas exhibited a layer of inflammatory cells on the surface of the suture material. The volume, density, and crimp pattern of these bands appeared to increase gradually in both groups by 8 and 16 weeks. Some treated repair tissues at 16 weeks had densely packed, highly

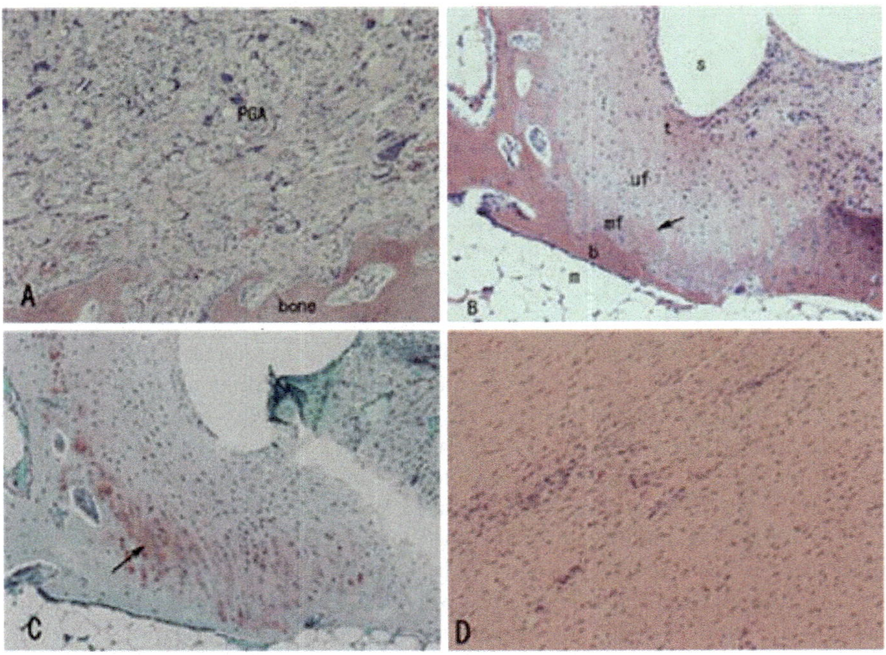

Fig. 10.7 Micrographs of specimens in PGA group. (**a**) At the PGA–bone interface at 4 weeks after the operation: *PGA* PGA fibers, *bone* trabecular bone. Hematoxylin and eosin, ×100. (**b**) At the PGA–bone interface at 16 weeks: *s* suture tract, *t* tendon, *uf* unmineralized fibrocartilage, *mf* mineralized fibrocartilage, *b* bone, *m* bone marrow, *arrow* tide mark. Hematoxylin and eosin, ×100. (**c**) At the PGA–bone interface at 16 weeks: *arrow* metachromasia indicating proteoglycan. Safranin-O, ×100. (**d**) At the PGA–tendon interface at 16 weeks. Hematoxylin and eosin, ×100. (From Yokoya et al. [50])

crimped fibers; these fibers were grouped in bundles along the axis of the tensile load.

Implants consisting of PGA sheets, a rapidly absorbable material, were used to replace completely resected infraspinatus tendon insertion sites in 33 adult Japanese white rabbits, and a well-arranged fibrocartilage layer was found at the regenerated tendon insertion sites; however, the sites of tendon insertion were mainly regenerated by type III collagen [51]. From the results of this experimental study, we concluded that the PGA sheet scaffold material allows for the regeneration of the tendon-to-tendon as well as the tendon-to-bone interface in an animal model. The PGA sheet is therefore a possible alternative scaffold material for tendon regeneration in cases of rotator cuff repair.

We hypothesized that it would be better to repair defects of the rotator cuff clinically according to the patch graft technique using a polyglycolic acid (PGA) sheet without sacrificing the autologous tissue, such as the fascia lata, and selecting a minimally invasive operative procedure, arthroscopic patch grafting.

Although some research has been reported regarding the regeneration of tendon insertion sites, these sites were regenerated with autologous tissues [52, 53], not artificial biomaterials. The tissue-engineering approach using biodegradable three-dimensional scaffolds offers more potential options for the treatment of severe tendon lesions. However, no studies have previously reported the regeneration of tendon insertion sites using artificial biomaterials [53–55]. Three-dimensional scaffolds should be biocompatible, highly porous, and biodegradable. The scaffold should permit cell invasion and easy attachment of cells and should provide an environment that is suitable for cell proliferation and differentiation. The cells must be allowed to secrete their own extracellular matrix components, promoting the formation of a tissue-like organization, while the scaffold itself tends to degrade as it synchronizes the organization of the extracellular matrix [56]. Polytetrafluoroethylene (PTFE), used as an artificial biomaterial for irreparable massive rotator cuff tears [7, 55], poly-L-lactate-epsilon-caprolactone (PLC), a synthetic scaffold possessing adequate flexibility, retractility, and a late absorbable speed [40, 41, 44], and polyglycolic acid (PGA), which shows relatively fast degradation and is the strongest absorbable monofilament available [45], are some of the most commonly used artificial biomaterials in experimental studies. Among them, PGA, which enhances cell–cell interactions at high cell densities and stimulates extracellular matrix production [12], appears to have the desired characteristics.

Tissue-engineering techniques using a biodegradable scaffold offer potential alternatives for recreating valid tendon-to-tendon and tendon-to-bone interfaces. In the present study, implants consisting of PGA sheets, a rapidly absorbable material, were used to replace completely resected infraspinatus tendon insertion sites in 33 adult Japanese white rabbits, and a well-arranged fibrocartilage layer was found at the regenerated tendon insertion sites. Based on the results of this experimental study, we concluded that the PGA sheet scaffold material allows for the regeneration of the tendon-to-tendon and tendon-to-bone interface in an animal model. PGA sheets are a possible alternative scaffold material for tendon regeneration in the setting of rotator cuff repair.

Based on these experimental data, we investigated the clinical results of arthroscopic PGA sheet patch grafts for irreparable rotator cuff tears. The results showed that the application of a patch graft with a PGA sheet, an artificial biomaterial, can improve the results of repair of irreparable rotator cuff tears in terms of postoperative pain control and short-term outcomes. The use of patches, either biological or artificial biomaterials, has been advocated to reduce the high-intensity rate, as supported by the rationale that collagenous scaffolds may improve tendon resiliency after repair, even if these materials are typically absorbed within a few weeks after implantation [57].

On the one hand, biological patches are mechanically weak [58] and rapidly resorbed upon implantation. On the other hand, biological patches provide a suitable environment for tissue repair [59, 60], whereas artificial biomaterials are biologically inert and thought to not provide the regenerative stimuli that support the healing process. Theoretically, the ideal patch for rotator cuff repair should combine the features of both biological and artificial biomaterial patches, serving as an inductive template to carry signals supporting tissue regeneration [60]. The quality of tendons has considerable limitations regarding torn rotator cuff tendons.

In an effort to augment the deficient rotator cuff tissue, and at the same time maintain the anatomic integrity of the shoulder, some surgeons incorporate biological tissue scaffolds into the cuff deficiency [61–64]. A porcine submucosa subintestinal graft, named Restore (DePuy, Warsaw, IN, USA), was found to increase pain and lead to poor tendon healing. Its clinical outcome in humans is in contrast to that seen in many preclinical animal studies, which suggests that the Restore graft may not be suitable for human rotator cuff repair [65].

The GraftJacket (Wright Medical Group, Memphis, TN, USA) is derived from the human dermis and is used as an interpositional graft in cases of massive and irreparable rotator cuff tears. Improvement in the UCLA (University of California Los Angeles) shoulder scores at the 2-year follow-up has been demonstrated. Furthermore, magnetic resonance has indicated tissue incorporation into the graft [66].

Synthetic scaffolds include polytetrafluoroethylene (PTFE) felts and polyester grafts. PTFE was found to improve pain scores in 30 patients with massive rotator cuff tears [63]. In particular, Teflon grafts (PTFE graft) provided satisfactory functional results and strength in 23 of 25 patients, again patients with massive rotator cuff tears, whereas Gore-Tex grafts (PTFE graft) improved the mean JOA score in 27 patients from 57.7 to 88.7 [66], and Dacron grafts (polyester) improved the Constant score in 15 of 17 patients. The Leeds–Keio graft (polyester) used in subscapular transposition augmentation shows superior clinical results to those obtained with augmentation grafts [64].

The chemical and physical properties of synthetic grafts can be controlled, although the trade-off is a lack of biocompatibility, which usually makes the graft nonabsorbable. In addition, a high rate of immune and inflammatory responses has been reported [67]. For these reasons, the PGA sheet may be an ideal patch, being absorbable and regenerative at this point. However, the satisfactory results reported here, as well as the extensive clinical experience and successful outcomes, prompt further studies.

The limitations of this study include the following: (1) the retrospective design, requiring further randomized prospective studies to ultimately assess the value of patch grafts in rotator cuff repair; (2) the lack of an a priori power analysis; and (3) the fact that no second-look arthroscopic surgeries or biopsies of the repair tissue were performed.

10.5 Conclusion

The 2-year clinical results of irreparable rotator cuff tears repair using arthroscopic patch grafts with a PGA sheet demonstrated an improved shoulder function and significantly lower high-intensity rate, compared with that observed in patients treated with a fascia lata patch. PGA sheets, an absorbable artificial biomaterial, may be an ideal patch, being absorbable and regenerative at this point.

The satisfactory results reported here, as well as the extensive clinical experience and successful outcomes, prompt further studies.

Conflicts of Interest The authors, their families, and any research foundations with which they are affiliated did not receive any financial payments or other benefits from any commercial entity related to the subject matter of this article.

Acknowledgments We are grateful to Brian Quinn for his critical reading of the manuscript.

References

1. Frankle M, Siegal S, Pupello D, Saleem A, Mighell M, Vasey M (2005) The reverse shoulder prosthesis for glenohumeral arthritis associated with severe rotator cuff deficiency: a minimum two-year follow-up study of sixty patients. J Bone Joint Surg Am 87:1697–1705
2. Celli L, Rovesta C, Marongiu MC, Manzieri S (1998) Transplantation of teres major muscle for infraspinatus muscle in irreparable rotator cuff tears. J Shoulder Elbow Surg 7:485–490
3. Gerber C (1992) Latissimus dorsi transfer for the treatment of irreparable tears of the rotator cuff. Clin Orthop Relat Res 275:152–160
4. Karas SE, Giachello TL (1996) Subscapularis transfer for reconstruction of massive tears of the rotator cuff. J Bone Joint Surg Am 78:239–245
5. Heikel HV (1968) Rupture of the rotator cuff of the shoulder: experiences of surgical treatment. Acta Orthop Scand 39:477–492
6. Ozaki J, Fujimoto S, Masuhara K, Tamai S, Yoshimoto S (1986) Reconstruction of chronic massive rotator cuff tears with synthetic materials. Clin Orthop Relat Res 202:173–183
7. Langer R, Vacanti JP (1993) Tissue engineering. Science 260:920–926
8. Awad HA, Butler DL, Harris MT et al (2000) In vitro characterization of mesenchymal stem cell-seeded collagen scaffolds for tendon repair: effects of initial seeding density on contraction kinetics. J Biomed Mater Res 51:233–240

9. Cao D, Liu W, Wei X, Xu F, Cui L, Cao Y (2006) In vitro tendon engineering with avian tenocytes and polyglycolic acids: a preliminary report. Tissue Eng 12:1369–1377
10. Awad HA, Butler DL, Boivin GP et al (1999) Autologous mesenchymal stem cell-mediated repair of tendon. Tissue Eng 5:267–277
11. Liu W, Chen B, Deng D, Xu F, Cui L, Cao Y (2006) Repair of tendon defect with dermal fibroblast engineered tendon in a porcine model. Tissue Eng 12:775–788
12. Lu L, Zhu X, Valenzuela RG, Currier BL, Yaszemski MJ (2001) Biodegradable polymer scaffolds for cartilage tissue engineering. Clin Orthop Relat Res 391:S251–S270
13. Kamath G, Galatz LM, Keener JD, Teefey S, Middleton W, Yamaguchi K (2009) Tendon integrity and functional outcome after arthroscopic repair of high-grade partial-thickness supraspinatus tears. J Bone Joint Surg Am 91:1055–1062
14. Nho SJ, Shindle MK, Adler RS, Warren RF, Altchek DW, MacGillivray JD (2009) Prospective analysis of arthroscopic rotator cuff repair: subgroup analysis. J Shoulder Elbow Surg 18:697–704
15. Verma NN, Bhatia S, Baker CL III et al (2010) Outcomes of arthroscopic rotator cuff repair in patients aged 70 years or older. Arthroscopy 26:1273–1280
16. Warrender WJ, Brown OL, Abboud JA (2011) Outcomes of arthroscopic rotator cuff repairs in obese patients. J Shoulder Elbow Surg 20:961–967
17. Boileau P, Brassart N, Watkinson DJ, Carles M, Hatzidakis AM, Krishnan SG (2005) Arthroscopic repair of full-thickness tears of the supraspinatus: does the tendon really heal? J Bone Joint Surg Am 87:1229–1240
18. Cole BJ, McCarty LP III, Kang RW, Alford W, Lewis PB, Hayden JK (2007) Arthroscopic rotator cuff repair: prospective functional outcome and repair integrity at minimum 2-year follow-up. J Shoulder Elbow Surg 16:579–585
19. Coleman SH, Fealy S, Ehteshami JR et al (2003) Chronic rotator cuff injury and repair model in sheep. J Bone Joint Surg Am 85:2391–2402
20. Galatz LM, Ball CM, Teefey SA, Middleton WD, Yamaguchi K (2004) The outcome and repair integrity of completely arthroscopically repaired large and massive rotator cuff tears. J Bone Joint Surg Am 86:219–224
21. Goutallier D, Postel JM, Lavau L, Bernageau J (1999) Impact of fatty degeneration of the supraspinatus and infraspinatus muscles on the prognosis of surgical repair of the rotator cuff. Rev Chir Orthop Reparatrice Appar Mot 85(7):668–676
22. Harryman DT 2nd, Mack LA, Wang KY, Jackins SE, Richardson ML, Matsen FA 3rd (1991) Repairs of the rotator cuff: correlation of functional results with integrity of the cuff. J Bone Joint Surg Am 73(7):982–989
23. Klepps S, Bishop J, Lin J et al (2004) Prospective evaluation of the effect of rotator cuff integrity on the outcome of open rotator cuff repairs. Am J Sports Med 32(7):1716–1722
24. Depalma AF, Callery G, Bennett GA (1949) Variational anatomy and degenerative lesions of the shoulder joint. Instr Course Lect 6:255–281
25. Codman EA (1938) Rupture of the supraspinatus. Am J Surg 42:603–606
26. Sher JS, Uribe JW, Posada A, Murphy BJ, Zlatkin MB (1995) Abnormal findings on magnetic resonance images of asymptomatic shoulders. J Bone Joint Surg Am 77:10–15
27. Tempelhof S, Rupp S, Seil R (1999) Age-related prevalence of rotator cuff tears in asymptomatic shoulders. J Shoulder Elbow Surg 8:296–299
28. Galatz LM, Ball CM, Teefey SA, Middleton WD, Yamaguchi K (2004) The outcome and repair integrity of completely arthroscopically repaired large and massive rotator cuff tears. J Bone Joint Surg Am 86-A(2):219–224
29. Nho SJ, Adler RS, Tomlinson DP et al (2009) Arthroscopic rotator cuff repair: prospective evaluation with sequential ultrasonography. Am J Sports Med 37(10):1938–1945
30. Gazielly DF, Gleyze P, Montagnon C (1994) Functional and anatomical results after rotator cuff repair. Clin Orthop Relat Res 304:43–53
31. Gerber C, Fuchs B, Hodler J (2000) The results of repair of massive tears of the rotator cuff. J Bone Joint Surg Am 82(4):505–515

32. Bedi A, Dines J, Warren RF, Dines DM (2010) Massive tears of the rotator cuff. J Bone Joint Surg Am 92(9):1894–1908
33. Gerber C, Wirth SH, Farshad M (2011) Treatment options for massive rotator cuff tears. J Shoulder Elbow Surg 20(2 suppl):S20–S29
34. Trappey GJ, Gartsman GM (2011) A systematic review of the clinical outcomes of single row versus double row rotator cuff repairs. J Shoulder Elbow Surg 20(2 suppl):S14–S19
35. Kim DH, Elattrache NS, Tibone JE et al (2006) Biomechanical comparison of a single-row versus double-row suture anchor technique for rotator cuff repair. Am J Sports Med 34 (3):407–414
36. Park MC, Cadet ER, Levine WN, Bigliani LU, Ahmad CS (2005) Tendon-to-bone pressure distributions at a repaired rotator cuff footprint using transosseous suture and suture anchor fixation techniques. Am J Sports Med 33(8):1154–1159
37. Sano H, Yamashita T, Wakabayashi I, Itoi E (2007) Stress distribution in the supraspinatus tendon after tendon repair: suture anchors versus transosseous suture fixation. Am J Sports Med 35(4):542–546
38. Bishop J, Klepps S, Lo IK, Bird J, Gladstone JN, Flatow EL (2006) Cuff integrity after arthroscopic versus open rotator cuff repair: a prospective study. J Shoulder Elbow Surg 15 (3):290–299
39. Yamada K, Miyamoto S, Takayama M et al (2002) Clinical application of a new bioabsorbable artificial dura mater. J Neurosurg 96:731–735
40. Jeong SI, Kim BS, Kang SW et al (2004) In vivo biocompatibility and degradation behavior of elastic poly(L-lactide-co-epsilon-caprolactone) scaffolds. Biomaterials 25:5939–5946
41. Shin'oka T, Matsumura G, Hibino N et al (2005) Midterm clinical result of tissue-engineered vascular autografts seeded with autologous bone marrow cells. J Thorac Cardiovasc Surg 129:1330–1338
42. Rodkey WG, Cabaud HE, Feagin JA, Perlik PC (1985) A partially biodegradable material device for repair and reconstruction of injured tendons: experimental studies. Am J Sports Med 13:242–247
43. Honda M, Morikawa N, Hata K et al (2003) Rat costochondral cell characteristics on poly(L-lactide-co-epsilon-caprolactone) scaffolds. Biomaterials 24:3511–3519
44. Bourne RB, Bitar H, Andreae PR, Martin LM, Finlay JB, Marquis F (1988) In vivo comparison of four absorbable sutures: Vicryl, Dexon Plus, Maxon, and PDS. Can J Surg 31:43–45
45. Grimmer JF, Gunnlaugsson CB, Alsberg E et al (2004) Tracheal reconstruction using tissue-engineered cartilage. Arch Otolaryngol Head Neck Surg 130:1191–1196
46. Kang SW, Son SM, Lee JS et al (2006) Regeneration of whole meniscus using meniscal cells and polymer scaffolds in a rabbit total meniscectomy model. J Biomed Mater Res A 78:659–671
47. Mahmoudifar N, Doran PM (2006) Effect of seeding and bioreactor culture conditions on the development of human tissue-engineered cartilage. Tissue Eng 12:1675–1685
48. Mizuno H, Roy AK, Zaporojan V, Vacanti CA, Ueda M, Bonassar LJ (2006) Biomechanical and biochemical characterization of composite tissue-engineered intervertebral disks. Biomaterials 27(3):362–370
49. Terada S, Yoshimoto H, Fuchs JR et al (2005) Hydrogel optimization for cultured elastic chondrocytes seeded onto a polyglycolic acid scaffold. J Biomed Mater Res A 75:907–916
50. Yokoya S, Yu M, Nagata Y, Deie M, Ochi M (2008) Tendon–bone insertion repair and regeneration using polyglycolic acid sheet in the rabbit rotator cuff injury model. Am J Sports Med 36:1298–1309
51. Ouyang HW, Goh JC, Lee FH (2004) Use of bone marrow stromal cells for tendon graft-to-bone healing: histological and immunohistochemical studies in a rabbit model. Am J Sports Med 32:321–327
52. Sano H, Kumagai J, Sawai T (2002) Experimental fascial autografting for the supraspinatus tendon defect: remodeling process of the grafted fascia and the insertion into bone. J Shoulder Elbow Surg 11:166–173

53. Dejardin LM, Arnoczky SP, Ewers BJ, Haut RC, Clarke RB (2001) Tissue-engineered rotator cuff tendon using porcine small intestine submucosa: histologic and mechanical evaluation in dogs. Am J Sports Med 29:175–184
54. Funakoshi T, Majima T, Iwasaki N et al (2005) Application of tissue engineering techniques for rotator cuff regeneration using a chitosan-based hyaluronan hybrid fiber scaffold. Am J Sports Med 33:1193–1201
55. Kimura A, Aoki M, Fukushima S, Ishii S, Yamakoshi K (2003) Reconstruction of a defect of the rotator cuff with polytetrafluoroethylene felt graft: recovery of tensile strength and histocompatibility in an animal model. J Bone Joint Surg Br 85:282–287
56. Hokugo A, Takamoto T, Tabata Y (2006) Preparation of hybrid scaffold from fibrin and biodegradable polymer fiber. Biomaterials 27:61–67
57. Badylak SF, Tullius R, Kokini K et al (1995) The use of xenogeneic small intestinal submucosa as a biomaterial for Achilles tendon repair in a dog model. J Biomed Mater Res 29 (8):977–985
58. Badylak S, Kokini K, Tullius B, Whitson B (2001) Strength over time of a resorbable bioscaffold for body wall repair in a dog model. J Surg Res 99(2):282–287
59. Beattie AJ, Gilbert TW, Guyot JP, Yates AJ, Badylak SF (2009) Chemoattraction of progenitor cells by remodeling extracellular matrix scaffolds. Tissue Eng Part A 15(5):1119–1125
60. Derwin KA, Badylak SF, Steinmann SP, Iannotti JP (2010) Extracellular matrix scaffold devices for rotator cuff repair. J Shoulder Elbow Surg 19(3):467–476
61. Rhee YG, Cho NS, Lim CT, Yi JW, Vishvanathan T (2008) Bridging the gap in immobile massive rotator cuff tears: augmentation using the tenotomized biceps. Am J Sports Med 36:1511–1518
62. Wong I, Burns J, Snyder S (2010) Arthroscopic GraftJacket repair of rotator cuff tears. J Shoulder Elbow Surg 19(Suppl):104–109
63. Kimura A, Okamura K, Fukushima S, Ishii S, Aoki M (2000) Clinical results of rotator cuff reconstruction with PTFE felt augmentation for irreparable massive rotator cuff tears. Shoulder Joint 24:485–488
64. Nada AN, Debnath UK, Robinson DA, Jordan C (2010) Treatment of massive rotator-cuff tears with a polyester ligament (Dacron) augmentation: clinical outcome. J Bone Joint Surg Br 92:1397–1402
65. Cho NS, Yi JW, Rhee YG (2009) Arthroscopic biceps augmentation for avoiding undue tension in repair of massive rotator cuff tears. Arthroscopy 25:183–191
66. Hirooka A, Yoneda M, Wakaitani S et al (2002) Augmentation with a Gore-Tex patch for repair of large rotator cuff tears that cannot be sutured. J Orthop Sci 7:451–456
67. Chen J, Xu J, Wang A, Zheng M (2009) Scaffolds for tendon and ligament repair: review of the efficacy of commercial products. Expert Rev Med Devices 6:61–73

Chapter 11
Superior Capsule Reconstruction for Irreparable Rotator Cuff Tears

Teruhisa Mihata

Abstract In 2007 we developed a superior capsule reconstruction for treating irreparable rotator cuff tears. This technique can restore shoulder function with pain relief and low complication rates (re-tear 7/180, 4 %; infection 2/180, 1.1 %; severe synovitis 3/180, 1.7 %; severe stiffness 3/180, 1.7 %). The presence of indications for this surgery is determined by preoperative MRI. Goutallier grades 3 and 4 (fatty infiltration equal to, or more than, muscle volume) are absolute indications. If the torn tendon is severely atrophied, degenerated, and thin in Goutallier grade 2, we recommend superior capsule reconstruction. During arthroscopy, the torn tendon is examined quality and mobility. If it cannot be made to reach the original footprint (i.e., it is an irreducible tear), a preoperative decision is made for superior capsule reconstruction. If the tendon can reach the original footprint after mobilization (i.e., it is a reducible tear), superior capsule reconstruction followed by rotator cuff repair over the reconstructed superior capsule is chosen. Factors prognostic of clinical outcome are the degree of graft healing and the level of deltoid function. Re-tear of the graft of the repaired infraspinatus tendon causes shoulder pain or decreased active elevation. In some patients, concomitant cervical spinal palsy worsens after surgery, resulting in poor shoulder function despite graft healing.

Keywords Irreparable • Reconstruction • Rotator cuff • Shoulder • Superior capsule

---

T. Mihata (✉)
Department of Orthopedic Surgery, Osaka Medical College, 2-7 Daigaku-machi, Takatsuki, Osaka 569-8686, Japan

Orthopaedic Biomechanics Laboratory, Long Beach VA Healthcare System and University of California, Irvine, CA, USA

First Towakai Hospital, Takatsuki, Osaka, Japan

Katsuragi Hospital, Kishiwada, Osaka, Japan
e-mail: tmihata@yahoo.co.jp; tmihata@osaka-med.ac.jp

K. Tamai et al. (eds.), *Advances in Shoulder Surgery*,
DOI 10.1007/978-4-431-55988-7_11

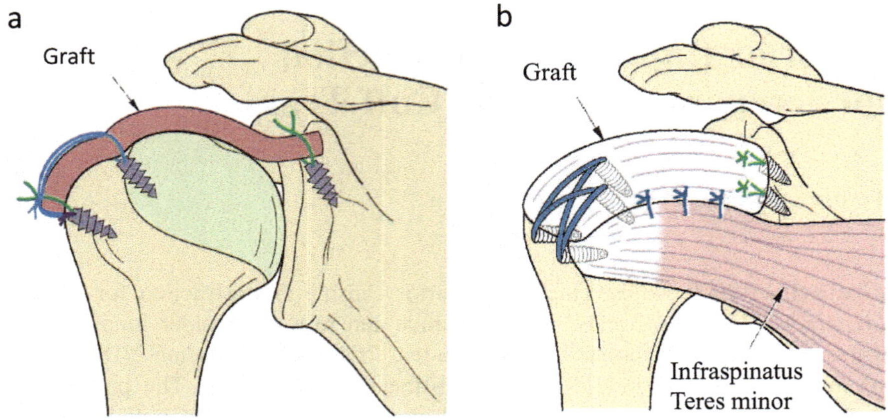

Fig. 11.1 Superior capsule reconstruction. We have developed a method of superior capsule reconstruction as a surgical treatment for irreparable rotator cuff tears. The graft is attached medially to the superior glenoid and laterally to the greater tuberosity. This is followed by side-to-side suturing between the graft and the infraspinatus or teres minor tendon. (**a**) Compression double-row repair technique. (**b**) SpeedBridge repair technique (Arthrex). (**a** from Mihata [7]; **b** from Mihata [8])

11.1 History, Outcomes, and Biomechanics

In 2007 we developed superior capsule reconstruction for the treatment of irreparable rotator cuff tears [1] (Fig. 11.1). The number of these procedures increased in our hospitals between 2007 and 2014, because superior capsule reconstruction can restore shoulder function with pain relief and a low rate of complications (re-tear 7/180, 4 %; infection 2/180, 1.1 %; severe synovitis 3/180, 1.7 %; severe stiffness 3/180, 1.7 %).

The clinical outcomes of the first 24 shoulders in 23 consecutive patients with irreparable rotator cuff tears (11 large tears, 13 massive tears) that underwent arthroscopic superior capsule reconstruction (ASCR) were first reported in 2013 [1]. Mean active elevation increased significantly from 84 to 148° ($P < 0.001$) and external rotation increased from 26 to 40° ($P < 0.01$). Acromiohumeral distance increased from 4.6 mm preoperatively to 8.7 mm postoperatively ($P < 0.0001$). Twenty patients (83.3 %) had no graft tear or no tendon re-tear during follow-up (24–51 months) (Fig. 11.2). The mean American Shoulder and Elbow Surgeons score improved from 23.5 to 92.9 points ($P < 0.0001$).

The biomechanical role of superior capsule reconstruction has been confirmed by a cadaveric study [2]. In that study, superior translation and subacromial contact pressure were significantly greater in simulated irreparable rotator cuff tears than in the intact condition (normal rotator cuff). After superior capsule reconstruction using a fascia lata allograft, superior translation and subacromial contact pressure were completely normalized to the intact level. Side-to-side sutures between the graft and residual rotator cuff tendons may improve force coupling in the shoulder

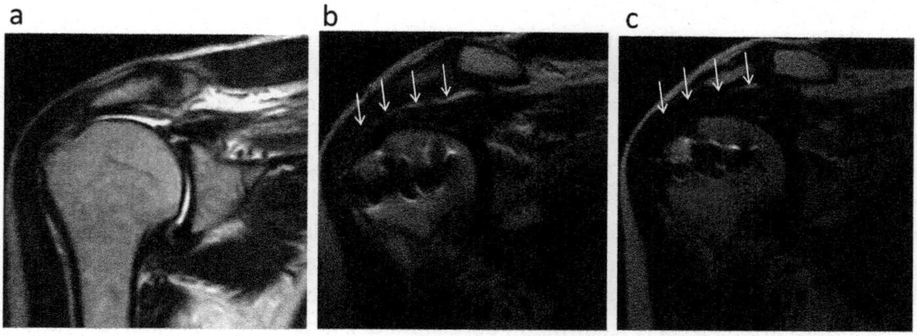

Fig. 11.2 MRI findings before and after superior capsule reconstruction. (**a**) Before surgery. The torn supraspinatus tendon was severely retracted, and the supraspinatus muscle was severely atrophied and infiltrated with fat. (**b**) One year after surgery. (**c**) Four years after surgery. The reconstructed superior capsule has become thicker (*white arrows*)

joint. Restoration of shoulder stability after superior capsule reconstruction improves deltoid function, resulting in increased active shoulder range of motion (especially elevation).

11.2 Indications and Prognostic Factors

Patient suitability for superior capsule reconstruction is determined by preoperative MRI. Goutallier grades 3 and 4 (fatty infiltration equal to, or more than, muscle volume) are absolute indications [3]. If the torn tendon is severely retracted, degenerated, and thin in Goutallier grade 2, we recommend superior capsule reconstruction.

The stage of osteoarthritis before surgery is classified by using the Hamada grade [4]. In this system, grade 1 is associated with minimal radiographic changes; grade 2 is characterized by narrowing of the subacromial space to less than 6 mm; grade 3 is defined as erosion and so-called acetabulization of the acromion caused by superior migration of the humeral head; grade 4 is associated with glenohumeral arthritis; and grade 5 is characterized by the presence of humeral head osteonecrosis. Irreparable rotator cuff tears with Hamada grades 1–3 are an absolute indication for ASCR. Whereas young patients with Hamada grade 4 are recommended for ASCR, elderly patients with Hamada grade 4 and all patients with Hamada grade 5 should have total shoulder arthroplasty with open surgical superior capsule reconstruction.

During arthroscopy, the torn tendon is examined for quality and mobility. If the torn tendon cannot be made to reach the original footprint (i.e., the tear is irreducible), a preoperative decision is made to perform superior capsule reconstruction alone. If the torn tendon can reach the original footprint after mobilization (i.e., the tear is reducible), superior capsule reconstruction followed by rotator cuff repair over the reconstructed superior capsule is chosen.

The factors prognostic of clinical outcome in superior capsule reconstruction are the degree of graft healing and the level of deltoid function. Re-tear of the graft of the repaired infraspinatus tendon causes shoulder pain or decreased active elevation. Some patients with irreparable rotator cuff tears have concomitant cervical spinal palsy. When patients already have severe deltoid atrophy and weakness from concomitant cervical spinal palsy, we do not recommend superior capsule reconstruction. However, we sometimes do superior capsule reconstructions in patients with slight or moderate deltoid weakness. In some patients the cervical spinal palsy deteriorates after surgery, resulting in poor shoulder function even when the graft is healed.

11.3 Surgical Technique

11.3.1 Measurement of Defect Size

Subacromial bursal tissue around the torn tendons is completely removed before measurement of the defect size. Degenerated (e.g., thin and weak) tendon tissue is also removed, because postoperative tear of the degenerated rotator cuff tendon worsens the postoperative outcome even when the reconstructed superior capsule remains intact. The defect size is then measured in the mediolateral (from the superior glenoid to the lateral edge of the greater tuberosity) and anteroposterior (from the anterior edge to the posterior edge of the torn tendon) directions (Fig. 11.3).

11.3.2 Deciding on Graft Size

Deciding on the correct graft size is the most important step in this surgery. If the graft is torn after surgery because it is too small, the clinical results will be poor.

11.3.2.1 Length in the Anteroposterior Direction

The anteroposterior length of the defect is measured without partial repair of the infraspinatus tendon. In our early cases, we performed a partial repair of the infraspinatus tendon before superior capsule reconstruction. However, we experienced postoperative re-tear of the repaired infraspinatus tendon even when the fascia lata graft had not been torn. The clinical results in such cases of partial re-tear are acceptable (approximately 50–70 % of the recovery achieved in cases

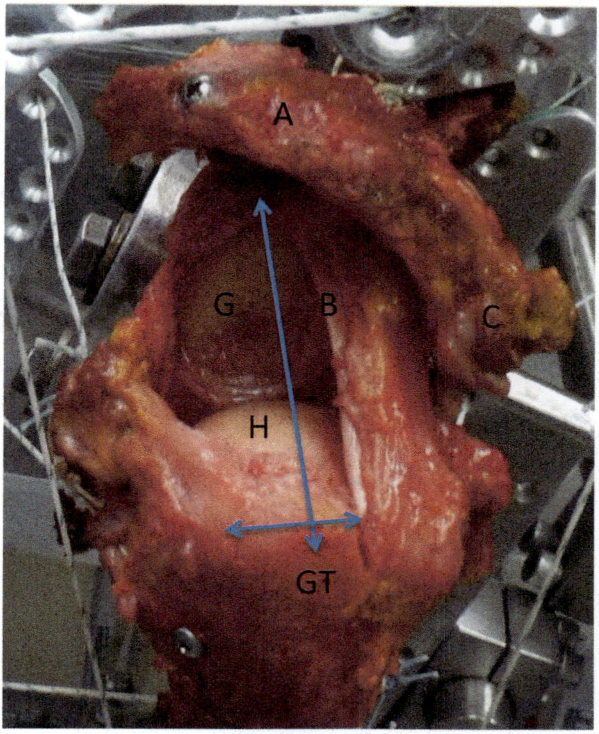

Fig. 11.3 Measurement of defect size. The size of the defect is measured in the mediolateral (from the superior glenoid to the lateral edge of the greater tuberosity) and anteroposterior (from the anterior edge to the posterior edge of the torn tendon) directions. *A* acromion, *B* biceps long head tendon, *C* coracoid process, *G* glenoid, *GT* greater tuberosity, *H* humeral head

where there is no re-tear) but not excellent. For this reason, we now omit the partial repair before measurement. Afterward, the graft length in the anteroposterior direction was determined to be exactly the same as the length of the defect without partial repair of the torn infraspinatus tendon.

11.3.2.2 Length in the Mediolateral Direction

To make a 10-mm footprint on the superior glenoid and allow for 5 mm of latitude in graft size, in the mediolateral direction the graft should be 15 mm longer than the distance from the superior glenoid to the lateral edge of the greater tuberosity. A graft that is too short, especially in the mediolateral direction, will re-tear, resulting in a poor clinical outcome.

11.3.2.3 Graft Thickness

The appropriate graft thickness for superior capsule reconstruction using the fascia lata is 6–8 mm. The average thickness of one layer of autologous fascia lata is

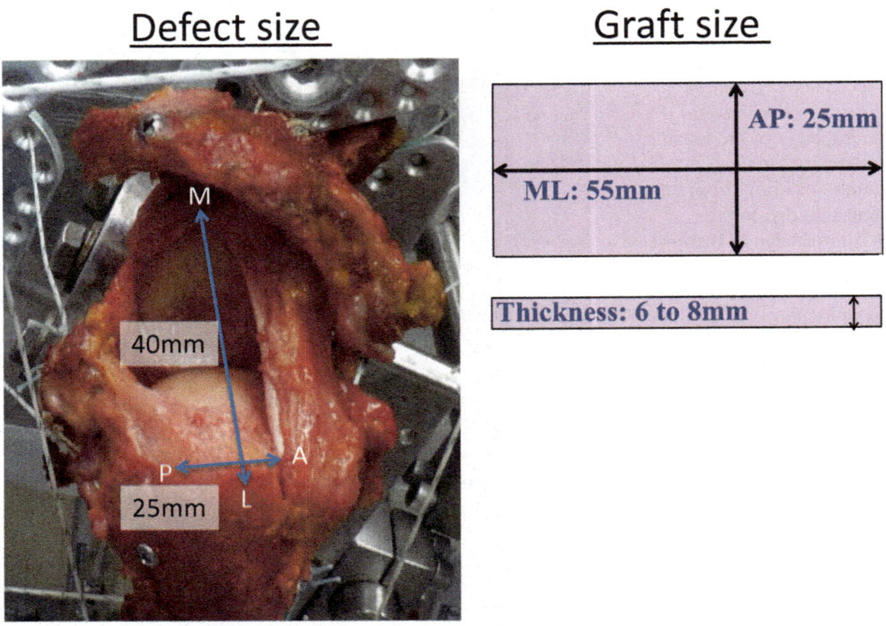

Fig. 11.4 Example. If the defect size is 25 mm anteroposteriorly and 40 mm mediolaterally, the graft should be 25 mm anteroposteriorly, 55 mm (40 + 15 mm) mediolaterally, and 6–8 mm thick

2–4 mm. Therefore, a graft thickness of 6–8 mm is achieved by folding the fascia lata twice or three times. If a fascia lata allograft is used for superior capsule reconstruction, approximately six to eight layers of fascia lata may be needed to give a graft 6–8 mm thick, because the allograft is thinner than an autograft.

11.3.2.4 Example

If the defect is 25 mm anteroposteriorly and 40 mm mediolaterally, the graft should be 25 mm in the anteroposterior direction, 55 mm (40 + 15 mm) in the mediolateral direction, and 6–8 mm thick (Fig. 11.4).

11.3.3 Harvesting the Fascia Lata and Making the Autograft

Fascia lata is harvested around the greater trochanter, taking care to include the posterior, thicker tissue. All fatty tissue should be removed from the graft (Figs. 11.5 and 11.6). The layers of fascia lata are united with nonabsorbable sutures very well to prevent delamination after surgery.

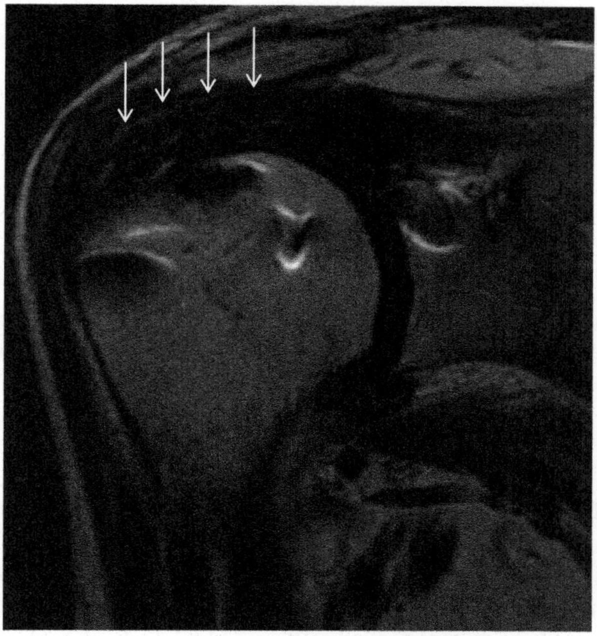

Fig. 11.5 Magnetic resonance imaging (MRI) findings 3 months after superior capsule reconstruction. When all fatty tissue on the graft was removed, T_2-weighted MRI showed that the graft area was of low intensity (*white arrows*)

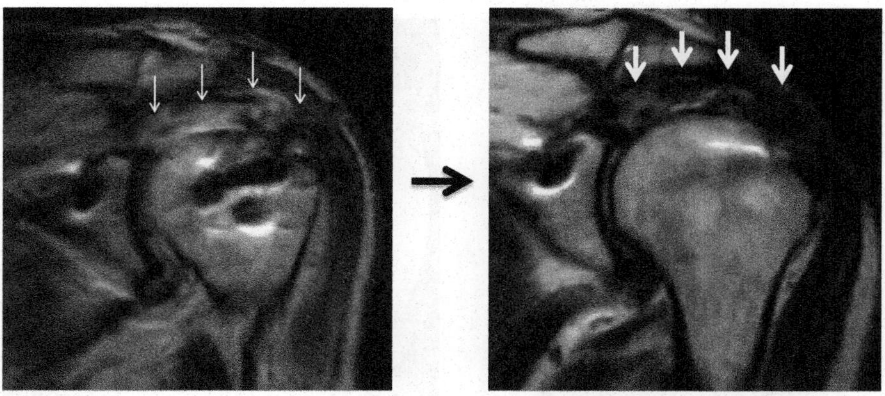

Fig. 11.6 MRI findings after superior capsule reconstruction. *Left:* When some of the fatty tissue was not removed during surgery, T_2-weighted MRI 3 months after surgery showed both low- and high-intensity areas in the graft (*white thin arrows*). *Right*: 1 year after surgery, the graft (*white thick arrows*) was thicker and the low-intensity area had increased on T_2-weighted MRI

11.3.4 Treatment of Associated Lesions

Subscapularis tears should be repaired. Biceps tenodesis or tenotomy is performed for biceps subluxation or dislocation.

11.3.5 Acromioplasty

Acromial spurs on the anterior, lateral, or medial side should be resected. The inferior surface of the acromion (to a thickness of 2 or 3 mm) should be resected to prevent subacromial impingement after surgery.

11.3.6 Anchor Placement on the Superior Glenoid

All soft tissue on the footprint of the superior glenoid should be removed to give a good bone bed before insertion of the suture anchors. Two 4.5-mm Corkscrew FT (Arthrex) anchors are inserted at the 10- or 11-o'clock and 11- or 12-o'clock positions on the glenoid of the right shoulder, and at the 12- or 1-o'clock and 1- or 2-o'clock positions of the left shoulder (Fig. 11.7).

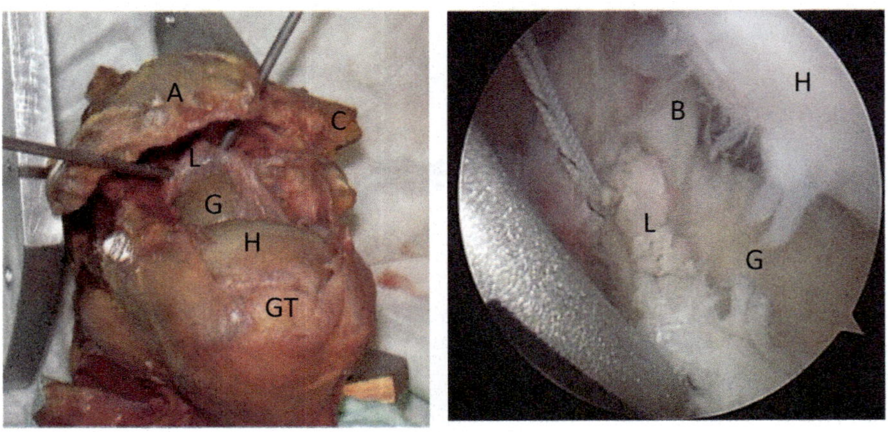

Fig. 11.7 Anchor placement on the superior glenoid. Two 4.5-mm Corkscrew FT (Arthrex) anchors are inserted at the 10 or 11-o'clock and 11 or 12-o'clock positions on the glenoid of the right shoulder. *Left:* cadaveric shoulder; *right*: posterior view of shoulder arthroscopy. *A* acromion, *B* biceps long head tendon, *C* coracoid process, *G* glenoid, *GT* greater tuberosity, *H* humeral head, *L* labrum

11.3.7 Anchor Placement on the Medial Footprint

All soft tissue on the footprint of the greater tuberosity should be removed. Two 4.75-mm SwiveLock (Arthrex) anchors with FiberTape (Arthrex) are inserted on the medial footprint of the greater tuberosity to make a SpeedBridge (Arthrex) (Fig. 11.1). When we fix the graft on the greater tuberosity using compression double-row repair technique, two 4.5-mm Corkscrew FT (Arthrex) anchors are inserted on the medial footprint (Figs. 11.1 and 11.9) [5, 6].

11.3.8 Insertion of Fascia Lata into the Subacromial Space

A 10-ml syringe is used as a cannula. Fiberwires (Arthrex) from the superior glenoid suture anchors are placed through the fascia lata in a mattress fashion when the graft is still outside the body (Fig. 11.8). After all Fiberwires have been placed through the fascia lata, one Fiberwire is tied while the graft is pushed into the subacromial space. The graft can then be inserted in its appropriate place on the glenoid. All sutures are then tied in the subacromial space.

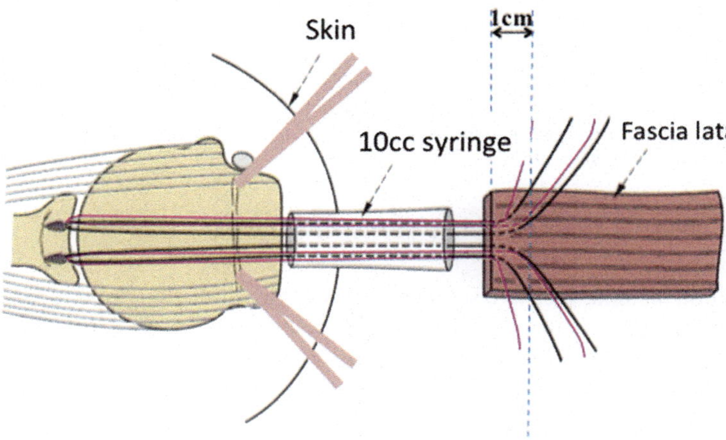

Fig. 11.8 Insertion of fascia lata into the subacromial space. A 10-ml syringe is used as a cannula. Fiberwires (Arthrex) from the superior glenoid suture anchors are placed through the fascia lata in a mattress fashion when the graft is still outside the body. After all Fiberwires have been placed through the fascia lata; one Fiberwire is tied while the graft is pushed into the subacromial space. The graft can then be inserted into its appropriate place on the glenoid. All sutures are tied in the subacromial space. (From Mihata [7])

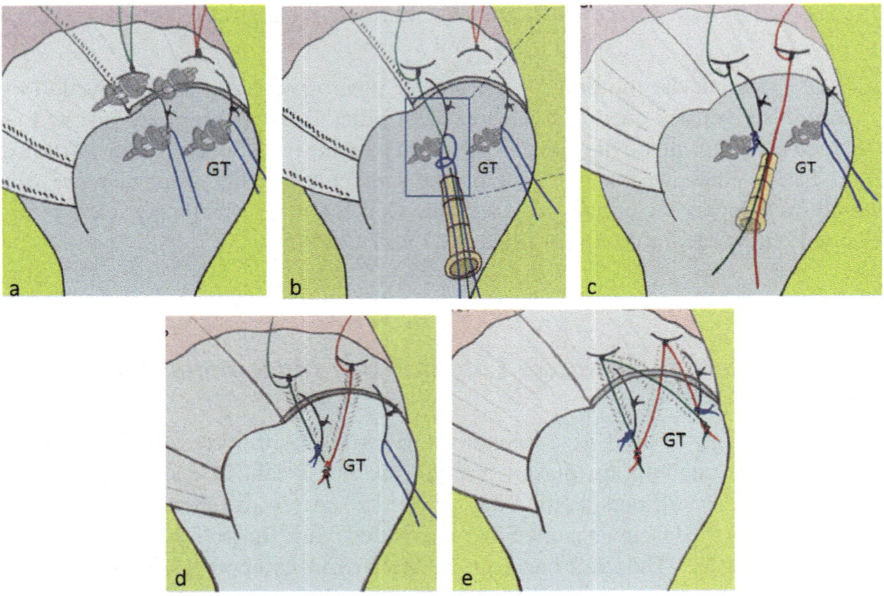

Fig. 11.9 The compression double-row repair technique (combination of the double-row and suture-bridge technique). (**a**) First, the conventional double-row repair is performed. After the knots were tied for the conventional double-row repair, the medial sutures were not cut because the suture limbs would be used to create suture bridges over the tendon. (**b**) The lateral suture is tied around the medial limb to create a loop for the suture bridge. (**c**, **d**) A suture limb from another medial suture is tied to the first medial suture limb with a nonsliding knot, which is called the "rotator cuff knot," thereby yielding two suture bridges from two medial suture limbs and the loop from both limbs of a single lateral suture. (**e**) The remaining medial suture limbs are then tied through loops of the lateral suture in the same procedure used for the first suture bridge. *GT* greater tuberosity. (From Mihata et al. [6])

11.3.9 Attachment to the Greater Tuberosity

Any fixation method, such as a suture bridge, double row, or single row, can be used to attach the graft to the greater tuberosity. My preference is the compression double-row repair [5, 6], which is one of the most secure fixations (Figs. 11.1 and 11.9), or SpeedBridge (Arthrex), which provides easy and secure fixation of the graft (Fig. 11.1).

11.3.10 Side-to-Side Suturing Between the Graft and the Infraspinatus Tendon or Teres Minor

Two or three sutures for posterior side-to-side suturing are placed between the graft and the infraspinatus tendon or teres minor (Fig. 11.1). Side-to-side suturing both anteriorly and posteriorly may cause postoperative shoulder stiffness, so it is best not to add anterior sutures in superior capsule reconstruction using fascia lata.

11.4 Postoperative Protocol

An abduction brace is used for 4 weeks after superior capsule reconstruction. After the immobilization period, passive and active-assisted exercises are initiated to promote scaption (scapular plane elevation). Eight weeks after surgery, patients begin to perform exercises to strengthen the rotator cuff and the scapular stabilizers. Physical therapists have assisted all our patients.

References

1. Mihata T, Lee TQ, Watanabe C, Fukunishi K, Ohue M, Tsujimura T, Kinoshita M (2013) Clinical results of arthroscopic superior capsule reconstruction for irreparable rotator cuff tears. Arthroscopy 29(3):459–470. doi:10.1016/j.arthro.2012.10.022,S0749-8063(12)01789-6 [pii]
2. Mihata T, McGarry MH, Pirolo JM, Kinoshita M, Lee TQ (2012) Superior capsule reconstruction to restore superior stability in irreparable rotator cuff tears: a biomechanical cadaveric study. Am J Sports Med 40(10):2248–2255, 0363546512456195 [pii] 10.1177/0363546512456195
3. Goutallier D, Postel JM, Bernageau J, Lavau L, Voisin MC (1994) Fatty muscle degeneration in cuff ruptures. Pre- and postoperative evaluation by CT scan. Clin Orthop Relat Res 304:78–83
4. Hamada K, Fukuda H, Mikasa M, Kobayashi Y (1990) Roentgenographic findings in massive rotator cuff tears. A long-term observation. Clin Orthop Relat Res 254:92–96
5. Mihata T, Fukuhara T, Jun BJ, Watanabe C, Kinoshita M (2011) Effect of shoulder abduction angle on biomechanical properties of the repaired rotator cuff tendons with 3 types of double-row technique. Am J Sports Med 39(3):551–556
6. Mihata T, Watanabe C, Fukunishi K, Ohue M, Tsujimura T, Fujiwara K, Kinoshita M (2011) Functional and structural outcomes of single-row versus double-row versus combined double-row and suture-bridge repair for rotator cuff tears. Am J Sports Med 39(10):2091–2098. doi:10.1177/0363546511415660 0363546511415660[pii]
7. Mihata T (2012) New surgical treatment for the massive rotator cuff tears: superior capsule reconstruction. J MIOS 63:43–49
8. Mihata T (2014) Superior capsule reconstruction for massive rotator cuff tears. Orthopaedics 27 (5):51–55

Chapter 12
Tendon Transfer for Massive Rotator Cuff Tear

Naoki Suenaga, Naomi Oizumi, Hiroshi Yamaguchi, Tomoya Matsuhashi, and Noboru Taniguchi

Abstract Tendon transfer is one of the useful procedures in patients with massive rotator cuff tears with or without arthritis of shoulder joint. When the case with tearing of two tendons of the rotator cuff has hypertrophied teres minor and subscapularis muscles without arthritis of the shoulder joint, partial subscapularis transfer, as reported by Cofield, would be a useful technique. If a case having tearing of three tendons of the rotator cuff has only hypertrophied teres minor muscle without arthritis of the shoulder joint, pectoralis major transfer underneath the conjoined tendon could obtain a good outcome. Cases with tears of three tendons of the rotator cuff having only hypertrophied subscapularis muscle, the so-called posterosuperior tear of the rotator cuff, without arthritis of the shoulder joint, need latissimus dorsi and teres major transfer. Furthermore, it is necessary to replace the humeral head by shoulder arthroplasty with using a smaller size of humeral head prosthesis in patients with shoulder arthropathy because of the reduced size of the original humeral head. In this chapter, Dr. Oizumi describes the so-called Cofield procedure, such as a partial subscapularis transfer, Dr. Yamaguchi explains the technique of pectoralis major muscle transfer, and Dr. Matsuhashi introduces the so-called Paavoleinen technique and the latissimus dorsi and teres major transfer from anterior approach. Finally, Dr. Taniguchi described the concept and technique of a smaller humeral head replacement with cuff reconstruction using muscle transfer in patients with cuff tear arthropathy.

N. Suenaga (✉) • N. Oizumi
The Upper Extremity Center of Joint Replacement and Endoscopic Surgery, Hokushin Orthopedic Hospital, 3 jou 3 chome, Kikusuimotomachi, Shiroishi-ku, Sapporo, Hokkaido 080-8638, Japan
e-mail: naokisuenaga@yahoo.co.jp

H. Yamaguchi
Rehabilitation Clinic Yamaguchi, Okinawa, Japan

T. Matsuhashi
Department of Orthopaedic Surgery, NTT East Sapporo Hospital, Hokkaido, Japan

N. Taniguchi
Department of Orthopaedic Surgery, University of Miyazaki, Miyazaki, Japan

K. Tamai et al. (eds.), *Advances in Shoulder Surgery*,
DOI 10.1007/978-4-431-55988-7_12

Keywords Rotator cuff • Irreparable rotator cuff tears • Muscle transfer • Humeral head replacement • Pectoralis major muscle transfer • Massive rotator cuff tear • Teres minor transfer • Cuff tear arthropathy

12.1 Partial Transfer of Subscapularis for Irreparable Massive Rotator Cuff Tear

12.1.1 Introduction

The transfer of the subscapularis (SSC) tendon in patients with irreparable massive rotator cuff tear was first reported by Cofield [1] in 1982. In his procedure, all of the SSC tendon was transferred to the defect of the supraspinatus (SSP) and infraspinatus (ISP) tendons in 26 cases including 13 cases with shoulder arthroplasty. In his series, pain decreased in 22 cases and shoulder abduction of 123°–130° was obtained. Following Cofield's report, Bigliani et al. [2] reported 11 cases of transfer of the upper one third of the SSC tendon to the defect of the SSP tendon. Karas et al. [3] reported 20 cases of the transfer of the upper one half to two thirds of the SSC tendon to the defect of the SSP and ISP tendons. Karas called attention to the fact that elevation decreased in some cases, although overall outcome was good (pain decreased in 19 cases; postoperative abduction was 152°). From the biomechanical point of view, Nakajima [4] reported a cadaver study of simulation of the transfer site of SSC tendon, with the result that transfer to the lateral and anterior part of the SSP defect maximizes the moment arm of the transferred tendon at abduction and that transfer of the upper 70 % of the SSC tendon was recommended. Based on these previous studies, the authors have performed partial transfer of subscapularis tendon for irreparable massive rotator cuff tears since 2009. Indication, surgical procedure, postoperative rehabilitation, and clinical outcomes of our procedure are introduced in this section.

12.1.2 Indication

Irreparable tear of supraspinatus (SSP) and infraspinatus (ISP) tendons with intact subscapularis (SSC) and teres minor (TM) is a good indication for this procedure (Fig. 12.1). In cases in which the TM tendon is not effective, which is usually predictable with lag of external rotation (discrepancy between active and passive external rotation), additional reconstruction of the posterior cuff defect, such as transfer of latissimus dorsi, should be considered.

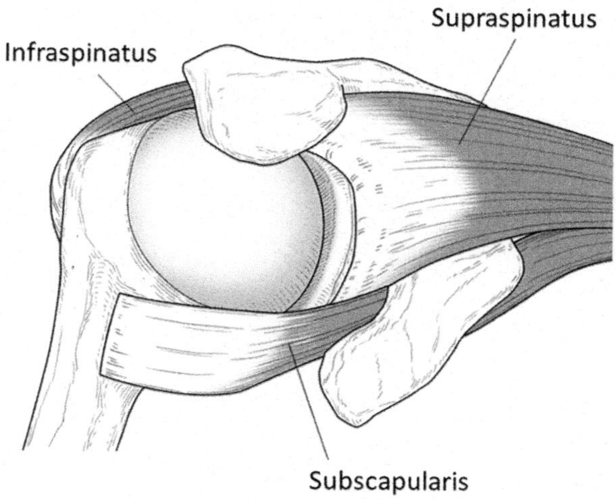

Fig. 12.1 Massive rotator cuff tear for partial subscapularis (SSC) tendon transfer. Supraspinatus (SSP) and infraspinatus (ISP) tendons are torn and medially retracted; SSC and teres minor (TM) tendons are intact

12.1.3 Surgical Procedure

The surgery is performed in a beach-chair position under general anesthesia with interscalene block.

Superior approach is used for this procedure. When sufficient exposure of the SSC is not obtained with the superior approach, the deltopectoral approach can also be used for harvesting the SSC tendon. In that case, the skin incision is extended as a combined curved incision of superior and deltopectoral approaches.

From the superior approach, the deltoid is divided between anterior and middle fibers. Care should be taken not to extend the split more than 4 cm distally to avoid axillary nerve injury. Anterior acromioplasty according to Neer's procedure and sufficient extra- and intraarticular mobilization of torn SSP and ISP tendons are performed. The long head of the biceps is completely or partially torn in most of these patients. Tenodesis with suture anchor at the bicipital groove, soft tissue tenodesis, or simple tenotomy is performed by the surgeon's preference.

The upper two thirds of the SSC tendon is subperiosteally detached from the lesser tuberosity after the release of the coracohumeral ligament (Fig. 12.2). The lower one third of SSC should be preserved to prevent anterior instability. Enough excursion of the SSC should be obtained by splitting SSC muscle belly proximally so that the SSC tendon can completely cover the cuff defect. The capsule can be released along the lateral rim of the labrum to gain further excursion. With sufficient mobilization, the SSC tendon usually can reach to the middle facet. Sufficient numbers of #2 nonabsorbable braids are passed through the SSC tendon with the Mason–Allen method to hold the tendon strongly. The upper border (yellow line in Figs. 12.2 and 12.3) of the transferred tendon is sutured to the remained SSP and ISP tendon if possible. The end (blue line in Figs. 12.2 and 12.3) and the lower border (red line in Figs. 12.2 and 12.3) of the transferred tendon is

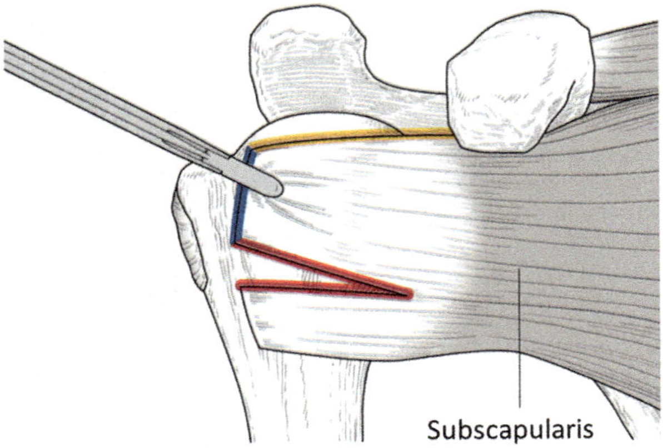

Fig. 12.2 Preparing SSC tendon for transfer. Upper two thirds of SSC tendon is detached from the lesser tuberosity

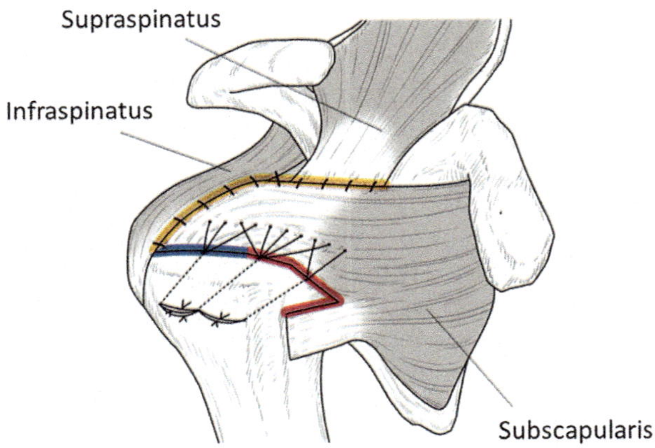

Fig. 12.3 Transfer of upper two thirds of SSC tendon. The upper border (*yellow line*) of the transferred tendon is sutured to the remaining SSP and ISP tendon. The end (*blue line*) and the lower border (*red line*) of the transferred tendon are sutured to the footprint at the greater tuberosity (GT) using the surface-holding method

sutured to the footprint at the greater tuberosity (GT) using the surface-holding method [5–7] (Fig. 12.4) as follows. A bone trough is made to create a medially advanced footprint, and suture anchors are inserted at the proximal edge of the bone trough. The anchor threads are passed through the transferred tendon and pulled out from the lateral edge of the bone trough to the distal cortex of the GT. Then, knots are tied on the surface of the cortex.

12.1.4 Postoperative Treatment

The shoulder is immobilized for 8 weeks with an abduction brace (AirBee brace G3; Ikeda, Japan). The postoperative rehabilitation protocol is shown in Table 12.1. The protocol may be modified according to the condition and intraoperative

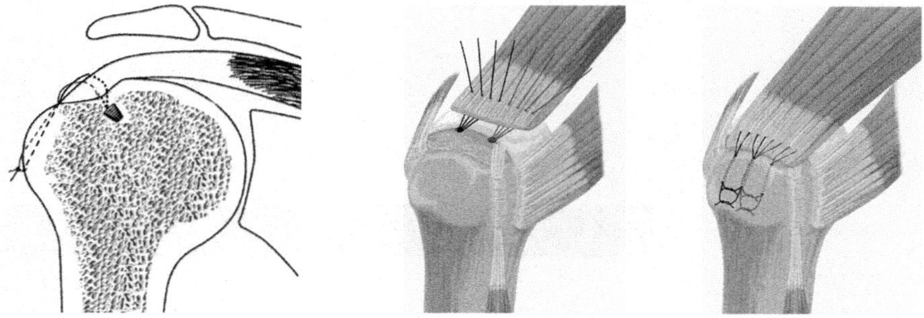

Fig. 12.4 Surface-holding. A bone trough is made to create a medially advanced footprint, and suture anchors are inserted at the proximal edge of the bone trough. The anchor threads were passed through the transferred tendon and pulled out from the lateral edge of the bone trough to the distal cortex of the GT. Then, knots are tied on the surface of the cortex

findings of each patient. Heavy labor or sports are permitted at 4–6 months after surgery.

12.1.5 Advantages and Tips of This Procedure

This procedure can be performed in the same surgical field with relatively simple technique and less complication of donor site compared to other procedures for irreparable massive cuff tears. It is also useful with shoulder arthroplasty. Tips to obtain satisfactory outcomes of this procedure follow. (1) Preoperative evaluation of quality of SSC is mandatory, including clinical evaluation and magnetic resonance imaging (MRI). (2) It is important to reconstruct the force couple by suturing transferred tendon not only to the greater tuberosity (GT) but also to the remaining SSP and ISP tendon as much as possible. (3) Patients with irreparable teres minor (TM) tendon are not indicated for this procedure. Indication for patients with anterior instability should be considered carefully.

12.1.6 Clinical Outcomes

Outcomes of 12 shoulders of 12 patients who underwent partial subscapularis transfer were evaluated. There were seven men and five women; average age at the time of surgery was 63.3 years (range, 47–77 years). The shoulder scoring system of the Japanese Orthopaedic Association (JOA score: 100 points) and active range of motion (ROM) were investigated. ROM of internal rotation was rated according to the JOA score (>T12, 6 points; L1–S, 4 points; buttock, 2 points; <lateral thigh, 0 points). The muscle strength of Internal Rotation (IR) was

Table 12.1 Postoperative rehabilitation protocol

	Day 1 (/)	Day 2 (/)	Week 1 (/)	Week 2 (/)	Week 4 (/)	Week 6 (/)	Week 8 (/)	Week 10 (/)	Week 12 (/)
							Brace off		
Finger grip ex. (100/day)									
Shoulder shrug, scapular ex. (30/day)									
Elbow ex. (30/day)									
Active external rotation ex. (30/day)		*							
Mobilizer					*				
Active ex. in flexion position @ supine position					*				
Target angle: Elevation					120°	150°	165°		170°
External rotation					30°	50°	70°		90°
Hanging ex. (15/day)					*				

(continued)

Table 12.1 (continued)

Resistant ex. (except for abduction, external rotation) (30/day)					■	■	■	■	■
D2 ex. @ supine position (50/day)							■	■	■
Anti-gravity active ex. (50/day)								■	■
Resistant abduction & external rotation ex. (30/day)									■

[a]Starting day may differ in each patient

measured using a hand-held dynamometer μTas MF-01 (Anima, Japan). Cuff integrity on MRI was assessed in ten shoulders using Sugaya's classification [8], and type 4 and 5 were defined as re-tear. The mean follow-up period was 16.8 months (range, 12–49 months). Statistical analysis was conducted using the Wilcoxon's signed-rank sum test ($P < 0.05$ as significant).

The JOA score significantly improved from preoperative 65.9 points (range, 36.0–79.5) to postoperative 89.5 points (73–100) ($P = 0.003$). Especially, pain score (30 points) remarkably improved, from 9.0 points to 28.6 points. Active shoulder flexion and external rotation were significantly improved from 126° (50–160°) to 142° (90–160°), and from 34° (10–60°) to 46° (30–60°), respectively ($P = 0.04$, $P = 0.02$). Pre- and postoperative IR score did not show significant difference (5.0 vs. 4.8). The average muscle power of IR (% of contralateral side) was 92.7 % preoperatively and 96.4 % postoperatively in first IR, and 82.3 % preoperatively and 90.5 % postoperatively in second IR; there were no significant differences. Postoperative MRI showed type 1 in six shoulders and type 3 in four shoulders. There was no repeat tear.

12.1.7 Conclusion

The partial transfer of SSC tendon for an irreparable massive rotator tear can provide satisfying pain relief and improvement of ROM without decrease of IR strength. The surgical procedure is relatively simple and less invasive compared to other procedures. This procedure can be one of the useful options for irreparable tear of SSP and ISP with intact subscapularis muscle.

12.2 Pectoralis Major Muscle Transfer for the Treatment of Irreparable Rotator Cuff Tears

In this chapter, we introduce our technique of pectoralis major muscle transfer for irreparable rotator cuff tears.

12.2.1 Patient Selection

Irreparable tear of supraspinatus (SSP) and subscapularis (SSC) tendon with or without infraspinatus (ISP) tendons is a good indication for this procedure. If the teres minor (TM) tendon is not effective, which is usually predictable with lag of external rotation (discrepancy between active and passive external rotation), additional reconstruction of posterior cuff defect, such as transfer of latissimus dorsi, should be considered.

The criteria for operative repair include (1) at least 6 months of failed nonoperative treatment except for the actual trauma, with the patient continuing to complain of subjectively unacceptable pain or disability or both; (2) patient needed/wanted to use the arm at or above the level of the head; (3) good motivation to comply with the postoperative treatment regimen; and (4) an absence of moderate to marked osteoarthritis (OA).

12.2.2 Laboratory Studies on Pectoralis Major Muscle Transfer

In some biomechanical studies, cuff tear shoulders without arthropathy showed certain patterns of stress distribution on the glenoid cavity according to the torn tendons [9–15]. Hisada et al. [11] reported that all cases with well-repaired cuffs changed stress distribution pattern postoperatively. Repair of the torn cuff tendon was expected to restore cuff function and to affect the kinematics of the glenohumeral joint, which then changed stress distributions in the joint. Therefore, this procedure can change stress distribution of the glenohumeral joint. It may also damage cartilage and promote OA. On the other hand, Konrad et al. [16] reported that anterior and superior stability of the glenohumeral joint were restored to values closer to those for the intact shoulder when the pectoralis major tendon was routed underneath, rather than above, the conjoint tendon. Therefore, the pectoralis major tendon, which is routed underneath, will be better except for the risk of musculocutaneous nerve injury.

12.2.3 *Surgical Technique*

Surgery is performed in a beach-chair position under general anesthesia with an interscalene block.

After the skin incision, the anterior approach was utilized. The deltoid was split between the anterior and middle fibers, and a portion of the anterior fibers was detached from the acromion. Anterior acromioplasty and resection of the coracoacromial ligament were performed. After evaluating the torn cuff, the deltopectoral approach was used to transfer the pectoralis major muscle. Extraarticular and intraarticular soft tissue was released to obtain sufficient mobility of the tendon. If tendons were overly retracted for reattachment to the greater and the lesser tuberosity with the arm at the side, medial attachment, that is, at approximately 10 mm, was employed. We attempted a primary repair with the surface-holding repair technique (Fig. 12.4) [5–7]. If the repair was not enough, we performed pectoralis major muscle transfer for covering the anterior or anterosuperior defect. Pectoralis major muscle transfer was performed as follows. The superior two third of the tendon was completely detached from the humerus and mobilized medially. The muscle fibers of the detached section of the tendon were split by blunt dissection from the clavicle and the sternum so that only the sternal part could be used for the transfer (Fig. 12.5). In the superficial cases, the tendon was transferred above the conjointed tendon, while in the underneath cases, the tendon was transferred under the conjointed tendon and anterior to the musculocutaneous nerve.

The tendon detached medially was sutured at the side of the supraspinatus, and the tendon detached laterally was sutured at the greater and the lesser tuberosity. A bone trough was made at approximately 1 cm proximal to the greater and the lesser tuberosity. Metal or absorbent suture anchors were placed on the proximal site of the “footprint” to enlarge the contact area of the tendon on the bony surface. Two or three threads from each anchor were pulled out to the lateral cortex and tied without tying on the tendon (Fig. 12.6).

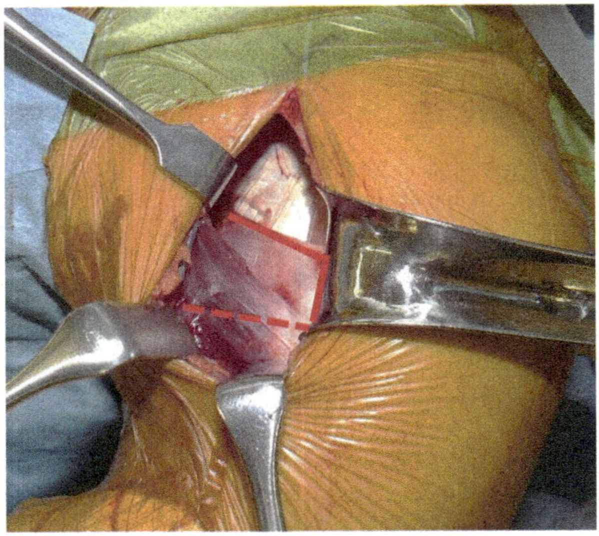

Fig. 12.5 The superior two thirds of the pectoralis major tendon is transferred

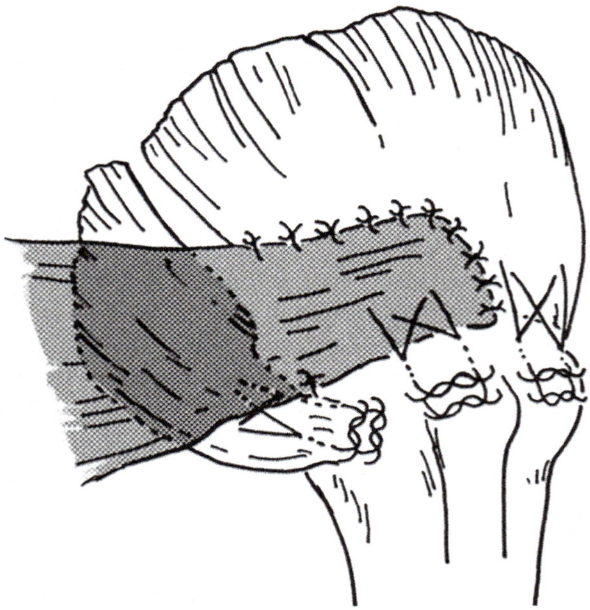

Fig. 12.6 The tendon detached medially was sutured at the side of supraspinatus, and the tendon detached laterally was sutured at the greater and the lesser tuberosity

12.2.4 Rehabilitation Protocol (Table 12.1)

An abduction pillow was used 8 weeks postoperatively. A systematic postoperative rehabilitation program was performed using passive range-of-motion (ROM)

exercises starting 2 weeks after the surgery. Active elevation in a sitting position from the adducted position of the shoulder was permitted starting at 10 weeks. Isometric cuff exercises were allowed from 12 weeks postoperatively. Heavy work or sports were permitted after 6 months postoperatively, after assessing the recovery of muscle strength and ROM.

12.2.5 *Outcomes*

We evaluated and compared clinical outcomes of the pectoralis major muscle transfer routed either above (superficial group) or under (underneath group) the conjointed tendon. Twenty-six patients (average age, 65.6 years) with anterosuperior rotator cuff tears were divided into the superficial group (11 shoulders) and the underneath group (15 shoulders). All patients were examined clinically using the Japanese Orthopaedic Association (JOA) score. Active ranges of motion and shoulder radiographs were assessed. A magnetic resonance image (MRI) was available for 20 shoulders. The average follow-up was 26.0 months.

Pectoralis major transfer achieved the following results. Jost et al. [13] reported that 25 of 30 shoulders (75 %) that were routed above the conjointed tendon had excellent or good results. The 12 shoulders with an isolated subscapularis tear had a higher mean postoperative relative Constant score than the 18 with a massive tear (79 % compared with 64 %). Galatz et al. [17] reported that 11 of 14 shoulders (79 %) that were routed underneath the conjoint tendon had satisfactory results. Resch et al. [18] reported that 9 of 12 shoulders (75 %) that were routed underneath the conjointed tendon had excellent or good results. Especially in four shoulders with subscapularis and supraspinatus tendon tear, four of four shoulders (100 %) had excellent results. In our results, a score greater than 80 points was defined as excellent and good results, Nine of 11 shoulders (82 %) in the superficial group and 14 of 15 shoulders (93 %) in the underneath group had good results.

Reported repair integrity of pectoralis major transfer is summarized literally as follows. Gavriilidis et al. [19] reviewed the postoperative MRI of 11 of 13 shoulders (85 %) and found intact tendons when the underneath procedure was performed. Lederer et al. [20] reported that 42 of 52 shoulders (81 %) showed no sign of degeneration or tear, and the area of insertion at the greater tuberosity showed good osseous integration of transferred tendon when the underneath procedure was performed. In total, 17 of 20 shoulders (85 %) had intact tendons, 5 of 7 shoulders (71 %) in the superficial group and 12 of 13 shoulders (92 %) in the underneath group.

Concordantly, our results are similar to the results of the latter studies. Clinically, there is no significant difference between two groups. However, according to MRI results, some advantages were identified in the underneath group.

12.2.6 Conclusions

Satisfactory clinical outcomes were obtained with pectoralis major transfer for irreparable anterosuperior tendon tear. Especially, pectoralis major muscle transfer routed under the conjointed tendon seemed a reliable treatment for irreparable anterosuperior tendon tear to obtain pain relief and function.

12.3 Teres Minor Tendon Transfer/Latissimus Dorsi Tendon Transfer for Irreparable Massive Rotator Cuff Tears

Massive rotator cuff tear impair function and inflict severe shoulder pain to affected patients. Before surgery, all tears had failed to respond to conservative treatment consisting of physical therapy and treatment with nonsteroidal antiinflammatory drugs for duration of at least 6 months.

12.3.1 Surgical Procedures

All patients received general anesthesia was positioned in the "beach-chair" position. A superior approach to the rotator cuff was performed. The deltoid was split between the anterior and middle thirds, and care was taken to preserve the origin and to protect the axillary nerve. However, a portion of the anterior or middle fibers was detached from their origin when greater exposure was necessary. The indication for various procedures of the Coracoacromial arch was decided depending on the preoperative examination, which included physical examination and systematic block tests by use of local anesthesia in the subacromial bursa and glenohumeral joint [21, 22]. As a result, an anterior acromioplasty described by Neer [23] and resection of the coracoacromial ligament was performed in all shoulders. The torn tendon was pulled out with no. 2 nonabsorbable sutures running through the edge of the tendon. The adhesions with the surrounding tissues were severe in all cases; therefore, careful and sufficient extraarticular and intraarticular releases were performed to obtain enough mobility of the tendon to pull it out for the repair. Extraarticular release included blunt and sharp dissection of adhesions of the cuff tendon with the bursa and capsule and excision of the coracohumeral ligament at the insertion to the coracoid process. Intraarticular releases of the cuff tendon and the capsule from the superior to anterior labrum were also performed. After sufficient releases and debridement of the tendon edge, the tendon was pulled out. If the tendon could not reach over the top of the humeral head, tendon transfer should be considered during surgery. In this chapter, teres minor tendon transfer, the so-called Paavoleinen's procedure, and latissimus dorsi and teres najor tendon transfer are proposed as the alterative surgery. Both procedures are performed in the "beach-chair" position.

12.3.2 Teres Minor Tendon Transfer

Assessment of the condition of teres minor muscle by using MRI findings should be done before surgery. To improve shoulder function, we exclude the shoulder with neurological disorder and the teres minor in severe fatty degeneration. Primary advantage of this procedure is that tendon transfer can be performed through the same superior skin incision. If any residual infraspinatus exist, the teres minor with any residual infraspinatus transfer is selected. The intact insertions of the teres minor and any residual infraspinatus were clearly marked on the tuberosity. A small oscillating saw or osteotome is then used to osteotomize a portion of the greater tuberosity of approximately 1.5 × 1.5 cm where the intact posterior cuff is attached (Fig. 12.7b). The bone fragment is ideally at least 5 mm in thickness. Fixation of the fragment was achieved with one 3.5-mm cortical screw (Fig. 12.7c) with suture anchors, which are used to augment the suture site and enlarge the contact area of the tendon with bony fragment. After enough irrigation is confirmed, the deltoid muscle is reattached to the acromion with nonabsorbable sutures passed through bone [24].

12.3.3 Latissimus Dorsi and Teres Major Tendon Transfer

To harvest the latissimus dorsi tendon, a V-shaped skin incision is made on the anterior axilla with abducted shoulder position. The incision should not be run over

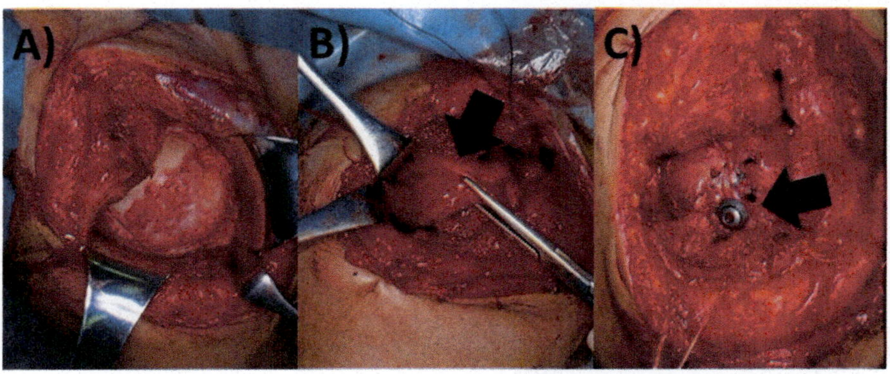

Fig. 12.7 (**a**) Superior part of the humeral head is exposed massively. (**b**) Teres minor tendon with bone pedicle is transferred to the footprint of supraspinatus tendon approximately (*arrow*). **c** Bone fragment is fixed with cortical screw (*arrow*). Suture anchors are used to augment the suture site and enlarge the contact area of the tendon with the bony fragment

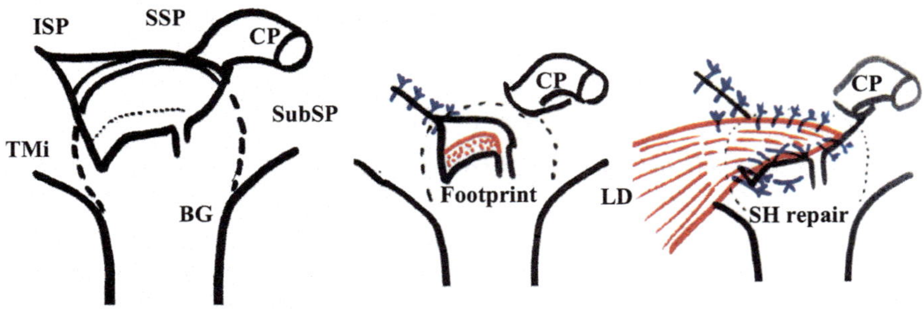

Fig. 12.8 The transferred latissimus dorsi tendon should be secured to the subscapularis tendon, residue tendons of supraspinatus/infraspinatus, and the greater tuberosity

the anterior border of the latissimus dorsi muscle. After retracting subcutaneous tissues and resecting the muscle fascia, the anterior and superior borders of the latissimus dorsi muscle can be defined. Then, the dissection is started from medial border carefully. To pull out the Latissimus dorsi tendon sufficiently, inferior muscular release should be done widely. During release muscle belly from surrounding tissue, the thoracodorsal nerve and artery should be handled with care. To maximize the tendon length for a tendon graft, the latissimus dorsi and teres major tendon should be released from the insertion site of the humeral shaft. The humerus should be internally rotated with shoulder abduction during the release to maximize the tendon length. Then, to pull out the tendons, the released tendons are reinforced by a no. 2 nonabsorbable running suture with a locking Krackow technique [25]. The muscular tunnel under the deltoid and over the long head of triceps is developed with blunt dissection. A long clamp is placed from the superior incision through the tunnel, and the tendons are pulled into the superior incision. The pulled-out tendons should cover the rotator cuff defect without excessive tension. The anterior edge of the tendon is secured to the subscapularis tendon edge and the lesser tuberosity (Fig. 12.8). The medial edge of the tendon is secured to the edge of the remaining portions of the supraspinatus and infraspinatus tendons. The lateral edge of the tendon is secured to the greater tuberosity. After enough irrigation is confirmed, the deltoid muscle is reattached to the acromion with nonabsorbable sutures passed through bone.

12.3.4 Rehabilitation Program After Surgery (Table 12.1)

An abduction brace is used for 8 weeks after surgery. A systematic rehabilitation program is carried out, with passive range-of-motion (ROM) exercises from 2 weeks after surgery, active ROM exercises from 10 weeks, and isometric cuff exercises from 12 weeks. Heavy work or sports were permitted after 6 months postoperatively, in principle, by assessing recovery of muscle strength and ROM.

12.4 Muscle Transfer with a Smaller Humeral Head Replacement in Patients with Cuff Tear Arthropathy

Rotator cuff tear arthropathy was originally described in 1983 by Neer et al. who described a massive rotator cuff tear as the initial event in the development of degenerative arthritis [26]. This arthropathy has at least three critical features: rotator cuff insufficiency, degenerative changes of the glenohumeral joint, and superior migration of the humeral head. In terms of rotator cuff sufficiency, this massive degenerative rotator cuff tear is usually irreparable and pain sometimes remains after the surgery. To treat the cuff tear arthropathy, reverse shoulder arthroplasty (RSA) has been widely used [27–30], and there are many reports showing that shoulder elevation and pain relief improved significantly following this procedure.

Nevertheless, the long-term result of RSA surgery was not favorable. The Constant-Murley score was less than 30 points in 72 % of patients after 10 years [28], and high rates of complications such as deltoid rupture, glenoid loosening, infection, neurological injury, dislocation, acromial fracture, and breakage of the prosthesis have been reported. Following these results, Boileau et al. suggested that the application of RSA should be limited to elderly patients over 70 years of age [31].

As an alternative treatment option for younger patients with cuff tear arthropathy who are not available for RSA, we have developed a strategy to use a smaller humeral head for humeral head replacement (HHR) including cuff reconstruction with or without muscle transfers. The advantages of this method are as follows. First, using a smaller head allows easier reconstruction of rotator cuff defect; we already found that the size of humeral head in cuff tear arthropathy patients is often enlarged (unpublished). Second, the small/thin head shifts the center of shoulder joint rotation medially that contributes to advance the lever arm of deltoid muscle. Third, passive range of motion can be expected to improve without the capsule resection that is usually performed during RSA; remaining capsule may contribute to joint stability. Fourth, the mismatch between humeral head with small size and glenoid with original size may yield a broad range of passive motion, followed by expected range of active motion when muscle power is regained.

12.4.1 Operative Indication

The indication of this surgery should be considered comprehensively, based on preoperative clinical findings, imaging, and operative findings. The elderly patients who maintain daily activity without severe pain, and the patients with severe osteoarthritis with upper migration of the humeral head, are not included in indication of this surgery; those patients should be treated with conservative therapy such as exercise for tendon function and range of motion, thermotherapy, nonsteroidal antiinflammatory drugs, and hyaluronic acid injection, etc. The patients who have reparable rotator cuff tear with glenohumeral arthropathy and have severe pain that sometimes causes sleeplessness may be good candidates for this surgery so long as they are eager to elevate the arm.

12.4.2 Indication for Humeral Head Replacement

The indication for humeral head replacement with smaller head is the cases of which the patients have osteoarthritic change of glenohumeral joint, irreparable tendon with upper migration and femoralization of humeral head, or subacromial bony erosion and articular eburnation of the humeral head showing subchondral sclerosis. Patients with good active range of motion despite arthritis and a massive rotator cuff tear (biomechanically balanced shoulder) can still have a good outcome from this surgery.

In contrast, the patients with Seebauer classification type IIB are not recommended for this procedure, because coracoacromial arch preservation is crucial for shoulder stability postoperatively. Those patients who are not able to participate in rehabilitation, have atrophy in all rotator cuff muscles (subscapularis, supraspinatus, infraspinatus, and teres minor), or have severe atrophic deltoid muscle (as seen in elderly patients who have had multiple surgeries in the past), should avoid this surgery; they are good candidates for RSA. In addition, elderly patients who are older than 70 years with massive anterosuperior cuff defects with insufficient coracoacromial arch are also recommended for RSA.

12.4.3 Indication for Tendon Transfer with Smaller Humeral Head Replacement for CTA

Tendon transfer with humeral head replacement is selected based on preoperative clinical findings as well as operative findings. In most cases of cuff tear arthropathy, the supraspinatus and infraspinatus tendons are torn and remarkably retracted, including severe degeneration and atrophy. During the surgery, when the rotator cuff tendon does not reach to the center of humeral head at 30° of shoulder abduction, even though tendon mobilization such as coracohumeral ligament resection, tendon release affected by adhesions, and capsular release are attempted, tendon transfer should be employed.

In this regard, our concept is to utilize remained healthy muscle rather than fatty degenerative muscles for ideal cuff reconstruction. In cases in which the subscapularis and teres minor tendons remained intact, two thirds of the superior aspect of the intact subscapularis muscle is used to suture with the teres minor tendon by side-to-side sutures and fixed laterally to the greater tubercle.

If the anterosuperior part of the rotator cuff including the subscapularis muscle is deficient, a pectoralis major transfer is used to cover the defect. If the posterosuperior part of the rotator cuff including the teres minor is deficient, a latissimus dorsi and teres major transfer is employed with an anterior approach.

12.4.4 Surgical Approach

All procedures are performed on patients in a beach-chair position under general anesthesia with a preoperative interscalene block.

A superior deltoid splitting approach is applied between the anterior and middle fibers with preservation of the coracoacromial arch. Approximately 5 mm of the lateral side of the acromion is resected to expose the humeral head and to remove osteophytes for successful deltoid muscle repair.

After resection of the humeral head at the level of the anatomic neck using an osteotome, with guidance provided by the collar of the trial stem, the trial stem is inserted with a 40° angle of retroversion, because the humeral head is expected to stay on the glenoid during shoulder elevation and to prevent anterosuperior escape of the head (Fig. 12.9).

Then, the coracohumeral ligament is resected and intra- and extraarticular mobilization of the cuff is performed, followed by attaching nonabsorbable thread in the edge of the tendon from posterior through anterior with a Mayson–Allen stitch. When partial rupture is found in the long head of the biceps, tenodesis is performed at the biceps groove and the tendon is resected in the joint.

To determine the size of the humeral head, a trial head that matches the resected head in diameter and thickness is employed; if the cuff repair seems to be difficult with this head, a thinner head with the same diameter is tried, and even a thinner

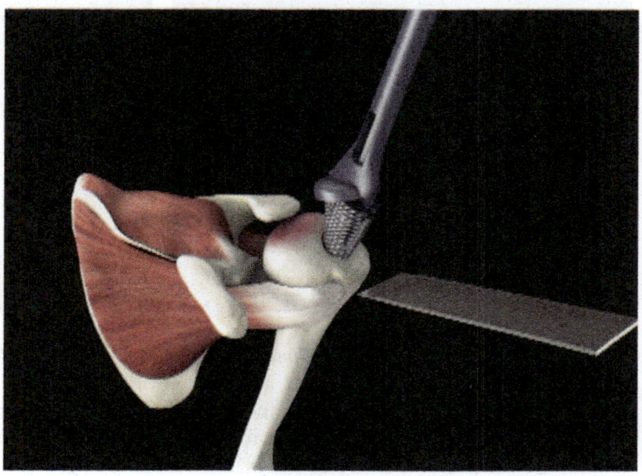

Fig. 12.9 Resection of humeral head at the level of anatomic neck using an osteotome with guidance provided by the collar of the trial stem inserted with a 40° angle of retroversion

head with smaller diameter (4 mm at most) is available unless incongruity and instability occur because of mismatch between the head and glenoid.

Next, the humeral stem is inserted following impaction bone grafting with cancellous bone from resected humeral head and an artificial bone tip. The greater tubercle may be shaved if that is higher than the humeral head by fluoroscopy examination.

Then, cuff repair is executed; in cuff tear arthropathy, in most cases the supraspinatus and infraspinatus tendons are torn and remarkably retracted, appearing with severe degeneration and atrophy that make rotator cuff repair difficult primarily, even though a smaller and thinner head is used. In these cases tendon transfers should be added.

If the anterosuperior part of the rotator cuff including the subscapularis was deficient, a pectoralis major transfer is performed to cover the defect, adding the deltopectoral approach and passing the pars sternocostalis of the pectoralis major tendon under the conjoined tendon. If the posterosuperior part of the rotator cuff including the teres minor was deficient, latissimus dorsi and teres major transfer, which is passed under the deltoid muscle, is executed with an anterior approach.

However, when the subscapularis and teres minor tendons remain intact, cuff repair may be attempted primarily. Two thirds of the superior aspect of the intact subscapularis muscle is detached subperiosteally (Fig.12.10a) and transferred anterosuperiorly, while the intact teres minor tendon is lifted posterosuperiorly. Then the teres minor and subscapularis tendons are sutured side to side and then sutured laterally to the greater tubercle, and finally the supraspinatus and infraspinatus tendons are sutured at the medial site of the transferred subscapularis and teres minor tendon (Fig. 12.10b). After the deltoid muscle is reattached to acromion with nonabsorbable thread, the skin is closed layer by layer and the surgery is completed.

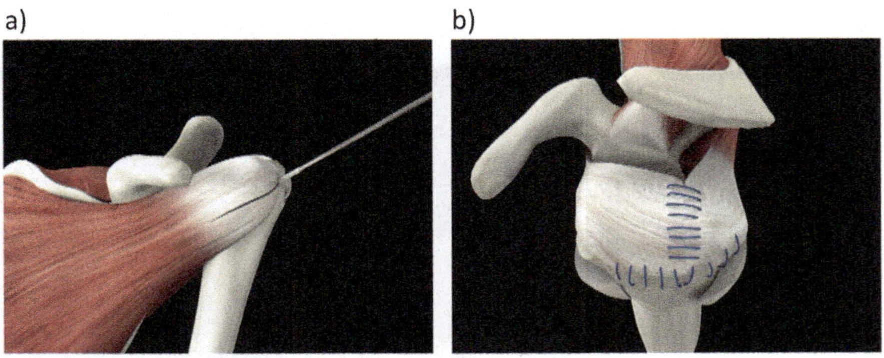

Fig. 12.10 Two thirds of the superior aspect of the intact subscapularis muscle is detached subperiosteally (**a**) and transferred anterosuperiorly; the intact teres minor tendon was lifted posterosuperiorly. Then, the teres minor and subscapularis tendons are sutured side to side and then sutured laterally to the greater tubercle, and finally the supraspinatus and infraspinatus tendons are sutured at the medial site of the transferred subscapularis and teres minor tendon (**b**)

12.4.5 *Postoperative Procedure*

An abduction pillow is used for 8 weeks postoperatively. Passive motion of the shoulder begins from 4 weeks after surgery. Active elevation in a sitting position from the adducted position of the shoulder is permitted after 10 weeks, and isometric cuff exercises are initiated at 12 weeks. The patients were allowed to resume heavy work after sufficient muscle strength was evident, along with range-of-motion (ROM) recovery, at 6 months or more postoperatively.

References

1. Cofield RH (1982) Subscapular muscle transposition for repair of chronic rotator cuff tears. Surg Gynecol Obstet 154:667–672
2. Bigliani LU, Cordasco FA, McLLveen SJ, Musso ES (1992) Operative repair of massive rotator cuff tears: long-term results. J Shoulder Elbow Surg 1:120–130. doi.org/10.1016/1058-2746(92)90089-L
3. Karas SE, Giachello TL (1996) Subscapularis transfer for reconstruction of massive tears of the rotator cuff. J Bone Joint Surg Am 78:239–245
4. Nakajima T, Liu J, Hughes RE, O'Driscoll S, An KN (1999) Abduction moment arm of transposed subscapularis tendon. Clin Biomech 14:265–270. doi.org/10.1016/S0268-0033(98)00075-8
5. Funakoshi T, Suenaga N, Sano H, Oizumi N, Minami A (2008) In vitro and finite element analysis of a novel rotator cuff fixation technique. J Shoulder Elbow Surg 17:986–992. doi.org/10.1016/j.jse.2008.06.002
6. Taniguchi N, Suenaga N, Oizumi N, Miyoshi N, Araki N, Chosa E (2014) Surface-holding repair: an original arthroscopic rotator cuff repair technique. J Shoulder Elbow Surg 23:620–627. doi.org/10.1016/j.jse.2014.01.007
7. Yamaguchi H, Suenaga N, Oizumi N, Hosokawa Y, Kanaya F (2011) Open repair for massive rotator cuff tear with a modified transosseous-equivalent procedure: preliminary results at short-term follow-up. J Orthop Sci 16:398–404. doi:10.1007/s00776-011-0092-9
8. Sugaya H, Maeda K, Matsuki K, Moriishi J (2007) Repair integrity and functional outcome after arthroscopic double-row rotator cuff repair. A prospective outcome study. J Bone Joint Surg Am 89:953–960. doi.org/10.2106/JBJS.F.00512
9. Anetzberger H, Schulz C, Pfahler M, Refior HJ, Müller-Gerbl M (2002) Subchondral mineralization patterns of the glenoid after tear of the supraspinatus. Clin Orthop 404:263–268. doi.org/10.1097/00003086-200211000-00040
10. Galatz LM, Connor PM, Calfee RP, Hsu JC, Yamaguchi K (2003) Pectoralis major transfer for anterior-superior subluxation in massive rotator cuff insufficiency. J Shoulder Elbow Surg 12:1–5. doi.org/10.1067/mse.2003.128137
11. Hisada Y, Suenaga N, Oizumi N, Nagai M, Minami A (2007) The long-term stress distribution at the glenoid cavity after a rotator cuff reconstruction using CT osteoabsorptiometry. Katakansetsu (Shoulder Joint) 31:597–600
12. Nagai M, Suenaga N, Oizumi N, Kato H, Yamane S, Minami A (2002) The stress distribution of the glenoid using by CT osteoabsorptiometry. Katakansetsu (Shoulder Joint) 26:541–544
13. Von Eisenhart-Rothe R, Müller-Gerbl M, Wiedemann E, Englmeier K, Graichen H (2008) Functional malcentering of the humeral head and asymmetric long-term stress on the glenoid: potential reasons for glenoid loosening in total shoulder arthroplasty. J Shoulder Elbow Surg 17:695–702. doi:10.1016/j.jse.2008.02.008

14. Yamaguchi H, Suenaga N, Oizumi N, Hisada Y, Matsuhashi T, Miyoshi N, Hosokawa Y, Kanaya F (2009) Stress distribution patterns at glenoid cavity and undersurface of acromion in patients with cuff tear arthropathy measured by CT osteoabsorptiometry. Katakansetsu (Shoulder Joint) 33:785–788
15. Yokoya S, Mochizuki Y, Omae H, Kikugawa K, Kashiwagi K, Natsu K et al (2006) Analysis of stress distribution of glenoid with DMSB (distribution of mineralization of subchondral bone plate) by CT osteoabsorptiometry. Katakansetsu (Shoulder Joint) 30:375–3758
16. Konrad GG, Sudkamp NP, Kreuz PC, Jolly JT, McMahon PJ, Debski RE (2007) Pectoralis major tendon transfers above or underneath the conjoint tendon in subscapularis-deficient shoulders. An in vitro biomechanical analysis. J Bone Joint Surg Am 89:2477–2484. doi.org/10.2106/JBJS.F.00811
17. Jost B, Puskas GJ, Lustenberger A, Gerber C (2003) Outcome of pectoralis major transfer for the treatment of irreparable subscapularis tears. J Bone Joint Surg Am 85:1944–1951
18. Resch H, Povacz P, Ritter E, Matschi W (2000) Transfer of the pectoralis major transfer for the treatment of irreparable rupture of subscapularis tendon. J Bone Joint Surg Am 82:372–382
19. Gavriilidis I, Kircher J, Mangosch P, Lichtenberg S, Habermeyer P (2010) Pectoralis major muscle transfer for the treatment of irreparable anterosuperior rotator cuff tears. Int Orthop 34:689–694. doi:10.1007/s00264-009-0799-9
20. Lederer S, Auffarth A, Bogner R, Tauber M, Mayer M, Karpik S et al (2011) Magnetic resonance imaging-controlled results of the pectoralis major tendon transfer for irreparable anterosuperior rotator cuff tears performed with standard and modified fixation techniques. J Shoulder Elbow Surg 20:1155–1162. doi:10.1016/j.jse.2011.01.023
21. Suenaga N, Minami A, Iwasaki N, Kaneda K (2000) Coracoacromial arch decompression in rotator cuff surgery. Int Orthop 24:212–216
22. Suenaga N, Minami A, Fukuda K, Kaneda K (2002) The correlation between bursoscopic and histologic findings of the acromion undersurface in patients with subacromial impingement syndrome. Arthroscopy 8:16–20
23. Neer CS II (1972) Anterior acromioplasty for the chronic impingement syndrome in the shoulder: a preliminary report. J Bone Joint Surg Am 54:41–50
24. Matsuhashi T, Suenaga N, Oizumi N, Funakoshi T, Iwasaki N, Minami A (2012) Transfer of teres minor with bone pedicle for irreparable posterior-superior rotator cuff tears. J Orthop Sci 17(5):538–544. doi:10.1007/s00776-012-0249-1
25. Krackow KA, Thomas SC, Jones LC (1986) A new stitch for ligament tendon fixation. J Bone Joint Surg Am 68:764–766
26. Neer CS 2nd, Craig EV, Fukuda H (1983) Cuff-tear arthropathy. J Bone Joint Surg Am 65:1232–1244
27. Boileau P, Watkinson D, Hatzidakis AM, Hovorka I (2006) Neer Award 2005. The Grammont reverse shoulder prosthesis: results in cuff tear arthritis, fracture sequelae, and revision arthroplasty. J Shoulder Elbow Surg 15:527–540. doi:10.1016/j.jse.2006.01.003
28. Favard L, Levigne C, Nerot C, Gerber C, De Wilde L, Mole D (2011) Reverse prostheses in arthropathies with cuff tear: are survivorship and function maintained over time? Clin Orthop Relat Res 469:2469–2475. doi:10.1007/s11999-011-1833-y
29. Guery J, Favard L, Sirveaux F, Oudet D, Mole D, Walch G (2006) Reverse total shoulder arthroplasty. Survivorship analysis of eighty replacements followed for five to ten years. J Bone Joint Surg Am 88:1742–1747. doi:10.2106/JBJS.E.00851
30. Werner CM, Steinmann PA, Gilbart M, Gerber C (2005) Treatment of painful pseudoparesis due to irreparable rotator cuff dysfunction with the Delta III reverse-ball-and-socket total shoulder prosthesis. J Bone Joint Surg Am 87:1476–1486. doi:10.2106/JBJS.D.02342
31. Boileau P, Chuinard C, Roussanne Y, Bicknell RT, Rochet N, Trojani C (2008) Reverse shoulder arthroplasty combined with a modified latissimus dorsi and teres major tendon transfer for shoulder pseudoparalysis associated with dropping arm. Clin Orthop Relat Res 466:584–593. doi:10.1007/s11999-008-0114-x

Chapter 13
Frozen Shoulder

Junji Ide

Abstract Diagnosis of frozen shoulder is based upon the recognition of the characteristic features of the pain and limitation of both active and passive elevation, external rotation, and internal rotation. The macroscopic and histological features of the capsular contracture are well defined; however, the underlying pathological processes remain poorly understood. Furthermore, clearly defined diagnostic criteria are lacking. Contracture may cause protracted disability. Most patients are still managed by medication of nonsteroidal antiinflammatory drugs and physiotherapy in primary care, and only the more refractory cases are referred for specialist intervention. Targeted therapy is not possible, and treatment remains predominantly symptomatic. However, during the past 10 years, more active interventions that may shorten the clinical course, such as manipulation under anesthesia and arthroscopic capsular release, have become more popular.

Keywords Frozen shoulder • Manipulation under anaesthesia • Arthroscopic capsular release • Continuous passive motion machine

13.1 Introduction

Frozen shoulder is a common disorder in orthopedic practice, characterized by pain in the shoulder and physical restriction of movements of the glenohumeral joint. Frozen shoulder is a term coined by Codman in 1934 [1], who described the common features of a slow onset of pain felt near the insertion of the deltoid muscle, inability to sleep on the affected side with restriction in both active and passive elevation and external rotation, yet with normal radiographic appearance. Synonyms include pe'riarthrite scapulohume'rale [2] and adhesive capsulitis [3]. Although identification of the syndrome rests on the recognition of characteristic clinical features, clearly defined diagnostic criteria are lacking. Frozen shoulder may arise spontaneously without an obvious preceding cause, or may be

---

J. Ide (✉)
Department of Advanced Joint Reconstructive Surgery, Department of Orthopaedic Surgery, Kumamoto University Hospital, 1-1-1 Honjo, Chuo-ku, Kumamoto 860-8556, Japan
e-mail: ide@kumamoto-u.ac.jp

K. Tamai et al. (eds.), *Advances in Shoulder Surgery*,
DOI 10.1007/978-4-431-55988-7_13

Table 13.1 Definition of frozen shoulder

Symptoms	True (deltoid insertion) shoulder pain
	Night pain of insidious onset
Signs	Painful restriction of active and passive motion
	Passive elevation less than 100°
	Passive external rotation less than 30°
	Passive internal rotation less than L5
	All other shoulder conditions excluded
Investigations	Plain radiographs normal
	Arthroscopy shows vascular granulation tissue in the rotator interval

Table 13.2 Classification of frozen shoulder

Primary/idiopathic frozen shoulder
An underlying etiology or associated condition cannot be identified
Secondary frozen shoulder
An underlying etiology or associated condition can be identified
Intrinsic
In association with rotator cuff disorders (tendinitis and partial-thickness or full-thickness tears), biceps tendinitis, or calcific tendinitis
Extrinsic
In association with previous ipsilateral breast surgery, cervical radiculopathy, chest wall tumor, previous cerebrovascular accident, or more local extrinsic problems, including previous humeral shaft fracture, scapulothoracic abnormalities, acromioclavicular arthritis, or clavicle fracture
Systemic
Diabetes mellitus, hyperthyroidism, hypothyroidism, hypoadrenalism, etc.

associated with local or systemic disorders. The need for detection in diagnosis has recently been emphasized, and a system of terminology and classification based on consensus would be advantageous. A survey of the members of the British Elbow and Shoulder Society overwhelmingly agreed with the definition of frozen shoulder as seen in Table 13.1 [4]. In the United States, Zuckerman proposed to classify frozen shoulder into primary and secondary, and subdivided secondary frozen shoulder into intrinsic, extrinsic, and systemic ones [5] (Table 13.2). Diabetes mellitus is the condition most commonly associated with frozen shoulder, secondary systemic frozen shoulder. Diabetics have a 10–20 % lifetime risk of developing a frozen shoulder [6], with a risk two to four times greater than the general population [7].

13.2 Natural History

Many studies suggest that frozen shoulder is a benign condition, passing through phases of pain, pain and stiffness, stiffness and resolution, and typically leading to a functional recovery after 2–3 years [8, 9]. However, it is now accepted that up to 50 % of patients continued to have mild pain or stiffness 7 years after the initial symptoms as well as a deficit in shoulder range of motion compared with the contralateral shoulder [10]. It is estimated that approximately 7–15 % have some degree of permanent loss of movement, although few have persistent functional disability [11].

13.3 Pathology

The most common cause of painful restriction of movement is an idiopathic frozen shoulder, which is characterized by an inflammatory contracture of the capsule and ligaments, which reduces the available intraarticular volume, limiting glenohumeral movement. Macroscopically, the capsule has a glassy appearance with acute vasculitis, inflammation, and thickening, progressing to a more indolent fibrotic appearance with time.

Ide and Takagi reported intraarticular findings at arthroscopic capsular release [12]. All 42 patients (44 shoulders) manifested reduced intraarticular volume and highly vascular papillary infolding of the synovium (Fig. 13.1). Pathological findings, categorized as traumatic and nontraumatic frozen shoulder, are shown in Table 13.3. Regardless of etiology, all shoulders had similar intraarticular findings.

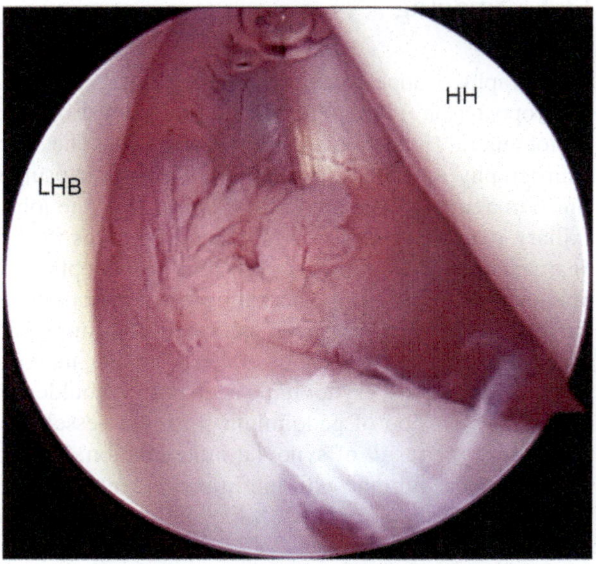

Fig. 13.1 Arthroscopic view of a right shoulder in patients with frozen shoulder from a posterior portal. Note the highly vascular papillary infolding of the synovium at rotator interval. LHB; long head of biceps tendon, HH; humeral head

Table 13.3 Arthroscopic findings of refractory frozen shoulder

	Nontraumatic ($n = 37$)	Traumatic ($n = 7$)
Highly vascular papillary infolding of		
Synovium	37 (100 %)	7 (100 %)
Rotator interval	36 (97 %)	7 (100 %)
LHB	25 (68 %)	6 (86 %)
Axillary pouch	22 (59 %)	4 (57 %)
Rotator cuff	21 (57 %)	2 (29 %)
Adhesion between LHB and rotator cuff	6 (16 %)	0 (0 %)
Incomplete rotator cuff tears	4 (11 %)	2 (29 %)
Labral lesions	3 (8 %)	1 (14 %)
Traumatic lesions of articular cartilage	0 (0 %)	0 (0 %)

After capsular release, capsule thickening was observed. The pathology of this condition is a soft tissue fibrosing and inflammation. There are no 'adhesions' within the joint. Future studies should be directed to give light on the initiator of inflammation, as well as of fibrosis, with the final aim to better treat or prevent frozen shoulder.

Histological examinations of synovial and capsular biopsies in patients with frozen shoulder demonstrate synovial hyperplasia with a normal underlying capsule (Fig. 13.2).

13.4 Imaging

Radiographic appearance is normal in patients with frozen shoulder. Anteroposterior radiograph in active elevation indicates that there is no glenohumeral joint movement (Fig. 13.3). The decrease of joint volume at arthrography indicates shortening of the joint capsule (Fig. 13.4). Magnetic resonance imaging (MRI) can detect thickening of the joint capsule. particularly in the axillary region [13, 14]. MRI also demonstrates thickening of the coracohumeral ligament [15]. MR arthrography may show obliteration of the subcoracoid fat triangle, resulting from shortening or fibrosis of the rotator interval capsule [15, 16]. Using dynamic MRI enhanced with intravenous gadolinium administration, Tamai et al. [17] demonstrated a greater increase of signal intensity in the glenohumeral joint synovium in frozen shoulder. This finding indicates an increased perfusion of gadolinium from the vessels to the synovium, which most probably is the result of synovial inflammation. The bone mineral density usually returns to near normal with the improvement of clinical symptoms [18]. A bone scan generally shows positive, which indicates increased local blood flow in frozen shoulder [19].

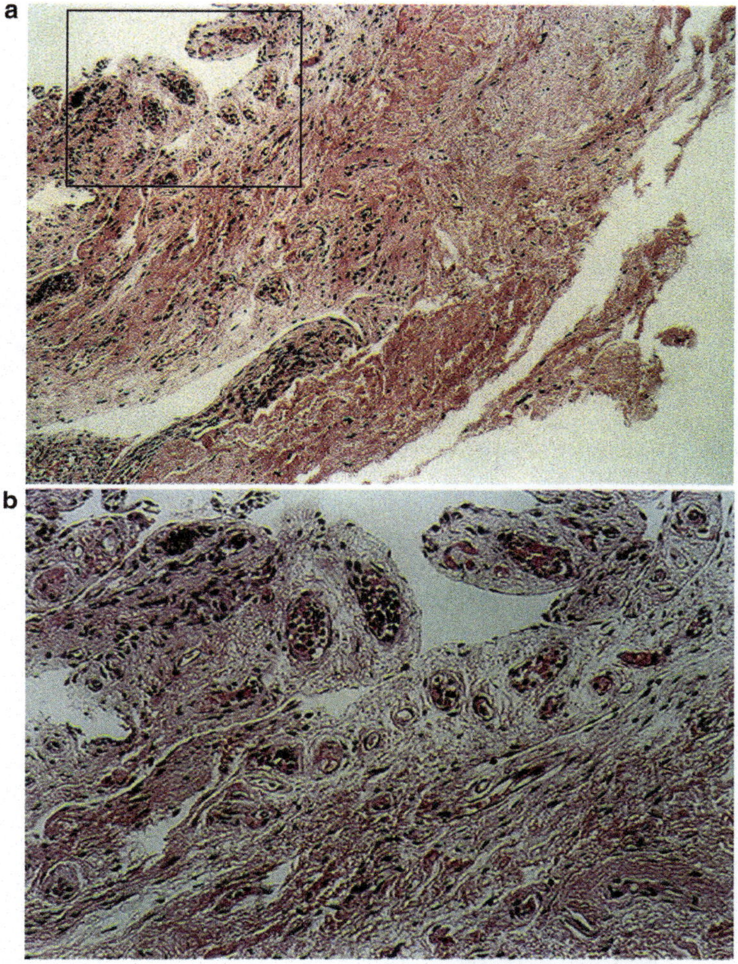

Fig. 13.2 Histological findings of synovial and capsular biopsies in patients with frozen shoulder demonstrate synovial hyperplasia with normal underlying capsule. (**a**) Hematoxylin and eosin staining, ×100. (**b**) Hematoxylin and eosin staining, ×400

13.5 Conservative Treatment

The goal of treatment is to relieve pain, restore movement, and regain function of the shoulder. There are many alternative forms of treatment for this condition, but evidence of their efficacy is not well established from clinical trials [20], and it is unclear if several interventions used in combination are better.

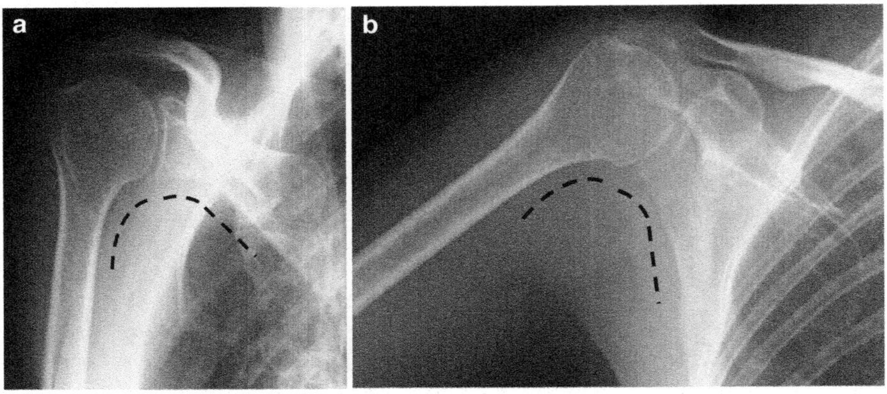

Fig. 13.3 (**a**) Radiographic appearance is normal in patients with frozen shoulder. (**b**) Anteroposterior radiograph in active elevation, indicating that there is no glenohumeral joint movement

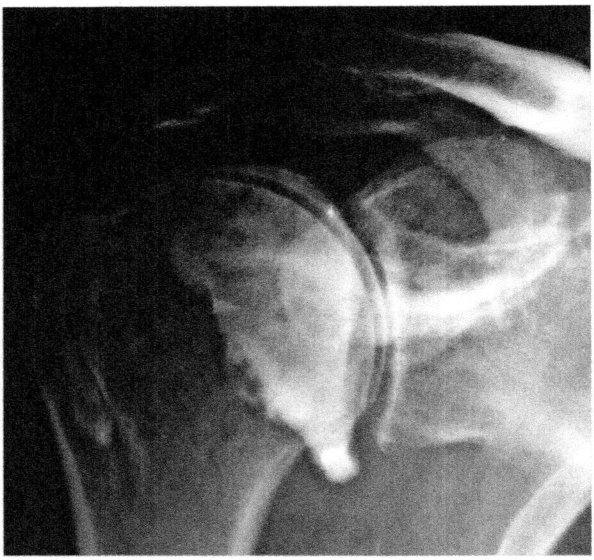

Fig. 13.4 Arthrography in patients with frozen shoulder, indicating the decrease of joint volume and shortening of the joint capsule

13.5.1 Physiotherapy

A recent Cochrane review concluded that the existing literature was insufficient to prove that physiotherapy alone was beneficial, with two small clinical trials concluding that physiotherapy alone did not offer any benefit when compared with no-treatment controls [21].

13.5.2 *Steroid Injection*

Although some studies have shown improvement with intraarticular steroid injection, others have found that this treatment produces little benefit [22]. A recent meta-analysis showed little evidence of benefit from steroid injection [23]. Steroid injections appear to provide earlier relief from pain, when compared with placebo, but whether this is sustained in the long term is unknown.

13.5.3 *Distension Arthrography*

This local anesthetic has the advantage of producing rapid improvement in movement, without recourse to a more interventional surgical procedure. Under fluoroscopic control, an arthrogram is initially performed to exclude a rotator cuff tear. The diagnosis of frozen shoulder is supported by the characteristic arthrographic appearance of a contracted capsule. Sterile water is then injected under pressure sufficient to cause capsular rupture. Data from a small placebo-controlled trial suggested that arthrographic distension provides significant short-term benefit, which is maintained in the medium term [24]. Further comparative studies are required to evaluate the efficacy of this technique.

13.5.4 *Manipulation Under Anaesthesia*

Manipulation under anesthesia (MUA) has been used extensively if physiotherapy fails. It has been successfully used alone or combined with a steroid injection or with an arthroscopic capsular release, and usually results in a rapid return of movement of the shoulder [25].

13.6 Surgical Treatment

My indications for arthroscopic treatment of shoulder stiffness are as follows [12]: limitation of active and passive range of motion, pain and dysfunction, at least 6 weeks of conservative treatment without progress, and symptoms for at least 3 months. Patients were subjected to arthroscopic capsular release if a closed manipulation did not restore at least 80 % of the range of motion of the normal, contralateral shoulder in all planes. It is my opinion that the major role of an arthroscopic treatment for shoulder stiffness is fast recovery and long-term efficacy.

I released the capsule using electrocautery from the anterior portal after diagnostic arthroscopy from the posterior portal in the lateral position. I did not release

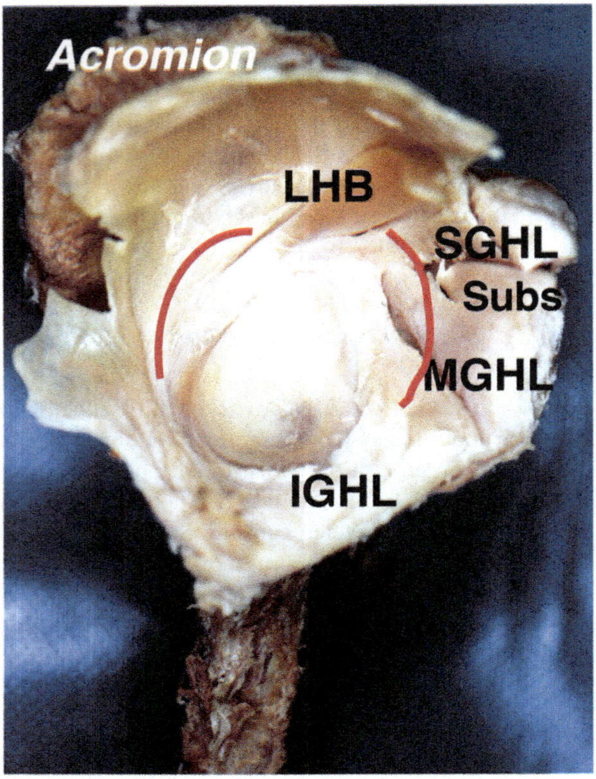

Fig. 13.5 Arthroscopic capsular release. Cadaveric specimen demonstrating capsular release (*red line*). Using electrocautery, we released the capsule including the superior glenohumeral ligament (*SGHL*) rotator interval, the middle glenohumeral ligament (*MGHL*), the anterior band of the inferior glenohumeral ligament (*IGHL*), the coracohumeral ligament extraarticularly, and/or the intraarticular portion of the subscapularis (*SubS*). To avoid axillary nerve injury, we did not release the inferior portion of the IGHL

the whole portion of the capsule, especially the inferior portion, if adequate range of motion was restored. A release of the superior and middle glenohumeral ligaments, the rotator interval, the coracohumeral ligament extraarticularly, or the intraarticular portion of the subscapularis was performed for loss of external rotation; a release of the anterior-inferior capsule including the anterior band of the inferior glenohumeral ligament was performed for loss of elevation; and a posterosuperior capsular release was performed for loss of internal rotation [12] (Fig. 13.5).

Preoperative pain and function of the shoulder joints in my patients were significantly improved at 4 weeks after the operation, and 91 % continued to be in good condition for a mean of 7.5 years [12]. There were no complications related to the arthroscopic procedure. I recommend selective arthroscopic capsular release for shoulder stiffness for which physiotherapy and manipulation under anesthesia have failed.

Intensive rehabilitation should begin immediately postoperatively with daily stretching exercises. Continuous passive motion (CPM) machines may also be useful to maintain movement, although controversy persists concerning the use of CPM machine exercise in patients with restricted shoulder motion. CPM exercise

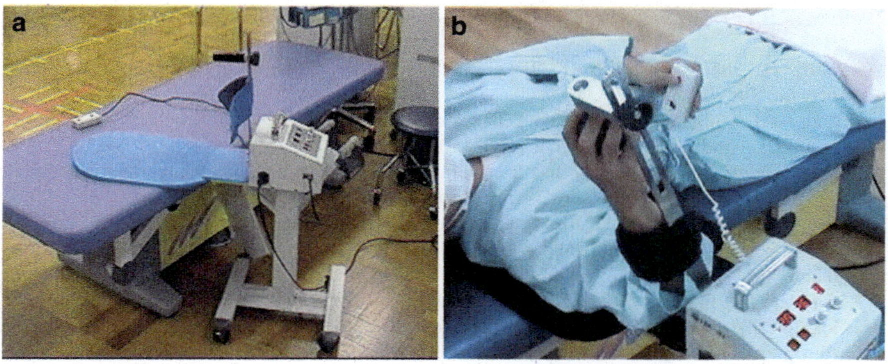

Fig. 13.6 (**a**) Continuous passive motion (CPM) machine providing for external and internal rotating motion of the shoulder joint (**b**) in abduction in the supine position, which supports scapular stability

may be useful in retaining the range of motion of the shoulder joint after restoring it by arthroscopic capsular release [12]. The CPM machine design in this study provides for external and internal rotating motion of the shoulder joint in abduction in the supine position, which supports scapular stability (Fig. 13.6).

The extent of capsular release depends on clinical judgement: some authors have advocated routinely performing a '360-degree' release [26], whereas others have adopted a more cautious approach [12, 27, 28]. Le Lievre and Murrell reported that shoulder range of motion at 7 years after 360° arthroscopic capsular release in patients with idiopathic adhesive capsulitis was equivalent to that in the contralateral shoulder, in contrast to results reported for nonoperative treatment [29]. Further investigation is needed to determine the optimal extent of the release.

References

1. Codman EA (1934) The shoulder. G. Miller, New York, pp 216–224
2. Duplay ES (1872) De la pe'riarthrite scapulohume'rale et des raideurs de l'epaule qui en son la consequence. Arch Gen Med 20:513–542
3. Neviaser JS (1945) Adhesive capsulitis of the shoulder. J Bone Joint Surg 27:211–222
4. Bunker TD, Schranz PJ (1998) Clinical challenges in orthopaedics: the shoulder. ISIS Medical Media, Oxford
5. Zuckerman JD, Rokito A (2011) Frozen shoulder: a consensus definition. J Shoulder Elbow Surg 20:322–325
6. Bridgman JF (1972) Periarthritis of the shoulder and diabetes mellitus. Ann Rheum Dis 31:69–71
7. Tighe CB, Oakley WS Jr (2008) The prevalence of a diabetic condition and adhesive capsulitis of the shoulder. South Med J 101:591–595
8. Grey RG (1978) The natural history of "idiopathic" frozen shoulder. J Bone Joint Surg Am 60:564

9. Reeves B (1975) The natural history of the frozen shoulder syndrome. Scand J Rheumatol 4:193–196
10. Shaffer B, Tibone JE, Kerlan RK (1992) Frozen shoulder. A long-term follow-up. J Bone Joint Surg Am 74:738–746
11. Binder AI, Bulgen DY, Hazleman BL, Roberts S (1984) Frozen shoulder: a long-term prospective study. Ann Rheum Dis 43:361–364
12. Ide J, Takagi K (2004) Early and long-term results of arthroscopic treatment for shoulder stiffness. J Shoulder Elbow Surg 13:174–179
13. Emig EW, Schweitzer ME, Karasick D, Lubowitz J (1995) Adhesive capsulitis of the shoulder. MR diagnosis. Am J Roentgenol 164:1457–1459
14. Gokalp G, Algin O, Yildirim N, Yazici Z (2011) Adhesive capsulitis: contrast-enhanced shoulder MRI findings. J Med Imaging Radiat Oncol 55:119–125
15. Gokalp MB, Pfirrmann CW, Gerber C, Hodler J, Zanetti M (2004) Frozen shoulder: MR arthrographic findings. Radiology 233:486–492
16. Zhao W, Zheng X, Liu Y, Yang W, Amirbekian V, Diaz LE, Huang X (2012) An MRI study of symptomatic adhesive capsulitis. PLoS One 7:e47277
17. Tamai K, Yamato M (1997) Abnormal synovium in the frozen shoulder. A preliminary report with dynamic magnetic resonance imaging. J Should Elbow Surg 6:534–543
18. Müller LP, Müller LA, Happ J, Kerschbaumer F (2000) Frozen shoulder: a sympathetic dystrophy? Arch Orthop Trauma Surg 120:84–87
19. Senocak O, Degirmenci B, Ozdogan O, Akalin E, Arslan G, Kaner B, Tasci C, Peker O (2002) Technetium-99m human immunoglobulin scintigraphy in patients with adhesive capsulitis: a correlative study with bone scintigraphy. Ann Nucl Med 16:243–248
20. Rookmoneea M, Dennis L, Brealey S et al (2010) The effectiveness of interventions in the management of patients with primary frozen shoulder. J Bone Joint Surg Br 92:1267–1272
21. Green S, Buchbinder R, Hetrick S (2003) Physiotherapy interventions for shoulder pain. Cochrane Database Syst Rev 2:CD004258
22. Robinson CM, Seah KT, Chee YH, Hindle P, Murray IR (2012) Frozen shoulder. J Bone Joint Surg Br 94:1–9
23. Buchbinder R, Green S, Youd JM (2003) Corticosteroid injections for shoulder pain. Cochrane Database Syst Rev 1:CD004016
24. Buchbinder R, Hoving JL, Green S, Hall S, Forbes A, Nash P (2004) Short course prednisolone for adhesive capsulitis (frozen shoulder or stiff painful shoulder): a randomised, double blind, placebo controlled trial. Ann Rheum Dis 63:1460–1469
25. Thomas WJ, Jenkins EF, Owen JM, Sangster MJ, Kirubanandan R, Beynon C, Woods DA (2011) Treatment of frozen shoulder by manipulation under anaesthetic and injection: does the timing of treatment affect the outcome? J Bone Joint Surg Br 93:1377–1381
26. Jerosch J (2001) 360 degrees arthroscopic capsular release in patients with adhesive capsulitis of the glenohumeral joint: indication, surgical technique, results. Knee Surg Sports Traumatol Arthrosc 9:178–186
27. Harryman DT 2nd (1993) Shoulders: frozen and stiff. Instr Course Lect 42:247–257
28. Warner JJ, Allen A, Marks PH, Wong P (1996) Arthroscopic release for chronic, refractory adhesive capsulitis of the shoulder. J Bone Joint Surg Am 78:1808–1816
29. Le Lievre HM, Murrell GA (2012) Long-term outcomes after arthroscopic capsular release for idiopathic adhesive capsulitis. J Bone Joint Surg Am 94:1208–1212

Chapter 14
Nerve Lesions Around the Shoulder

Naoyuki Ochiai

Abstract The shoulder girdle, composed of the scapula, the humerus, and the clavicula, is held on the trunk mainly by outer muscles and connects skeletally to the trunk only at the sternoclavicular joint: that is the main reason why the shoulder joint in the broad sense has a quite large range of motion. The shoulder joint in the narrow sense consists of the humerus and the scapula. The inner and outer muscles control its movement. Lesions of the nerves that innervate the outer and inner muscles disturb the complex but harmonious movements of the shoulder girdle, and the scapulohumeral rhythm is lost.

In this chapter, relative popular and clinically important nerve lesions are covered; not only the topics to which Japanese orthopedic surgeons have contributed but also current important issues are introduced.

Keywords Peripheral nerve injuries • Flail shoulder • Winging scapula • Misdirection • Nerve repair

14.1 Axillary Nerve Lesions

14.1.1 Anatomy

The axillary nerve diverges from the posterior cord of the brachial plexus just distal to the coracoid process, passes posteriorly through the quadrilateral space and just inferior to the shoulder joint capsule, and turns laterally around the humeral neck under the deltoid. It has fifth and sixth cervical nerve root components and innervates the teres minor and the deltoid and also the lateral cutaneous area of the shoulder. However, in quite a few cases it innervates no cutaneous area. The fact is important because absence of sensory loss does not guarantee that the axillary nerve is intact.

N. Ochiai (✉)
Kikkoman General Hospital, 100 Miyazaki, Noda, Chiba 728-0005, Japan
e-mail: ochiainaoyuki@ob.md.tsukuba.ac.jp

K. Tamai et al. (eds.), *Advances in Shoulder Surgery*,
DOI 10.1007/978-4-431-55988-7_14

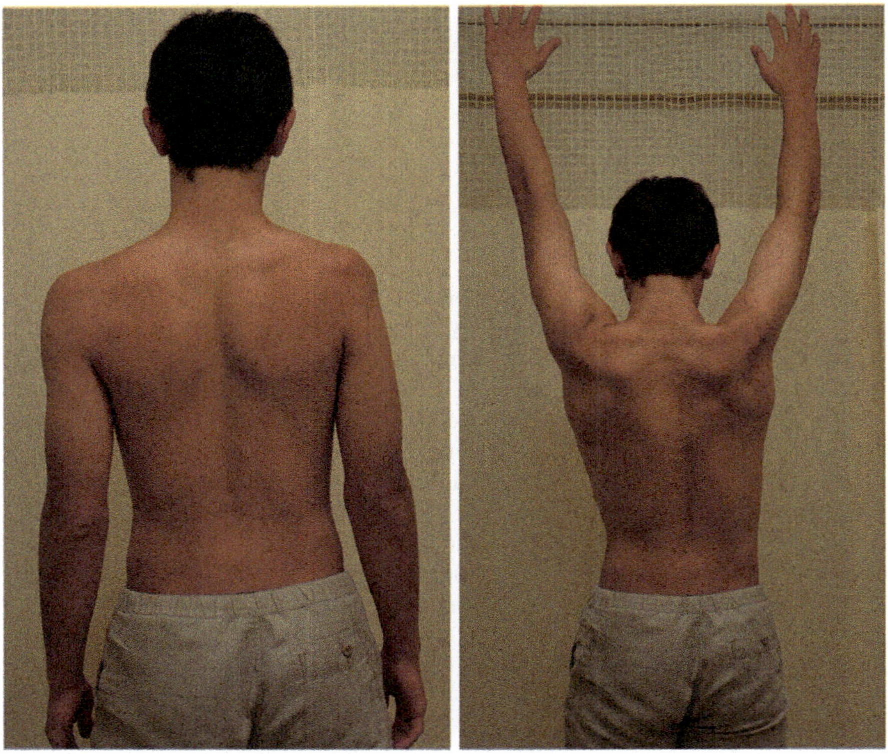

Fig. 14.1 Even though the right axillary nerve is paralyzed, the patient can abduct his right shoulder joint fully

14.1.2 Clinical Symptoms and Signs

The deltoid is not only a strong abductor but also a flexor and an extensor of the shoulder joint. However, in isolate paralysis of the axillary nerve, if the suprascapular nerve is intact, the patient can abduct the shoulder joint completely (Fig. 14.1). To avoid misdiagnosis, it is important to verify the deltoid atrophy and no muscle contraction in visual examination and palpation. Fujihara et al. proposed the "akimbo test" [1]: patients with axillary nerve paralysis cannot place their pronated hands on the iliac crest with abduction in the coronal plane and internal rotation of the shoulder joint because the posture eliminates compensation of the biceps brachii and the supraspinatus.

In axillary nerve injury, the teres minor, an external rotator, is also paralyzed but the infraspinatus compensates for the paralysis.

Generally, sensory disturbance appears at the lateral small area of the shoulder.

14.1.3 Causes of Paralysis

Axillary nerve injury occurs so often as a complication of shoulder joint dislocation. Fortunately, the nerve suffers generally from lesion in continuity, which means neurapraxia or axonotmesis. Manual reduction of the dislocation follows spontaneous recovery of the paralysis within several months. An isolate axillary paralysis also supervenes on severe contusion around the shoulder. In this case, even though without dislocation, the axillary nerve often ruptures between its fork from the posterior cord and the quadrilateral space. Surgical intervention such as free nerve grafting or nerve transfer is required [2, 3].

Recently, iatrogenic injuries of the axillary nerve have increased: first, ligation of the nerve under arthroscopic surgery for rotator cuff repair; second, thermal damage by radiofrequency for shrinkage of the joint capsule [4]; third, traction injury by reverse type of total shoulder arthroplasty [5]; and fourth, by drilling screw holes in MIPO (minimum invasive plate osteosynthesis) technique for proximal humeral shaft fracture [6]. Surgeons should pay much more attention to avoiding nerve injury during such surgery.

Deltoid paralysis appears also as a part of signs in the neuralgic amyotrophy, in which typical severe pain around the neck, shoulder, and upper arm precedes and continues 1 week or more. Just after the pain subsides, shoulder girdle muscles become paralyzed and develop severe atrophy. Usually the paralysis recovers within 1 year or more.

14.1.4 Treatments

In a complete paralysis after trauma, monthly electromyography is essential. If reinnervation potentials are not recorded within 4 months, surgical exploration is mandatory.

Good results can be expected by free sural nerve grafting, if surgical intervention is performed at least within 6 months, ideally within 4 months [7]. It will take 1.5 years until complete recovery. Recently, funicular transfer of the motor branch to the long head of the triceps brachii of the radial nerve to the distal stump of the axillary nerve is becoming popular. This procedure shortens the reinnervation time, because axonal regeneration distance is shortened.

Nishijima et al. described the “swallow-tail sign” to detect early recovery, in which the initial recovery of the posterior part of the deltoid, owing to the anatomic course of the nerve, starts in extension of the glenohumeral joint [8].

In case of no indication for nerve repair, shoulder functions are reconstructed by muscle and tendon transfer. The multiple muscle transfer of Saha is the basic concept of various methods [9]. Transferring the trapezius, the latissimus dorsi, and the clavicular head of the pectoralis major are representative.

14.2 Suprascapular Nerve Lesions

14.2.1 Anatomy

The suprascapular nerve diverges from the upper trunk of the brachial plexus at the posterior triangle, passes inferolaterally along the omohyoid to the suprascapular notch. Through the notch under the transverse ligament, the nerve traverses the supraspinous fossa and runs posteroinferiorly along the spinoglenoid notch to the infraspinous fossa. It has fifth and sixth cervical nerve root components and innervates the supraspinatus and the infraspinatus and also the glenohumeral capsule.

14.2.2 Clinical Symptoms and Signs

The supraspinatus and the infraspinatus are important parts of the rotator cuff muscles and act as the steering muscles of the humeral head. In acute traumatic paralysis the patient cannot abduct the shoulder joint and feels weakness in external rotation. In this situation rupture of the rotator cuff should be distinguished from paralysis with magnetic resonance imaging (MRI) (Fig. 14.2). However, in gradually developed paralysis, the patient can abduct the shoulder joint by compensatory action of other muscles. When muscle atrophy progresses, the infraspinous fossa becomes concave in appearance; however, supraspinous atrophy cannot be detected because it is hidden by the trapezius.

In the early phase of entrapment syndrome of the nerve, the patient complains of shoulder girdle pain.

14.2.3 Causes of Paralysis

Isolated suprascapular nerve paralysis is very rare. The overthrow motions in various kinds of sport performance induce entrapment neuropathy at the scapular or spinoglenoid notch where the nerve is repetitively compressed or stretched. Isolated infraspinatus paralysis occurs in volleyball or baseball players. Cummins et al. insist entrapment neuropathy is caused by the spinoglenoid ligament [10]. However, Ferrtti explains repetitive traction injury of the motor branch by eccentric contraction of the infraspinatus during sports performance [11].

The ganglion from the posterior shoulder joint capsule causes localized compression neuropathy of the nerve. Depending on its location, both supraspinatus and infraspinatus paralysis or isolated infraspinatus paralysis develops.

Recently, iatrogenic injuries of the suprascapular nerve have been reported [12]: first, by drilling holes for anchoring sutures during arthroscopic surgery for SLAP

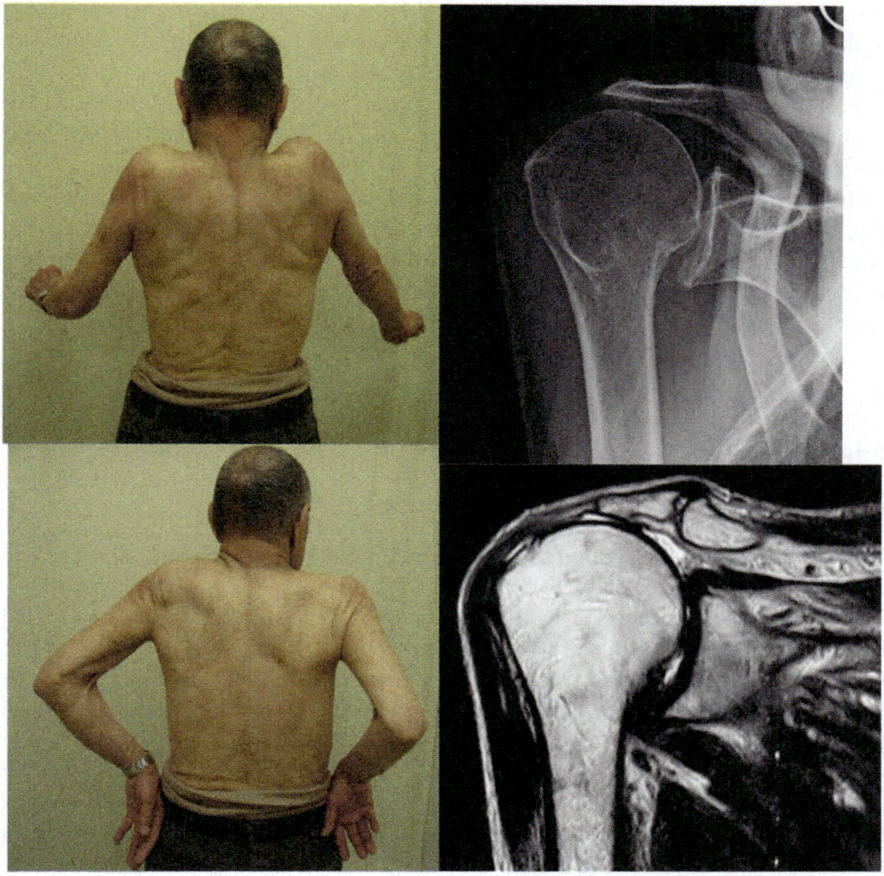

Fig. 14.2 This patient cannot abduct both shoulder joints but takes the akimbo posture. Both infraspinatus show severe atrophy. Magnetic resonance imaging (MRI) shows complete rupture of the rotator cuff. *EMG* verified nonneurogenic

lesion [13, 14]; and second, by drilling for fixation of the reverse type of total shoulder arthroplasty [15].

In addition, massive rupture of the rotator cuff itself also induces traction injury to the nerve [16].

14.2.4 Treatments

Neurolysis is indicated for entrapment neuropathy in which resection of the transverse ligament and/or spinoglenoid ligament and bony plasty of the scapular notch and the spinoglenoid notch are performed. However, the overuse syndrome in sport activity is usually asymptomatic. If the athletes can continue their performance without difficulties, the muscle shows complete atrophy, and the lesion is old, surgeons should be cautious in operative intervention.

Ganglion is resected by conventional method or arthroscopically. In the SLAP lesion with ganglion, not only resection of ganglion but also repairing the lesion itself is essential [17].

In the traumatic brachial plexus injury, nerve repair by direct neurorrhaphy or free nerve grafting is indicated. Recently, nerve transfer using a part of the accessory nerve has become popular. Ando showed the motor branch of the accessory nerve is transferred without paralysis of the upper part of the trapezius [18].

14.3 Combined Injury of the Axillary and Suprascapular Nerves

This type of injury is a subgroup of the traumatic brachial plexus injuries. The author reviewed retrospectively the files of axillary nerve injuries in Tokyo University Hospital for more than 30 years previously and found half of so-called solitary axillary nerve injuries were accompanied by incomplete paresis of the suprascapular nerve, which was proved by electromyographic findings [19]. The author was impressed by Seddon's textbook, which mentioned the combined injuries even though in a few words [20].

Thereafter, the author found a small group of patients who could not abduct the shoulder joint; however, they showed the biceps brachii and the brachioradialis were normal or slightly weak if at all. They were diagnosed as suffering from a lesion in continuity of C5,C6 type brachial plexus injuries (BPI). However, the prognosis of the shoulder was poor. The author supposed the lesions were simultaneous injuries of the suprascapular and axillary nerves from the former investigation. In 1983 the author explored and found rupture of the nerves at their fork respectively from the plexus. Alnot described the results of nerve grafting in the suprascapular nerve as being unforeseeable [21].

The author and colleagues found that the suprascapular nerve lesions spread from the fork of the upper trunk to the terminal at the infraspinatus and also exist at multiple sites as resulting from traction injuries. Hence, it is mandatory to explore the whole course of the nerve for success in nerve grafting. The author developed a new approach for nerve grafting for both axillary and suprascapular nerves and achieved excellent results [2, 22] (Fig. 14.3).

In severe BPI such as the total type, as many functions as possible must be reconstructed; however, resources of donor nerves are limited. Suzuki et al. then described reconstruction of the supraspinatus as being enough for shoulder stabilization [23]. However, in case of combined injury restricted in the axillary and suprascapular nerves, repair of both nerves is essential for strong shoulder function.

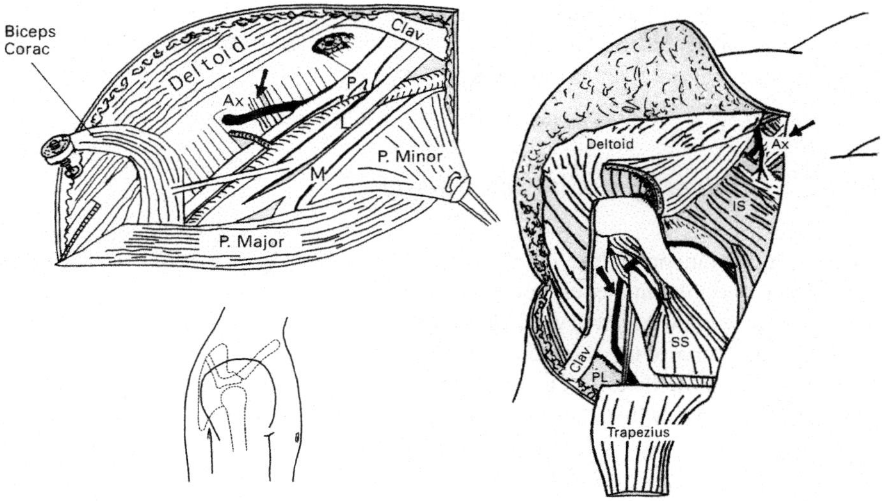

Fig. 14.3 New approach for full exposure of the axillary and suprascapular nerves. *Left above*: anterior approach for the axillary nerve. *Right*: posterior approach for the suprascapular nerve. *Left below*: Skin incision. (From Ochiai et al. [22], Figs. 14.1, 14.2, 14.3, with permission)

For the differential diagnosis between the combined nerve injuries from the C5,C6 type BPI, the discrepancy of muscle power is an important clue; that is, the deltoid and the infraspinatus shows [0] in manual muscle testing (MMT), even though the biceps brachii and brachioradialis remain almost normal [24].

Monthly electromyography is essential in the course of treatment. If reinnervation potentials are not recorded in the deltoid and the infraspinatus within 4 months, surgical exploration is mandatory.

Good result can be expected by free sural nerve grafting, if surgical intervention is performed at least within 6 months, ideally within 4 months. As Mikami et al. described reinnervation of both the supraspinatus and the infraspinatus is not essential, at least the infraspinatus must be reinnervated for good shoulder function [2]. If recovery of the infraspinatus is poor, the author prefers to transfer the latissimus dorsi to the infraspinatus insertion of the humerus.

14.4 Musculocutaneous Nerve Lesions

14.4.1 Anatomy

The musculocutaneous nerve diverges from the lateral cord of the brachial plexus under the pectoralis minor, passes laterally through the coracobrachialis and between the biceps brachii and the brachialis, and finally becomes the lateral cutaneous nerve of the forearm. It has fifth and sixth cervical nerve root components and innervates the coracobrachialis, the biceps brachii, and the brachialis muscles and also the lateral cutaneous area of the forearm. In an extremely rare case it has also a seventh cervical nerve root component.

14.4.2 Clinical Symptoms and Signs

The musculocutaneous nerve innervates elbow flexors. However, in isolate paralysis of the musculocutaneous nerve, the brachioradialis innervated by the radial nerve works even though it is weak as an elbow flexor, especially in forearm neutral position. The pronator teres and the common flexors in the forearm also compensate for paralyzed elbow flexors. The phenomenon is called Steindler's effect.

Generally, sensory disturbance appears at the lateral narrow area of the forearm.

14.4.3 Causes of Paralysis

Isolate paralysis of the musculocutaneous nerve is extremely rare. There is a report that in weight lifters repetitive strong contraction of elbow flexors damages the motor branches in the muscles themselves [25]. Musculocutaneous nerve injury occurs often as a part of the BPI.

Recently, iatrogenic injuries of the musculocutaneous nerve have increased. First, during transfer of the part of the coracoid process with conjoint tendons (Latarjet procedure, Bristow procedure) for stabilization of the shoulder joint, transient paralysis of the musculocutaneous nerve occurs [26]; second, drilling screw holes in MIPO (minimum invasive plate osteosynthesis technique) of the humeral shaft fracture [27]; and third, mal-positioning of the upper extremity during total shoulder arthroplasty [28]. Surgeons must pay much more attention to avoid nerve injury during these surgeries.

Biceps brachii paralysis appears also as a part of syndromes in neuralgic amyotrophy.

14.4.4 Treatments

In neuralgic amyotrophy and in weight lifters, there is no need for surgical intervention to the nerve. A good prognosis can be expected.

In complete paralysis after trauma, nerve repair such as neurorrhaphy or free nerve grafting is indicated. In the BPI including birth palsy, free nerve grafting and nerve transfer of the intercostal nerves, the accessory nerves, the phrenic nerves, medial pectoral nerve, and a funicule of the ulnar nerve or median nerve are indicated case by case. It is better to repair the nerve within 6 months after trauma.

If more than 6 months pass after trauma, muscle transfer of the latissimus dorsi, the pectoralis major, Steindler procedure, or free vascularized muscle transplantation is indicated.

14.5 Accessory Nerve Lesions

14.5.1 Anatomy

The accessory nerve, the XIth cranial nerve, arises from the medulla and upper cervical spinal cord, and leaves the cranial cavity through the jugular foramen and runs under the digastrics, sending a motor branch to the sternocleidomastoid, into the posterior triangle of the neck where the nerve runs superficially on the fascia carpet of the posterior triangle. It then descends deeply along the trapezius to innervate its upper, middle, and lower part.

14.5.2 Clinical Symptoms and Signs

The main clinical features are atrophy of the trapezius, dull pain around the shoulder, and limited active shoulder abduction. Because the trapezius is an anti-gravity muscle, the impaired shoulder drops. It is difficult to shrug the shoulder against resistance. During forward elevation of the upper extremity, especially under resistance, winging of the posteromedial corner of the scapula stands out [29]. During abduction the lower angle of the scapula rotates anterolaterally, the distance between the spinal process and the medial border of the scapula widens, and contraction of the clavicular head of the pectoralis major is marked.

14.5.3 Causes

Accessory nerve injury is mainly iatrogenic during biopsy of the cervical lymph nodes in the posterior triangle, and sometimes accompanies the BPI. In these cases only the trapezius is paralyzed and the sternocleidomastoid is intact. In idiopathic paralysis not only the trapezius but also the sternocleidomastoid are paralyzed. However, the author has no experience.

14.5.4 Treatment

Clean-cut injury of the accessory nerve and the iatrogenic one should be repaired by end-to-end suture or free nerve grafting within 1 year after injury [30, 31]. Teboul et al. reported that if repair is within 20 months after the injury and the patient younger than 50 years of age, good results can be expected from a repair of the accessory nerve [32]. In the case in which more than 1 year passed since injury, it is important to train muscles around the shoulder girdle to compensate for the paralyzed trapezius. If impairment is strong, reconstruction of shoulder abduction is indicated with Eden–Lange muscle transfer in which the levator scapulae is transferred to the acromion and the rhomboid to the lateral edge of the infraspinous fossa [33].

14.6 Long Thoracic Nerve Lesions

14.6.1 Anatomy

The long thoracic nerve is composed from the fifth, sixth, and seventh cervical nerve root components. The motor branch diverges from each nerve root at the exit from the intervertebral foramen. The branches from the fifth and sixth cervical nerve root run laterally through the scalenus medius, and the branch from the seventh cervical nerve root runs laterally anterior to the scalenus medius. These three branches join to form the long thoracic nerve and descend dorsal to the brachial plexus along the thoracic wall innervating the serratus anterior. From an anatomic point of view, the nerve is liable to repetitive traction injuries during sport performance.

14.6.2 Clinical Symptoms and Signs

The main clinical feature is a winging scapula during anterior elevation of the upper extremity because the paralyzed serratus anterior cannot fix the medial border of the scapula to the thoracic wall. The patient cannot push the shoulder girdle anteriorly.

14.6.3 Causes

In sport performance, repetitive motion in rotation and lateral bending of the neck toward the opposite direction, elevation of the upper extremity, and anteropulsion of the shoulder causes traction injury to the nerve because freedom of the nerve is relatively restricted between the scalenus medius and the branch to the upper part of the serratus anterior.

Serratus anterior paralysis appears also as a part of signs in neuralgic amyotrophy.

14.6.4 Treatment

Generally, isolated paralysis of the long thoracic nerve is treated nonsurgically and a good prognosis can be expected. In a case refractory to nonsurgical treatment, surgical intervention is indicated. As the static method, there is a scapulopexy in which the scapular medial border is fixed to the spinous process of the fourth, fifth, sixth, and seventh thoracic vertebrae with fascial bund from the fascia lata. As the dynamic method, the pectoralis minor or a part of the pectoralis major is transferred to the scapular body [34].

However, Nath et al. and LeNail et al. reported neurolysis was effective in the entrapment neuropathy of the long thoracic nerve [35, 36]. Tomaino reported a case in which medial pectoral nerve transfer to the long thoracic nerve was effective [37].

14.7 Brachial Plexus Injuries

14.7.1 Anatomy

The anterior branches of the four cervical nerve roots (C5–C8) and one thoracic nerve root (D1) forms the brachial plexus just beyond the scalene muscles. The posterior branches, coming from each nerve root just after their exit from the intervertebral foramen, innervates paravertebral muscles and cutaneous sensation of the posterior part of the neck and shoulder girdle.

The upper two anterior branches join to form the upper trunk, the anterior branch of the C7 root continues as the middle trunk, and the lower two anterior branches unite into the lower trunk. All three trunks proceed distally behind the clavicle and each separates into anterior and posterior divisions. The three posterior divisions unite to form a posterior cord behind the subclavian artery. It separates the subscapular nerve, the thoracodorsal nerve, the axillary nerve, and continues as the radial nerve. The subscapular nerve innervates the subscapularis and the teres major.

The upper two anterior divisions unite to form the lateral cord locating lateral to the subclavian and axillary artery. It separates the lateral pectoral nerve, then the musculocutaneous nerve just distal to the coracoid process, and continues as the part of median nerve. The lateral pectoral nerve innervates the clavicular head of the pectoralis major and the pectoralis minor.

The lower anterior division continues as the medial cord medial to the subclavian and axillary artery. It separates the medial pectoral nerve and the part of the median nerve, then continues as the ulnar nerve. The medial pectoral nerve innervates the sternal head of the pectoralis major and the pectoralis minor.

The long thoracic nerve is composed of the branches from C5, C6, and C7 roots. The nerve proceeds distally in the neck behind the brachial plexus, continues along the thoracic wall, and innervates the serratus anterior. The C5 root also divides off the dorsal scapular nerve. It continues distally in the neck behind the brachial plexus along the medial border of the scapula. It innervates the levator scapulae and the rhomboid major and minor. The suprascapular nerve comes from the upper trunk in the posterior triangle of the neck.

14.7.2 Clinical Symptoms and Signs

The author analyzed muscle paralytic patterns of several types of the BPI classified based on the myelogram and the intraoperative recording of the somatosensory evoked potential in 33 cases. The results are as follows [38, 39].

14.7.2.1 C5,C6 Type Injuries

The supraspinatus, the infraspinatus, the deltoid, the biceps brachii, the brachialis, the brachioradialis, and the supinator are paralyzed. Active abduction and external rotation of the shoulder are impaired. Active flexion of the elbow and supination of the forearm are also impossible. There is dull sensation over the cutaneous area of the shoulder and the lateral part of the forearm.

14.7.2.2 C5, C6, C7 Type Injuries

Adding to the clinical picture of C5,C6 type injuries, C5,C6,C7 type injuries show paralysis of the serratus anterior and the clavicular head of the pectoralis major. In the one thirds the triceps brachii, the extensor carpi radialis, the extensor digitorum communis, and the extensor pollicis longus are paralyzed.

The flexor carpi radialis paralyzes less than MMT (2) in 100 % and MMT (0) in 70 %. Paralysis of the flexor carpi radialis and the clavicular head of the pectoralis major are important signs of C7 root injury. The flexor digitorum superficialis, the flexor digitorum profundus, the flexor pollicis longus, and intrinsic muscles do not become paralyzed.

There is dull sensation over the lateral part of the arm, the forearm and the thumb, and the index and the long fingers. If the anesthetic area spreads into the lateral part of arm and forearm and the thumb, it suggests C5,C6,C7 injuries.

14.7.2.3 C5, C6, C7, C8 Type Injuries

All muscles of the shoulder girdle including the pectoralis major and upper arm are paralyzed.

The extensor digitorum communis is paralyzed in 100 %, the extensor carpi radialis in 80 %, and the flexor carpi radialis in 100 %. The muscles preserving more than MMT (3) are the extensor pollicis longus in 60 %, the flexor digitorum superficialis in 50 %, the flexor digitorum profundus in 70 %, the flexor pollicis longus in 80 %, the abductor pollicis brevis in 80 %, the abductor digiti minimi in 60 %, and the first interossei dorsalis in 50 %.

If the anesthetic area spreads into the lateral part of arm and forearm to the ring finger, it suggests C5, C6, C7, C8 injuries. However, the dermatome varies in every body. The author experienced that even a C5, C6, C7, C8 type injured case had no anesthetic area.

14.7.2.4 Total Root Avulsion Type Injuries

Entire muscles of the shoulder girdle and extremity become paralyzed except the trapezius. The extremity loses sensation, except the medial small area of the upper arm which is innervated by the intercostobrachial cutaneous nerve from D2 cord segment.

14.7.2.5 Subclavical Lesions

14.7.2.5.1 Posterior Cord Injury

The clinical sign is a mixture of the axillary nerve paralysis and high lesion of the radial nerve. The patient cannot elevate the shoulder and loses the extensors of the elbow, wrist, and fingers. There is dull sensation over the lateral part of the shoulder and the dorsum of the first web.

14.7.2.5.2 Lateral Cord Injury

The biceps brachii and the brachialis innervated by the musculocutaneous nerve are paralyzed; however, patients can flex their elbow because the brachioradialis compensates for paralyzed elbow flexors. The pronater teres innervated by the part of the median nerve (C5, C6 components) is paralyzed and the wrist flexor weakens slightly.

There is dull sensation over the lateral part of the forearm, the thumb, and the index finger.

14.7.2.5.3 Medial Cord Injury

The muscles innervated by the median and the ulnar nerve except the pronator teres and the flexor carpi radialis are paralyzed. There is numbness over the hand and the medial part of the forearm.

14.7.3 Causes of Paralysis

Open penetrating wounds of the brachial plexus rarely occur in civilian life. Closed injuries of the brachial plexus are usually caused by mechanisms that forcefully widen the interval between the head and shoulder and stretch the elements of the brachial plexus, causing varying degree of injuries, such as root avulsion from the cord to the neurapraxia. The properties in stretched injuries are completely different from clean-cut injuries. In the former neural elements injured in various grades are scattered in a wide area along the plexus as if a straw rope is stretched. In Japan, motorcycle accidents are the most common causes. Others are the birth palsy caused by manipulating infants in delivery and contact sports such as rugby. Transient compression palsy occurs in a case of carrying a heavy rucksack and malpositioning the upper extremity during general anesthesia, etc. Nontraumatic causes are irradiation, neural tumor, neuritis, and psychosomatic lesions.

14.7.4 Diagnosis

Determination of the exact site of the lesion in the involved roots is important, because if the roots are avulsed from the cord, that is, a preganglionic lesion, a spontaneous recovery is impossible and surgical repair of the roots cannot be performed. By contrast, in postganglionic lesions where nerve roots are injured at the extraforaminal region, repairing the plexus is possible by surgical intervention.

To reach the correct diagnosis, detailed medical history and physical examination including MMT, sensory disturbance area, Tinel's sign, Horner's sign, and whether there are fractures such as the transverse process of the seventh cervical vertebra, the scapula, and ribs are essential. After classifying the paralysis pattern, using electrophysiological examination and MRI-myelogram or conventional myelogram and myelo-CT, degrees of injury in each nerve root are speculated. If at least one root appears avulsed, surgical exploration should be indicated. Surgical exploration is important for confirming the degree and the location of the lesions of not only the nerve root but also the whole brachial plexus and for planning the reconstruction of neural lesions and function of the extremity.

14.7.5 Treatments

In this textbook, topics are limited to reconstruction of the shoulder joint.

14.7.5.1 For C5,C6 type injuries, if the lesions are postganglionic and within 6 months post trauma, then free nerve graftings between C5 or C6 nerve roots and the suprascapular nerve, the axillary nerve, and the musculocutaneous nerve are indicated [7]. If the lesions are preganglionic, a motor branch of the accessory nerve to the middle and lower part of the trapezius is transferred to the suprascapular nerve, and a motor branch of the radial nerve to the long head of the triceps brachii is transferred to the axillary nerve. The musculocutaneous nerve is neurotized by intercostal nerve crossing directly [40, 41], ulnar nerve or median nerve funicular transfer [42, 43], or the phrenic nerve transfer [44]. The author prefers intercostal nerve crossing, because the ulnar nerve funicular transfer cannot avoid co-contracture between elbow flexion and hand intrinsic muscles or gripping movement, and proposed a new method for diameter mismatched neurorrhaphy [45] (Fig. 14.4). Concerning reconstruction of the shoulder joint, Suzuki et al. insists that the priority is in the repair of the suprascapular nerve to the axillary nerve for abduction of the shoulder joint and that repair of the long thoracic nerve is important in the C5,C6,C7 type injuries to stabilize the scapula for harmonizing performance in the shoulder joint [23].

For C5 or C6 type injuries, if delayed more than 6 months post trauma, Saha's multiple muscles transfer or arthrodesis are indicated for the shoulder joint. The modified Steindler procedure or the latissimus dorsi transfer or the pectoralis major transfer is standard for the elbow flexorplasty.

14.7.5.2 For C5,C6,C7 type and C5,C6,C7,C8 type injuries and total root avulsion within 6 months post trauma, the accessory nerve transfer to the suprascapular nerve or arthrodesis is indicated to stabilize the shoulder joint and the intercostal nerve crossing to the musculocutaneous nerve for elbow flexor reconstruction. If delayed more than 6 months post trauma, for elbow flexor reconstruction the vascularized free muscle transfer is indicated [46].

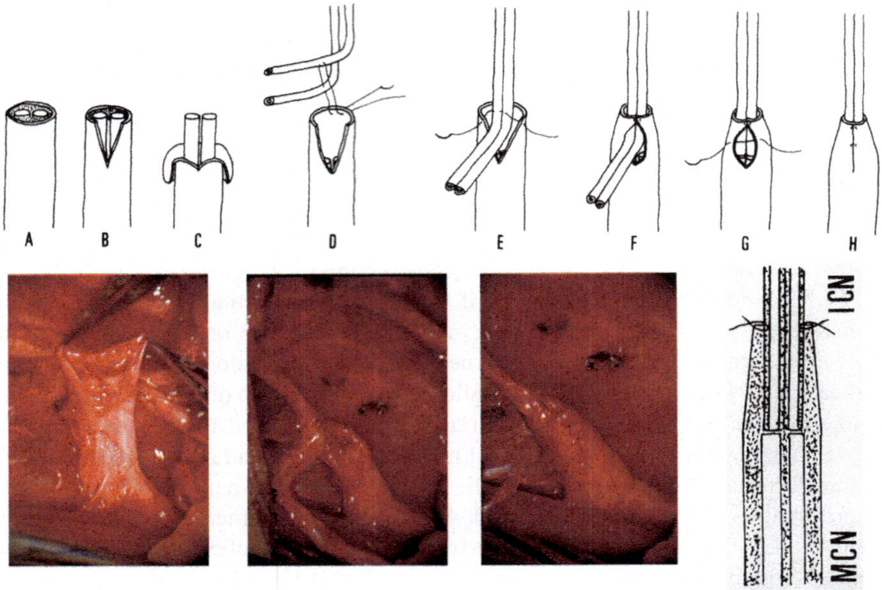

Fig. 14.4 A new technique for mismatched nerve suture. (Modified from J Hand Surg Br 18-B, Figs. 14.1 and 14.2)

14.8 Obstetrical Brachial Plexus Palsy

14.8.1 Concepts

Paralysis of the upper limb resulting from traction injury to the brachial plexus at delivery has decreased with the advent of improved obstetrical techniques. However, victims have not yet been eliminated. The injury to nerves may vary from slight stretching (neurapraxia or axonotmesis) to complete rupture (neurotmesis or root avulsion). From the natural recovery process, Kondo speculated that mechanisms of brachial plexus injuries are different between vertex delivery and breech delivery, as follows [47].

In a difficult vertex delivery, usually the infant is large and the body weight is more than 4000 g at birth. Because of disproportion between the head and body, the shoulder is impacted in the pelvic brim. The brachial plexus is injured when the shoulder is delivered by forced lateral flexion of the head and neck. Because the plexus is presumed to lie on the arc centering at the sternoclavicular joint or the first dorsal spine, the upper part of the plexus far from the center is liable to be stretched much more and injured more severely than the lower part of the plexus during the manipulation of lateral bending. As even severe cases regain some activities in the muscles innervated by the upper part of the plexus, the lesions seem to be intraneural and postganglionic in type, that is, Sunderland type 3 to 4 injuries, where misdirected reinnervation so often occurs.

In breech delivery, the birth palsy occurs in an immature baby to a large baby, that means the paralysis does relate to the manipulation during delivery rather than the figure of the infant. Traction is applied on the brachial plexus in Veit–Smellie procedure by pulling down the bilateral shoulder girdle to free the obstructed after-coming head. The traction force parallel to the axis of the neck acts as a shearing force to the plexus. The upper part of the plexus is liable to be injured much more severely than in the vertex delivery, that is, results in neurotmesis or root avulsion where no recovery is expected. Root avulsion occurs so often in the case accompanied by phrenic nerve paralysis. Sometimes bilateral BPI occur. These facts support the hypothesis of the mechanism already described.

It is generally agreed that lesions of the upper plexus are by far the most common. However, the lower plexus is sometimes at risk during a difficult breech delivery when traction is applied to the legs or trunk with the after-coming arm or arms fixed in a fully abducted position and also during difficult vertex delivery when traction is applied to a fully abducted prolapsed arm [48].

14.8.2 Clinical Symptoms and Signs

Immediately after birth the extremity exhibits a flaccid paralysis; as time passes, some muscles regain varying degrees of power. Fracture of the clavicula and separation of proximal epiphysis of the humerus must be differentiated by roentgenogram. The paralytic typing should be judged at 3 months after birth, when the plexus recovers from neurapraxia and the best possible assessment of the damage can be made.

14.8.2.1 Upper Type (C5,C6,(C7) Type)

The flexion, abduction, external rotation of the shoulder joint, flexion of the elbow joint, and supination of the forearm are impaired. If the C7 component is injured also, the elbow extensor and forearm extensors become weak; especially, the extensor carpi radialis is characteristically impaired. The waiter's tip position is a typical sign; the limb is adducted and internally rotated at the shoulder joint, extended at the elbow joint, and the forearm is pronated and flexed at the wrist joint, because the antagonistic muscles are paralyzed in each joint.

Sensory disturbance, if any, exists over the posterolateral aspect of the shoulder.

14.8.2.2 Total Type (C5–D1 Type)

The extremity exhibits a completely flaccid paralysis or weak finger flexors.

14.8.3 Prognosis

The quality of the recovery is greatly influenced by the severity of the injury [45].

In vertex delivery, if the deltoid and biceps brachii resume muscle contraction within 1 month, complete recovery is expected. If the deltoid and the biceps brachii show no muscle contraction, and however the extensors of wrist and finger initiate contraction until 3 months, almost complete recovery is expected. If the extensors of wrist and finger show no muscle contraction at 3 months, muscles innervated by the upper part of the plexus run into co-contraction and smooth movements of the shoulder and elbow joints are unexpected. If the deltoid and the biceps brachii resume no muscle contraction at 6 months, co-contraction appears in whole muscles of the extremity and finger functions are also impaired.

In breech delivery, if phrenic nerve palsy is accompanied or the deltoid and biceps brachii show no muscle contraction within 3 months, prognosis is poor. If the extensors carpi radialis shows muscle contraction within 3 months, complete recovery is expected. When the muscles innervated by the upper part of the plexus start muscle contraction after 5 months, they show co-contraction, and smooth movements of the shoulder and elbow joints are unexpected.

14.8.4 Treatment

Joint movements should be maintained with early physical therapy, and joint contractures should be prevented. Treatment must be conservative in the initial stages until the best possible assessment of the damage can be made at 3–6 months.

In the fourth quarter of the twentieth century, development of excellent microsurgical technique made it possible to resume neurosurgical intervention into obstetrical BPI. The operative targets are mainly the function of the shoulder and elbow joints. Operative intervention is practicable at 3 to 6 months on the basis of the prognostic judgment.

The operative procedures for neural reconstruction of the shoulder and elbow function are the same as the procedures in the adult BPI, that is, neurotization of the suprascapular nerve, the axillary nerve, and the musculocutaneous nerve by free nerve grafting or transferring of the accessory nerve, intercostal nerves, and the funiculus of the ulnar, median, radial, and medial pectoral nerves [49–52].

In older children, the Sever or L'Episcopo procedure is indicated for releasing the adducted and internally rotated shoulder joint. The trapezius and the latissimus dorsi transfer are indicated for abduction of the shoulder joint. The Steindler procedure is indicated for elbow flexion.

If co-contracture of the biceps brachii and the triceps brachii hinder the smooth movement of the elbow joint, intercostal nerve transfer to the musculocutaneous nerve is effective to regain smooth elbow function [53].

References

1. Fujihara Y, Doi K, Dodakundi C et al (2012) Simple clinical test to detect deltoid muscle dysfunction causing weakness of abduction – "akimbo" test. J Reconstr Microsurg 28:375–379
2. Mikami Y, Nagano A, Ochiai N et al (1997) Results of nerve grafting for injuries of the axillary and suprascapular nerves. J Bone Joint Surg Br 79:527–531
3. Hems TE, Mahmood F (2012) Injuries of the terminal branches of the infraclavicular brachial plexus: patterns of injury, management and outcome. J Bone Joint Surg Br 94:799–804
4. Greis PE, Burks RT, Schickendantz MS et al (2001) Axillary nerve injury after thermal capsular shrinkage of the shoulder. J Shoulder Elbow Surg 10:231–235
5. Lädermann A, Lübbeke A, Mélis B et al (2011) Prevalence of neurologic lesions after total shoulder arthroplasty. J Bone Joint Surg Am 93(14):1288–1293
6. Riemer BL, D'Ambrosia R (1992) The risk of injury to the axillary nerve, artery, and vein from proximal locking screws of humeral intramedullary nails. Orthopedics 15:697–699
7. Ochiai N, Nagano A, Sugioka H et al (1996) Nerve grafting in brachial plexus injuries. Results of free grafts in 90 patients. J Bone Joint Surg Br 78:754–758
8. Nishijima N, Yamauro T, Fujio K et al (1995) The swallow-tail sign: a test of deltoid function. J Bone Joint Surg Br 77:152–153
9. Saha AK (1967) Surgery of the paralyzed and flail shoulder. Acta Orthop Scand 97 ((suppl)):5–90
10. Cummins CA, Bowen M, Anderson K et al (1990) Suprascapular nerve entrapment at the spinoglenoid notch in a professional baseball pitcher. Am J Sports Med 27:810–812
11. Ferrtti A, De Carli A, Fontana M (1998) Injury of the suprascapular nerve at the spinoglenoid notch. The natural history of infraspinatus atrophy in volleyball players. Am J Sports Med 26:759–763
12. Boardman ND 3rd, Cofield RH (1999) Neurologic complications of shoulder surgery. Clin Orthop Relat Res 368:44–53
13. Shisido H, Kikuchi S (2001) Injury of the suprascapular nerve in shoulder surgery: an anatomic study. J Shoulder Elbow Surg 10:372–376
14. Kim SH, Koh YG, Sung CH et al (2010) Iatrogenic suprascapular nerve injury after repair of type II SLAP lesion. Arthroscopy 26:1005–1008
15. Molony DC, Cassar Gheiti AJ, Kennedy J et al (2011) A cadaveric model for suprascapular nerve injury during glenoid component screw insertion in reverse-geometry shoulder arthroplasty. J Shoulder Elbow Surg 20:1323–1327
16. Boykin RE, Friedman DJ, Higgins LD et al (2010) Suprascapular neuropathy. J Bone Joint Surg Am 92:2348–2364
17. Fehrman DA, Orwin JF, Jennings RM (1995) Suprascapular nerve entrapment by ganglion cysts: a report of six cases with arthroscopic findings and review of the literature. Arthroscopy 11:727–734
18. Ando M (1993) Reconstruction for brachial injury by the accessory nerve: anatomy of the accessory nerve and its innervation of the trapezius. J Jpn Orthop Assoc 67:911–918
19. Ochiai N, Yagi I, Nagano A et al (1981) Axillary nerve injury. Orthop Surg 32:612–616 (in Japanese)
20. Sir Herbert Seddon (1972) Surgical disorders of the peripheral nerves. Churchill Livingstone, Edinburgh, p 176
21. Alnot JY (1999) Paralytic shoulder secondary to post-traumatic peripheral nerve lesions in the adult. Acta Orthop Belg 65:10–22
22. Ochiai N, Nagano A, Mikami Y et al (1997) Full exposure of the axillary and suprascapular nerves. J Bone Joint Surg Br 79:532–533
23. Suzuki K, Doi K, Hattori Y et al (2007) Long-term results of spinal accessory nerve transfer to the suprascapular nerve in upper-type paralysis of brachial plexus injury. J Reconstr Microsurg 23:295–299

24. Ochiai N, Nagano A, Nakagawa T et al (1990) Combined injuries of axillary and suprascapular nerves; its differential diagnosis from C5, C6 type of brachial plexus injury. Orthop Surg Traumatol 33:693–699 (in Japanese)
25. Bird JS et al (1996) Acute focal neuropathy in male weight lifters. Muscle Nerve 19:897–899
26. Shah AA, Butler RB, Romanowski J et al (2012) Short-term complications of the Latarjet procedure. J Bone Joint Surg Am 94:495–501
27. Apivatthakakal T, Patiyasikan S, Luevitoonvechkit S (2010) Danger zone for locking screw placement in minimally invasive plate osteosynthesis (MIPO) of humeral shaft fractures: a cadaveric study. Injury 41:169–172
28. Nagda SH, Rogers KJ, Sestokas AK et al (2007) Neer Award 2005: peripheral nerve function during shoulder arthroplasty using intraoperative nerve monitoring. J Shoulder Elbow Surg 16: S2–S8
29. Chan PK, Hems TE (2006) Clinical signs of accessory nerve palsy. J Trauma 60:1142–1144
30. Ogino T, Sugawara M, Minami A et al (1991) Accessory nerve injury: conservative or surgical treatment? J Hand Surg Br 16:531–536
31. Okinaga S, Nagano A, Ochiai N et al (1992) Treatment for iatrogenic accessory nerve palsies. J Jpn Soc Surg Hand 8:977–980 (in Japanese)
32. Teboul F, Bizot P, Kakkar R et al (2004) Surgical management of trapezius palsy. J Bone Joint Surg Am 86-A:1884–1890
33. Wiater JM, Bigliani LU (1999) Spinal accessory nerve injury. Clin Orthop Relat Res 368:5–16
34. Wiater JM, Flatow EL (1999) Long thoracic nerve injury. Clin Orthop Relat Res 368:17–27
35. Nath RK, Lyons AB, Bietz G (2007) Microneurolysis and decompression of long thoracic nerve injury are effective in reversing scapular winging: long-term results in 50 cases. BMC Musculoskelet Disord 8:25
36. Le Nail LR, Bacle G, Marteau E et al (2014) Isolated paralysis of the serratus anterior muscle: surgical release of the distal segment of the long thoracic nerve in 52 patients. Orthop Traumatol Surg Res 100(4 suppl):S243–S248
37. Tomaino MM (2002) Neurophysiologic and clinical outcome following medial pectoral to long thoracic nerve transfer for scapular winging: a case report. Microsurgery 22:254–257
38. Ochiai N, Tsuyama N, Nagano A et al (1984) The root distribution in the motor innervation of the upper extremity: an analysis of 33 brachial plexus injuries. J Jpn Soc Surg Hand 1:535–539 (in Japanese)
39. Ochiai N, Nagano A, Okinaga S et al (1984) Investigation of the significance of the sensory disturbance in traumatic brachial plexus injuries. J Jpn Soc Surg Hand 4:157–160 (in Japanese)
40. Tsuyama N, Hara T (1973) Intercostal nerve transfer in the treatment of brachial plexus injuries of root-avulsion type. In: Orthopaedic Surgery and Traumatology. Proceedings of the Twelfth Congress of the International Society of Orthopaedic Surgery and Traumatology, Tel Aviv. Amsterdam, Excerpta Medica, 291:351–353
41. Nagano A, Tsuyama N, Ochiai N et al (1989) Direct nerve crossing with the intercostal nerve to treat avulsion injuries of the brachial plexus. J Hand Surg Am 14:980–985
42. Oberlin C, Beal D, Leechavengvongs S et al (1994) Nerve transfer to biceps muscle using a part of ulnar nerve for C5-6 avulsion of the brachial plexus: anatomical study and report of four cases. J Hand Surg 19A:232–237
43. Kawai H, Akita S (2004) Shoulder muscle reconstruction in the upper type of the brachial plexus injury by partial radial nerve transfer to the axillary nerve. Tech Hand Up Extrem Surg 8:51–55
44. Zheng MX, Qiu YQ, Xu WD et al (2012) Long-term observation of respiratory function after unilateral phrenic nerve and multiple intercostal nerve transfer for avulsed brachial plexus injury. Neurosurgery 70:796–801
45. Ochiai N, Mikami Y, Yamamoto S et al (1993) A new technique for mismatched nerve suture in direct intercostal nerve transfers. J Hand Surg Br 18-B:318–319

46. Akasaka Y, Hara T, Takahashi M (1991) Free muscle transplantation combined with intercostal nerve crossing for reconstruction of elbow flexion and wrist extension in brachial plexus injuries. Microsurgery 12:346–351
47. Kondo T (1980) Obstetrical paralysis. Orthop Surg 31:625–630 (in Japanese)
48. Sir Sunderland S (1978) Nerves and nerve injuries, 2nd edn. Churchill Livingstone, Edinburgh, pp 878–880
49. Kawabata H, Shibata T, Matsui Y et al (2001) Use of intercostal nerves for neurotization of the musculocutaneous nerve in infants with birth-related brachial plexus palsy. J Neurosurg 94:386–391
50. Kawabata H, Kawai H, Masatomi T, et al (1994) Accessory nerve neurotization in infants with brachial plexus birth palsy. Microsurgery 15:768–772
51. Ladak A, Morhart M, O'Grady K et al (2013) Distal nerve transfers are effective in treating patients with upper trunk obstetrical brachial plexus injuries: an early experience. Plast Reconstr Surg 132:985e–992e
52. Blaauw G, Slooff AC (2003) Transfer of pectoral nerves to the musculocutaneous nerve in obstetric upper brachial plexus palsy. Neurosurgery 53:338–341
53. Kawano K, Nagano A, Ochiai N et al (2007) Restoration of elbow function by intercostal nerve transfer for obstetrical paralysis with co-contraction of the biceps and the triceps. J Hand Surg Eur 32:421–426

Chapter 15
Proximal Humeral Fractures: Classification and Treatment

Kazuya Tamai, Yuichiro Yano, Katsuhisa Yoshikawa, and Jun'ichiro Hamada

Abstract Proximal humeral fractures account for 4–5 % of all fractures, with the higher incidence in women. The AO/ASIF system and the Neer's four-segment classification are used to record the fracture anatomy. The Neer's classification is more appropriate to provide an anatomic basis for guiding treatment regimens.

Generally, conservative treatments can achieve satisfactory healing in minimally displaced and most two-part surgical neck fractures. Surgery is indicated if surgical neck displacement exceeds 20 mm. Intramedullary nails and locking plates are most commonly used. The surgeon should pay attention to the possible varus deformity at the surgical neck. Greater tuberosity fractures are surgically treated if the displacement exceeds 5 mm. A tension band wiring is recommended in elderly patients. Three-part fractures are treated with osteosynthesis employing pins and wires, intramedullary nails, or locking plates. However, hardware complications are not uncommon in patients older than 60 years. In four-part valgus impacted fractures, it is important to elevate the head fragment superiorly for reduction rather than to pull the greater tuberosity inferiorly. For four-part fractures, hemiarthroplasty is the primary treatment of choice, but postoperative functional recovery is unsatisfactory. Although reverse shoulder arthroplasty looks promising, its use should be reserved for elderly patients.

Keywords Proximal humeral fractures • Classification • Treatment

K. Tamai (✉) • Y. Yano • K. Yoshikawa
Department of Orthopaedic Surgery, Dokkyo Medical University School of Medicine, 880 Kitakobaytashi, Mibu, Tochigi 321-0293, Japan
e-mail: ktamai@dokkyomed.ac.jp

J. Hamada
Department of Orthopaedic Surgery, Kuwano Kyoritsu Hospital, Fukushima, Japan

K. Tamai et al. (eds.), *Advances in Shoulder Surgery*,
DOI 10.1007/978-4-431-55988-7_15

15.1 Epidemiology

Proximal humeral fractures account for 4–5 % of all fractures, occurring in women more than twice as frequently as in men, with the highest incidence in women aged 80–89 years [9]. Proximal humeral fractures are reported in the Japanese population three to four times less frequently than in Caucasian populations, suggesting interracial variations [20]. Eighty-seven percent of this fracture type in adults resulted from falls from a standing height (low trauma energy) [3]. One population-based Norwegian study showed that the 10-year absolute risks of proximal humeral fractures in women aged 70 years or older were in the range of 5 %–7 % [2]. In older white women, proximal humeral fractures increased the risk of a subsequent hip fracture by more than five times in the first year after their occurrence [8]. One case-control study showed that individuals who left their houses more frequently had a significantly lower risk of proximal humeral fractures [20].

The literature shows that proximal humeral fractures occur at a high incidence in the fragile bones of elderly individuals with low levels of physical activity. Consequently, the surgeon should select the optimal therapeutic modality while taking into account the bone quality of the patient.

15.2 Fracture Anatomy

The Arbeitsgemeinschaft für Osteosynthesefragen/Association for the Study of Internal Fixation (AO/ASIF) and Neer classification systems are commonly used for characterizing fractures of the proximal humerus.

According to the AO/ASIF system [3], proximal humeral fractures are divided into three major types: extraarticular unifocal (type A), extraarticular bifocal (type B), and intraarticular (type C) fractures. These groups are further divided into subgroups based on displacement, dislocation, and the severity and location of impact (Fig. 15.1). Type A, type B, and type C fractures involve no, partial, and total impairment of the vascular supply to the humeral head, respectively. Despite its somewhat cumbersome nature, this coding system is popular in trauma surgery for reasons of its systematic approach to classifying different long bone fractures.

Neer's four-segment classification system [30] defines humeral fractures based on changes to the following four segments: humeral head, greater tuberosity, lesser tuberosity, and shaft. A fracture part is considered displaced if it is separated by more than 1 cm or if angulation between two segments exceeds 45°. A displaced fracture is categorized as two part, three part, or four part, depending on the number of segments involved. When a fracture causes only a small amount of displacement (i.e., <1 cm or <45°), it is termed a minimally displaced (one-part) fracture. In such cases, damage to soft tissue and blood supply is minimal. This classification scheme is easy to use and provides an anatomic basis for guiding treatment regimens. In his

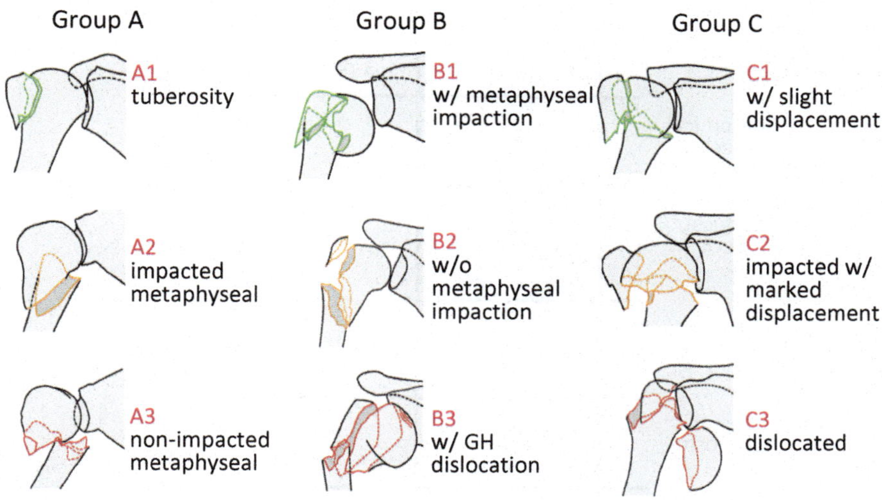

Fig. 15.1 AO/ASIF classification of proximal humeral fractures. Fractures are divided into extraarticular unifocal (type A), extraarticular bifocal (type B), and intraarticular (type C) groups. These groups are further divided into subgroups based on displacement, dislocation, and the severity and location of impact. Type A, type B, and type C fractures involve no, partial, and total impairment of the vascular supply to the humeral head, respectively. (Redrawn form the AO Surgery reference. https://www2.aofoundation.org/wps/portal/surgery)

2002 revision of this classification system, Neer introduced the valgus-impacted four-part fracture [32] (Fig. 15.2). This revised classification is more reasonable than the original one. We reviewed a total of 509 cases in a multicenter survey, and found that 98 % of them were classified into any category of the revised Neer classification [44]. This study confirmed the clinical utility of this system. The remaining 2 % could not be strictly assigned to any of the revised Neer fracture categories, but all were four-part equivalent fractures.

Generally, humeral fractures are evaluated using a trauma series, a set of three radiographs taken at right angles to each other [31] (Fig. 15.3). These X-rays can be obtained with the affected arm supported to minimize the patient's pain. Computed tomography (CT) scans, in particular three-dimensional CT, are useful for cases with complex fracture lines.

15.3 Principles of Treatment

Both the AO Foundation [37] and Neer [31] proposed principles for treating proximal humeral fractures (Tables 15.1 and 15.2). Their guidelines complement one another and are not mutually exclusive.

Neer proposed different treatment approaches based on the presence or absence of displacement (criteria: 1 cm of separation or 45° of angulation). However, he did

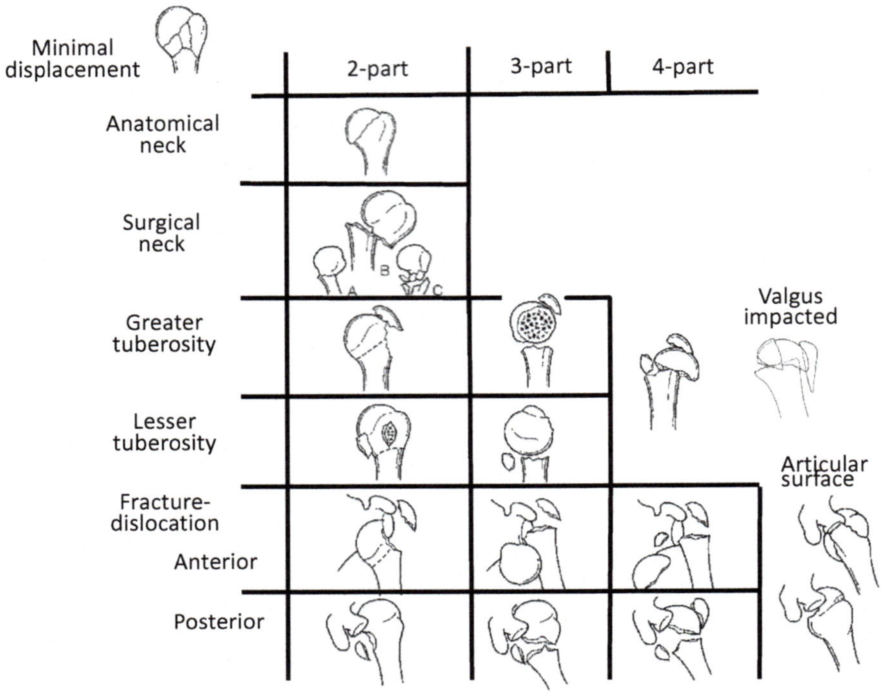

Fig. 15.2 Revised four-segment classification of Neer. This system is based on how the four segments, that is, the humeral head, greater tuberosity, lesser tuberosity, and shaft, are separated. A segment is considered displaced if it is separated by more than 1 cm or if angulation between two segments exceeds 45°. A displaced fracture is categorized as two part, three part, or four part, depending on the number of segments involved. The four-part valgus impacted fracture was added in the 2002 revision of this classification system. (Redrawn from Neer [32])

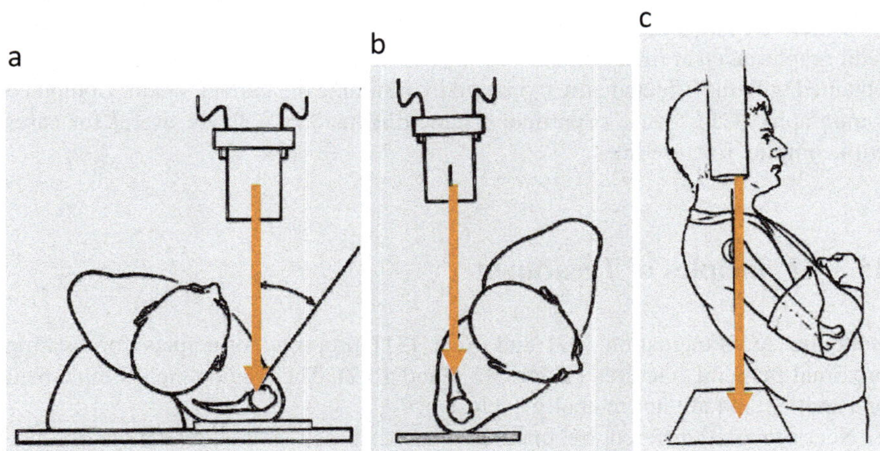

Fig. 15.3 Trauma series. A combination of anteroposterior (**a**), scapular Y (**b**), and Velpeau axillary (**c**) views can be obtained with the affected arm supported. (Redrawn from Neer [31])

Table 15.1 Indications for conservative and operative treatment

Conservative treatment is preferred in:
Elderly patients
Patients with significant comorbidities
Minimally displaced fractures
Surgical treatment in indicated in (20 % of patients):
Younger, or active older patients
At least one of the following occurs:
Tuberosities displaced more than 5 mm
Shaft fragment displaced more than 20 mm
Head fragment angulation greater than 45°

Source: Rüedi et al. [37]

Table 15.2 Treatment according to four-segment classification

Minimal displacement
Passive exercises progressing to active exercises as continuity permits
Two-part
Closed treatment, except for greater tuberosity and some shaft displacements
Three-part
Open reduction, internal fixation, and cuff repair, except prosthesis is now preferred in older patients and greater tuberosity three-part displacement with frail head attachments
Four-part
Prosthesis to replace the head with accurate fixation of the tuberosities and cuff repair

Source: Neer [31]

not suggest that all displaced fractures should be treated operatively. Regarding two-part surgical neck fractures, for example, he suggests primarily conservative management, and the AO Foundation recommends surgery if displacement exceeds 20 mm.

Concerning greater tuberosity fractures, Neer indicates surgery for two-part fractures, and the AO Foundation proposes surgery if displacement of 5 mm or more is present. In contrast to the approach for surgical neck fractures, surgery should be considered for greater tuberosity fractures even if they are classified as minimally displaced according to Neer's classification system.

15.4 Methods of Treatment

This section discusses fracture fixation approaches based on the revised Neer classification.

15.4.1 Minimally Displaced Fractures (One-Part Fractures)

One-part fractures, excluding those of the greater tuberosity, can be managed conservatively. Rehabilitation programs begin within 1 week after injury, starting with stooping and pendulum exercises, and gradually shifting to self-assisted passive exercises and active antigravity exercises. Generally, conservative treatments can achieve satisfactory healing in this type of fracture, even in patients with osteoporosis. The efficacy of early physiotherapy has been well documented, and immediate mobilization within 1 week of trauma is known to improve functional outcome [10, 14, 22, 26].

However, a one-part fracture with a fracture line in the surgical neck can be very unstable, sometimes developing into a two-part fracture if managed inadequately (Fig. 15.4).

The surgeon should use a screw or tension band wiring for internal fixation for a greater tuberosity fracture with 5 mm or greater displacement.

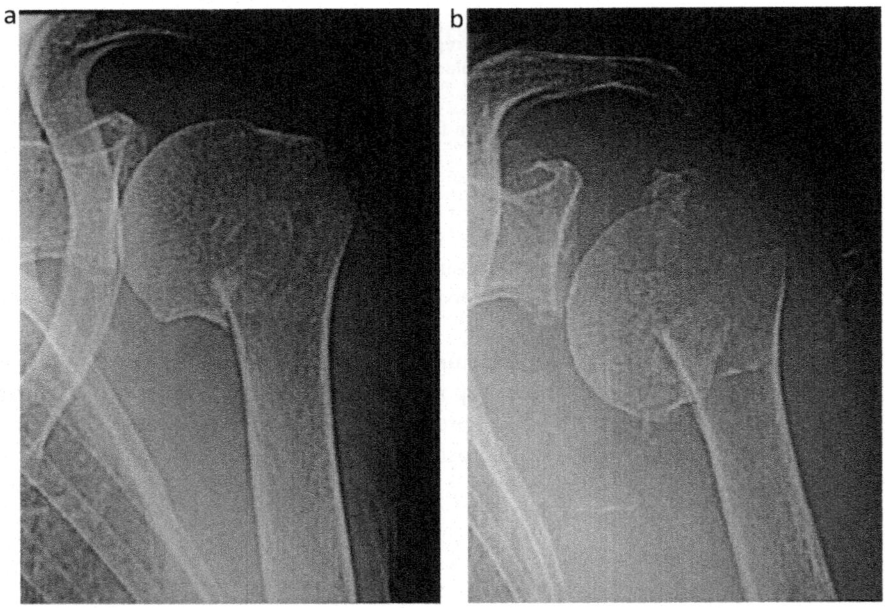

Fig. 15.4 One-part fracture in a 75-year-old woman. An X-ray immediately after injury showed a minimally displaced fracture (**a**), which was immobilized in an arm sling for conservative treatment. However, 1 week later, the humeral head was noted to be displaced and in a varus position, thus categorized as a two-part fracture (**b**). This change probably occurred because isometric contraction of the deltoid muscle pulled the humeral shaft upward, producing varus stress and destroying the lateral part of the humeral head

15.4.2 Two-Part Surgical Neck Fractures

Conservative management is indicated for surgical neck fractures if the head fragment is in contact with the shaft fragment. Because the surgical neck diameter is in the range of 30–40 mm, fractures involving displacement of approximately 20 mm or less can be treated conservatively. After 3 weeks of external fixation, patients begin physical rehabilitation programs (Fig. 15.5).

Surgery is indicated if the fracture involves no contact between the fragments or if the displacement worsens during conservative care. Intramedullary nails and plates are most commonly used for fixation of this fracture type. Occasionally, surgeons may employ the Kapandji procedure [24] (and variations thereof [33]), bundled pin fixation [45], and the Ender nailing technique [34], which are categorized as elastic fixation methods.

The surgeon should recognize the possibility that a surgical neck fracture may give rise to varus deformity, as shown in Fig. 15.4. Therefore, patients under conservative management should undergo radiographic evaluation twice per week in the first 2 to 3 weeks after injury. A lateral tension band may be used to counteract the varus stress. In the absence of medial column support, varus deformity may develop in cases where locked plating is used to treat proximal humerus

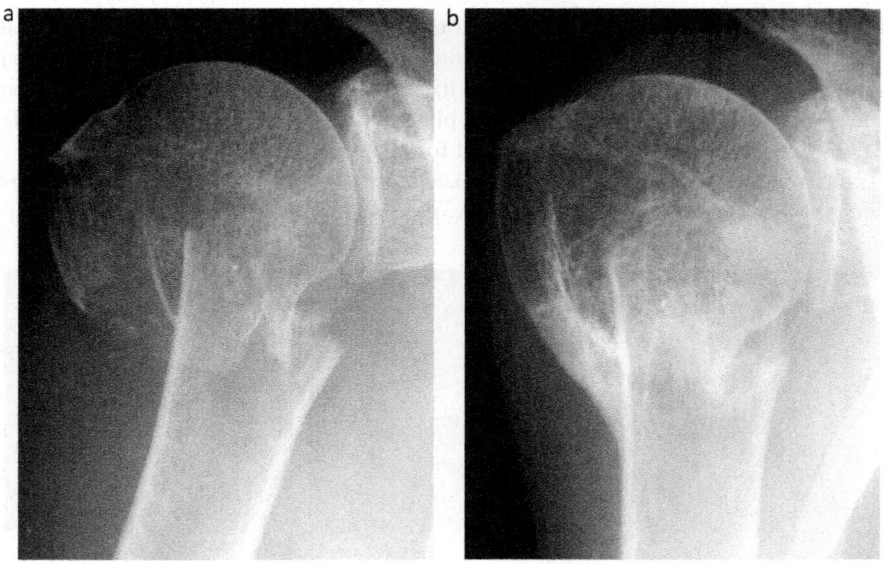

Fig. 15.5 Two-part surgical neck fracture in a 78-year-old woman. Although the X-ray immediately after the injury showed a surgical neck displacement exceeding 1 cm, the humeral head was impacted over the upper end of the shaft, suggesting a rather stable fracture (**a**). Conservative treatment resulted in bony union 8 weeks after the injury as well as satisfactory shoulder function (**b**)

fractures [17]. To prevent varus deformity, placement of a locked screw or endosteal strut augment [18] can be effective.

15.4.3 Two-Part Greater Tuberosity Fractures

In these fractures, the rotator cuff muscles act to displace the greater tuberosity. Proactive surgical management is recommended, because insufficient bony fusion and residual displacement may result in compromised abduction force and subacromial impingement. Use of screw fixation in elderly patients increases the risk of breaching the bone. A tension band wiring technique, whereby a soft wire is passed under the rotator cuff tendons, is recommended (Figs. 15.6 and 15.7).

15.4.4 Three-Part Fractures

As a general rule, three-part fractures are treated with osteosynthesis. Major approaches include pin and wire fixation (including the use of screws), the Resch method [36], bone suturing or wiring, intramedullary nailing, and locking plate fixation (Fig. 15.7). The surgeon should select the optimal method based on the fracture pattern, degrees of comminution and osteoporosis, the patient's general state, and other factors, with a primary interest in minimizing invasiveness (often leading to the choice of elastic internal fixation) or maximizing the initial fixation force (e.g., intramedullary nailing or plate fixation). Minimally invasive plate osteosynthesis (MIPO) is recommended for plate fixation [16, 27].

Intramedullary nailing has yielded excellent outcomes, although complications such as backing out of screws, screw protrusion into the glenohumeral joint,

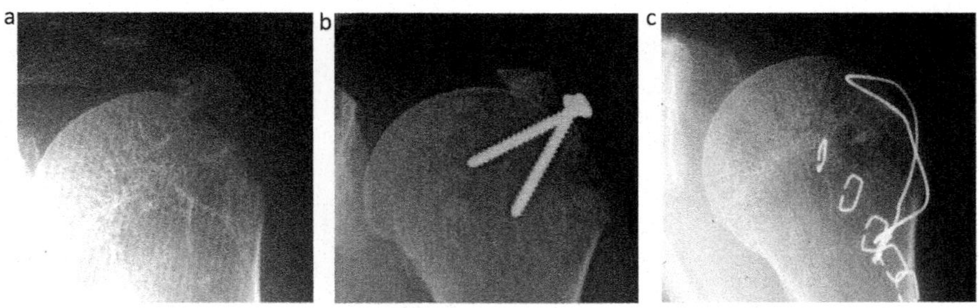

Fig. 15.6 Two-part greater tuberosity fracture in a 72-year-old woman. The X-ray immediately after the injury showed superior displacement of the greater tuberosity (**a**). Screw fixation of the greater tuberosity resulted in cut-out of the bone from the screws (**b**). At reoperation, tension band wiring with a soft wire passed under the rotator cuff tendons yielded stability of the tuberosity fragment (**c**). Screw fixation of the greater tuberosity fracture should be employed in young patients only

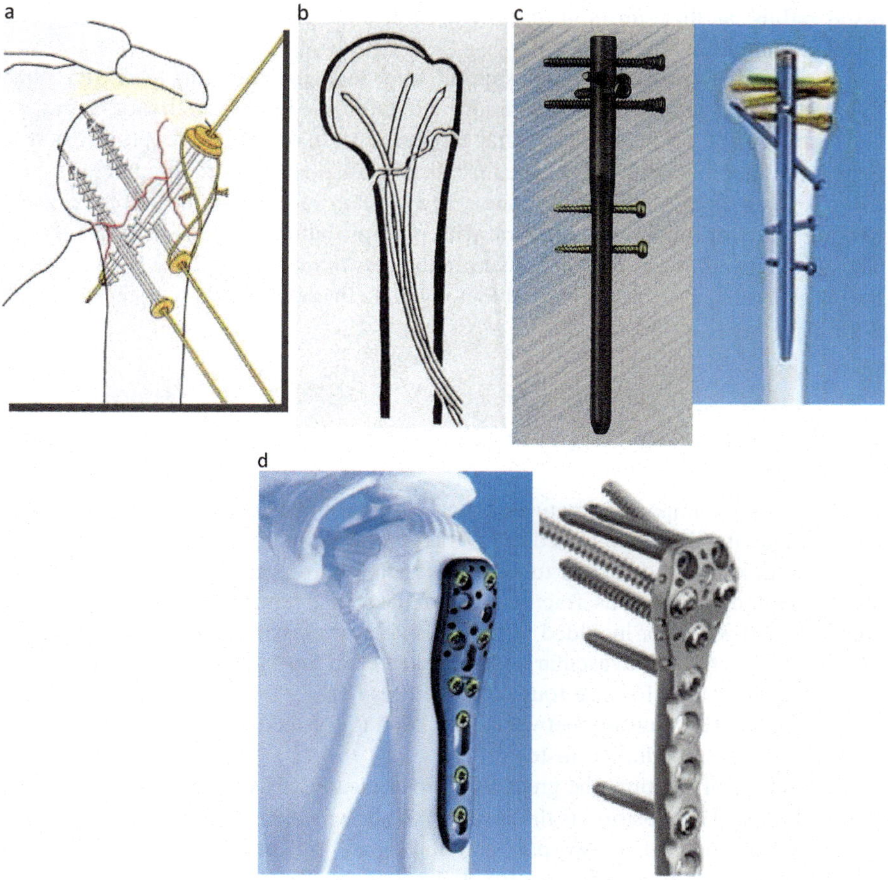

Fig. 15.7 Methods of osteosynthesis for two-part surgical neck and three- or four-part fractures. (**a**) Pin and wire fixation. (**b**) Kapandji procedure. (**c**) Intramedullary straight nail: Targon PH-P (*left*) and MultiLoc (*right*). (**d**) Locking plate: PHILOS (*left*) and NCB-PH (*right*)

tuberosity displacement, and osteonecrosis were reported in 20–30 % of treated patients [11, 19, 28]. Locking plate fixation is effective for patients with severe osteoporosis. However, complications such as screw cut-out, humeral head perforation, and varus displacement were reported in 13–36 % of treated patients [1, 17, 35]. Such complications were reported at higher rates in patients older than 60 years [35]. The humeral head has a higher bone mineral density in its medial part, particularly at the periarticular zone, as compared to other parts [47]. To ensure implant stability, therefore, it is recommended that the surgeon insert screws sufficiently deep into the medial part of the humeral head using an implant that allows for variable angles of screw insertion, such as the polyaxial locking plate [38]. It may be helpful to preoperatively determine the bone mineral density at the distal radius, as this shows an excellent correlation with the bone quality of the proximal humerus [46, 48].

Compromised medial cortical support may lead to reduction loss after plate fixation. Fibula allograft augmentation and inferomedial screw fixation may be necessary for fractures without medial support [28]. In severely osteoporotic bones, displaced fractures are at a significant risk of redisplacement if the greater tuberosity is fixed using the locking plate/screw system alone. It is desirable to use a locking plate for tuberosity reduction with multiple suture eyelets along its margin. These eyelets allow the surgeon to suture the soft tissue to the plate. Alternatively, the surgeon may use a conventional locking plate in combination with tension band wiring.

15.4.5 Four-Part Valgus Impacted Fractures

Four-part valgus impacted fractures are characterized by (i) valgus impaction of the head fragment, (ii) an angulated head fragment maintaining some congruity with the glenoid, and (iii) detached tuberosities remaining in proximity to the head and shaft fragments [23]. This fracture pattern was first reported by a group of AO surgeons and was later included in the revised Neer classification [32]. In this type of fracture, the rates of avascular necrosis have been reported at 8 % to 26 %, which are much lower than for true four-part fractures (21–75 %) [12]. This difference is attributable to the congruity between the shaft and the medial aspect of the head, as well as the intact medial periosteal hinge.

In this type of fracture, the greater tuberosity is located superiorly relative to the humeral head. This position is the result of the downward translocation of the head fragment, as opposed to two-part and three-part greater tuberosity fractures in which the greater tuberosity is retracted superiorly by the force created by the attached rotator cuff muscles (Fig. 15.8). It is therefore important, in four-part valgus impacted fractures, to elevate the head fragment superiorly for reduction rather than to pull the greater tuberosity inferiorly.

15.5 Four-Part Fractures

Hemiarthroplasty is the primary treatment of choice for this type of proximal humeral fracture. However, postoperative functional recovery is unsatisfactory in 30–40 % of treated patients, with a mean active flexion of approximately 90° [25]. Several parameters have been shown to bring better outcome of prosthetic replacement in acute proximal humeral fractures, including surgical operation within 14 days of injury, preserving lateral humeral offset, and avoiding tuberosity-related complications [13]. To enhance postoperative tuberosity consolidation while preventing bone resorption, secure fixation of the tuberosities is

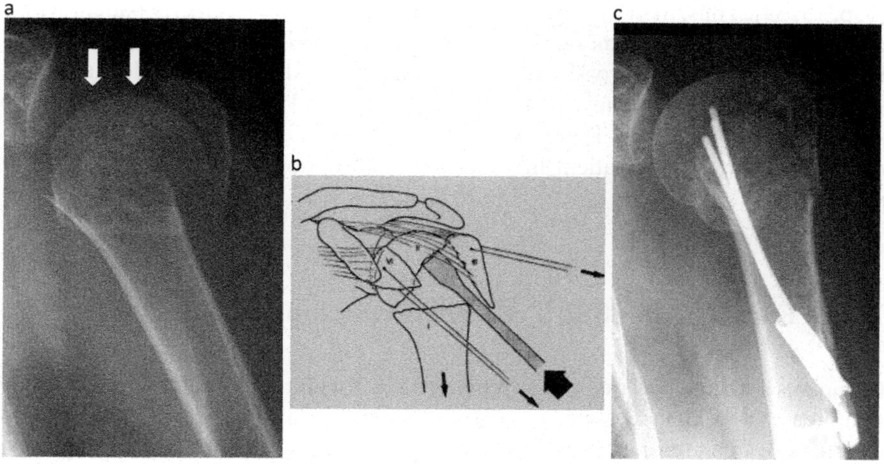

Fig. 15.8 Four-part valgus impacted fracture in a 75-year-old woman. The X-ray immediately after injury showed an impacted and low-positioned humeral head relative to the greater tuberosity (**a**), which usually results from an axial compression force onto the humeral head (*arrows*). Therefore, in treating this type of fracture, elevation of the humeral head is essential (**b**) (redrawn from Jakob et al. [23]). In this patient, a small elevator was used through a small incision to anatomically reduce the humeral head, which was fixated with the All-in-one nail, a kind of bundled intramedullary pins, inserted from the deltoid tuberosity (**c**)

necessary. For this purpose, use of fracture-dedicated shoulder prostheses is recommended, such as those having a window through which a graft can be inserted to create a bone bridge between the tuberosities [40].

It is controversial whether avascular necrosis risk can be predicted on the basis of fracture pattern. In a study evaluating predictors of fracture-induced humeral head ischemia, Hertel et al. found that the length of the posteromedial metaphyseal extension of the head fragment and the integrity of the medial soft tissue hinge were among the most relevant variables suggesting ischemia [21]. On the other hand, they later showed that intraoperative blood flow to the humeral head was unrelated to the incidence of postoperative avascular necrosis [4]. These and other studies indicate that there is currently no consensus regarding the predictability of avascular necrosis based on fracture pattern. We may reasonably consider that four-part fractures should preferably be treated with osteosynthesis rather than hemiarthroplasty, the latter of which is unlikely to ensure predictable, positive outcomes.

Reverse shoulder arthroplasty (RSA) is increasingly being used for acute four-part fractures of elderly patients traditionally treated with hemiarthroplasty. RSA generally provide satisfiable forward elevation, improved functional scores, and pain relief because it is less reliant on a functioning rotator cuff and healing of the tuberosities. Studies that compared RSA with hemiarthroplasty indicate better outcome in RSA in terms of active forward elevation (90°–120° versus 50°–80°), functional and quality of life (QOL) scores, and the number of revision surgeries

[5, 6, 15, 39]. Thus, there is a clear indication for an RSA in an elderly patient with a comminuted proximal humeral fracture with osteoporotic bone. However, it should be noted that the RSA works only with a functional deltoid, that adequate bone stock is required to achieve satisfactory results, and that long-term follow-up studies are still lacking. Therefore, the use of an RSA for fractures should be reserved for an elderly patient in which no other option will attain a satisfactory result.

15.6 Factors Affecting Treatment Outcome

Clinicians should be aware of poor prognostic factors for proximal humeral fracture treatment: these include old age, comorbidity, and associated glenohumeral dislocation [43]. In addition, factors associated with social independence are important predictors of mortality and function. An epidemiological study of 629 elderly patients demonstrated a significantly increased risk of poor outcome in individuals not living in their own home (e.g., institutionalized), not participating in recreational activities, not able to accomplish their own shopping, or not able to dress themselves [7]. Moreover, initial varus angulation of the humeral head (as compared to valgus angulation) and insufficient reduction of tuberosity displacement resulted in poor functional outcome [41–43]. Taking such risk factors into account, the surgeon should use a broad perspective when determining the most appropriate treatment modality (Fig. 15.9) [29].

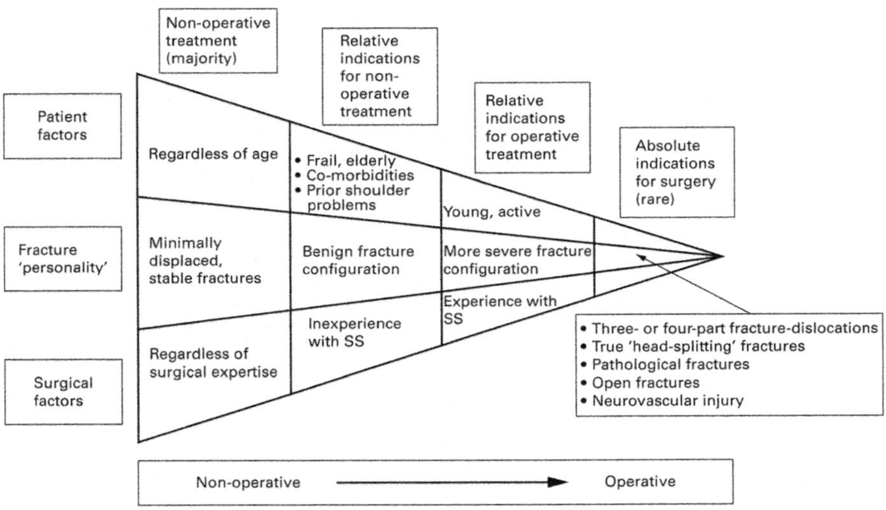

Fig. 15.9 Flowchart showing therapeutic decision making for proximal humeral fractures. Patients' factors (age, comorbidities, etc.), fracture personality (displacement, comminution, etc.), and surgeon's experience should be considered. (From Murray et al. [29])

References

1. Agudelo J, Schurmann M, Stahel P et al (2007) Analysis of efficacy and failure in proximal humeral fractures treated with locking plates. J Orthop Trauma 21:676–681
2. Ahmed LA, Schirmer H, Bjørnerem A et al (2009) The gender- and age-specific 10-year and lifetime absolute fracture risk in Tromsø, Norway. Eur J Epidemiol 24:441–448
3. AO surgery reference. https://www2.aofoundation.org/wps/portal/surgery
4. Bastian JD, Hertel R (2008) Initial post-fracture humeral head ischemia does not predict development of necrosis. J Shoulder Elbow Surg 17:2–8
5. Boyle MJ, Youn S-M, Frampton CMA et al (2013) Functional outcomes of reverse shoulder arthroplasty compared with hemiarthroplasty for acute proximal humeral fractures. J Shoulder Elbow Surg 22:32–37
6. Chalmers PN, Slikker W III, Mall NA et al (2014) Reverse total shoulder arthroplasty for acute proximal humeral fracture: comparison to open reduction: internal fixation and hemiarthroplasty. J Shoulder Elbow Surg 23:197–204
7. Clement ND, Duckworth AD, McQueen MM et al (2014) The outcome of proximal humeral fractures in the elderly. Predictors of mortality and function. Bone Joint J 96-B:970–977
8. Clinton J, Franta A, Polissar NL et al (2009) Proximal humeral fracture as a risk factor for subsequent hip fractures. J Bone Joint Surg Am 91:503–511
9. Court-Brown CM, Garg A, McQueen MM (2001) The epidemiology of proximal humeral fractures. Acta Orthop Scand 72:365–371
10. Court-Brown CM, McQueen MM (2002) Impacted varus (A2.2) proximal humeral fracture. Prediction of outcome and results of nonoperative treatment in 99 patients. Acta Orthop Scand 75:736–740
11. Cuny C, Scarlat MM, Irrazi M et al (2008) The telegraph nail for proximal humeral fractures: a prospective four-year study. J Shoulder Elbow Surg 17:539–545
12. DeFranco MJ, Brems JJ, Williams GR Jr et al (2006) Evaluation and management of valgus impacted four-part proximal humerus fractures. Clin Orthop 442:109–114
13. Demirhan M, Kilicoglu O, Altinel L et al (2007) Prognostic factors in prosthetic replacement for acute proximal humerus fractures. J Orthop Trauma 17:181–188
14. Gaebler C, McQueen MM, Court-Brown CM (2003) Minimally displaced proximal humeral fractures. Epidemiology and outcome in 507 cases. Acta Orthop Scand 74:580–585
15. Gallinet D, Clappaz P, Garbuio P et al (2009) Three or four parts complex proximal humerus fractures: hemiarthroplasty versus reverse prosthesis: a comparative study of 40 cases. Orthop Traumatol Surg Res 95:48–55
16. Gallo RA, Zeiders GJ, Altman GT (2005) Two-incision technique for treatment of complex proximal humerus fractures. J Orthop Trauma 19:734–740
17. Gardner MJ, Weil Y, Barker JU et al (2007) The importance of medial support in locked plating of proximal humerus fractures. J Orthop Trauma 21:185–191
18. Gardner MJ, Boraiah S, Helfet DL et al (2008) Indirect medial reduction and strut support of proximal humerus fractures using an endosteal implant. J Orthop Trauma 22:195–200
19. Gradl G, Dietze A, Arndt D et al (2007) Angular and sliding stable antegrade nailing (Targon PH) for the treatment of proximal humeral fractures. Arch Orthop Trauma Surg 127:937–944
20. Hagino H, Fujiwara S, Nakashima E et al (2004) Case-control study of risk factors for fractures of the distal radius and proximal humerus among the Japanese population. Osteoporos Int 15:226–230
21. Hertel R, Hempfing A, Stiehler M et al (2004) Predictors of humeral head ischemia after intracapsular fracture of the proximal humerus. J Shoulder Elbow Surg 13:427–433
22. Hodgson SA, Mawson SJ, Stanley D (2003) Rehabilitation after two-part fractures of the neck of the humerus. J Bone Joint Surg Br 85-B:419–422

23. Jakob RP, Miniaci A, Anson PS et al (1991) Four-part valgus impacted fractures of the proximal humerus. J Bone Joint Surg Br 73-B:295–298
24. Kapandji A (1989) Osteosynthesis using the "palm-tree" nail technic in fractures of the surgical neck of the humerus. Ann Chir Main 8:39–52 (in French)
25. Lanting B, MacDermid J, Drosdowech D et al (2008) Proximal humeral fractures. A systematic review of treatment modalities. J Shoulder Elbow Surg 17:42–54
26. Lefevre-Colau MM, Babinet A, Hayad F et al (2007) Immediate mobilization compared with conventional immobilization for the impacted nonoperatively treated proximal humeral fracture. A randomized controlled trial. J Bone Joint Surg Am 89-A:2582–2590
27. Lill H, Hepp P, Rose T et al (2004) The angle stable locking-proximal-humerus-plate (LPHP) for proximal humeral fractures using a small anterior-lateral-deltoid-splitting-approach. Technique and first results. Zentralbl Chir 129:43–48 (in German)
28. Linhart W, Ueblacker P, Grossterlinden L et al (2007) Antegrade nailing of humeral head fractures with captured interlocking screws. J Orthop Trauma 21:285–294
29. Murray IR, Amin AK, White TO et al (2011) Proximal humeral fractures. Current concepts in classification, treatment and outcomes. J Bone Joint Surg Br 93-B:1–11
30. Neer CS II (1970) Displaced proximal humeral fractures. Part I: classification and evaluation. J Bone Joint Surg Am 52:1077–1089
31. Neer CS II (1990) Shoulder reconstruction. Saunders, Philadelphia, pp 363–398
32. Neer CS II (2002) Four-segment classification of proximal humeral fractures: purpose and reliable use. J Shoulder Elbow Surg 11:389–400
33. Ogawa K, Kobayashi S, Ikegami H (2011) Retrograde intramedullary multiple pinning through the deltoid "V" for valgus-impacted four-part fractures of the proximal humerus. J Trauma 71:238–244
34. Ogiwara N, Aoki M, Okamura K et al (1996) Ender nailing for unstable surgical neck fractures of the humerus in elderly patients. Clin Orthop Relat Res 330:173–180
35. Owsley KC, Gorezyca JT (2008) Displacement/screw cutout after open reduction and locked plate fixation of humeral fractures. J Bone Joint Surg Am 90-A:233–240
36. Resch H, Povacz P, Fröhlich R et al (1997) Percutaneous fixation of three- and four-part fractures of the proximal humerus. J Bone Joint Surg Br 79:295–300
37. Rüedi TP, Buckley RE, Moran CG (2007) AO principles of fracture management, 2nd edn. Thieme Publishers, New York
38. Schiuma D, Plecko M, Kloub M et al (2013) Influence of peri-implant bone quality on implant stability. Med Eng Phys 35:82–87
39. Sebastiá-Forcada E, Cebrián-Góomez R, Lizaur-Utrilla A et al (2014) Reverse shoulder arthroplasty versus hemiarthroplasty for acute proximal humeral fractures. A blinded, randomized, controlled. J Shoulder Elbow Surg 23:1419–1426
40. Sirveaux F, Roche O, Molé D (2010) Shoulder arthroplasty for acute proximal humerus fracture. Orthop Traumatol Surg Res 96:683–694
41. Smith AM, Mardones RM, Sperling JW et al (2007) Early complications of operatively treated proximal humeral fractures. J Shoulder Elbow Surg 16:14–24
42. Solberg BD, Moon CN, Franco DP et al (2009) Locked plating of 3- and 4-part proximal humerus fractures in older patients. The effect of initial fracture pattern on outcome. J Orthop Trauma 23:113–119
43. Tamai K (2009) Classification and treatment of proximal humeral fractures. J Jpn Orthop Assoc 83:999–1009 (in Japanese)
44. Tamai K, Ishige N, Kuroda S et al (2009) Four-segment classification of proximal humeral fractures revisited. A multicenter study on 509 cases. J Shoulder Elbow Surg 18:845–850
45. Tamai K, Ohno W, Takemura M et al (2005) Treatment of proximal humeral fractures with a new intramedullary nail. J Orthop Sci 10:180–186
46. Wilson J, Bonner TJ, Head M et al (2009) Variation in bone mineral density by anatomical site in patients with proximal humeral fractures. J Bone Joint Surg Br 91:772–775

47. Yamada M, Briot J, Pedrono A et al (2007) Age- and gender-related distribution of bone tissue of osteoporotic humeral head using computed tomography. J Shoulder Elbow Surg 16:596–602
48. Yano Y, Tamai K, Yoshikawa K et al (2012) Differences in bone mineral density (BMD) between the proximal humerus and other measurement sites. Katakansetsu (Shoulder Joint) 36:881–883 (in Japanese)

Chapter 16
Reverse Shoulder Arthroplasty

Kenji Takagishi, Atsushi Yamamoto, Hitoshi Shitara, Tsuyoshi Ichinose, Tsuyoshi Sasaki, and Noritaka Hamano

Abstract Severe cuff deficiency and destruction of glenohumeral joint may lead to a painful and pseudo-paralyzed shoulder. In this situation an anatomic total shoulder prosthesis yields a limited clinical result or may even be contraindicated because of glenoid loosening. Early models for reverse shoulder prosthesis were developed to address the drawbacks of conventional shoulder prostheses have failed because of an underlying design flaw. The reverse prosthesis designed by Grammont has introduced new innovations that have led to its success. The Grammont prosthesis imposes a new biomechanical environment for the deltoid muscle to act, thus allowing it to compensate for the deficient rotator cuff muscles. Although new prostheses have been developed to improve on Grammont's original design, they continue to follow Grammont's core principles. Accumulated experience with reverse shoulder arthroplasty has led to expanded surgical indications, including cuff tear arthropathy, massive rotator cuff tears, fracture sequelae, rheumatoid arthritis, acute fractures, tumors or as a revision procedure for failed prostheses. The complication rates has increased with the increasing indications. Longer follow-up studies are required to assess the survival of the prosthesis and the functional performance over time, and it has been recommended to limit its use to elderly patients, basically those aged over 70 years.

Keywords Rotator cuff tear • Prosthesis • Cuff tear arthropathy

16.1 Introduction

The original type of anatomic total shoulder arthroplasty (TSA) was developed by Neer [1], who reported an excellent outcome of TSA for rheumatoid and osteoarthritic shoulders. Conventional arthroplasty was improved by a modular-type prosthesis, which could be separated into humeral and stem parts in 1986 [2].

K. Takagishi (✉) • A. Yamamoto • H. Shitara • T. Ichinose • T. Sasaki • N. Hamano
Department of Orthopaedic Surgery, Graduate School of Medicine, Gunma University, 3-39-22 Showa, Maebashi, Gunma 371-8511, Japan
e-mail: ktakagishi@gunma-u.ac.jp

K. Tamai et al. (eds.), *Advances in Shoulder Surgery*,
DOI 10.1007/978-4-431-55988-7_16

A newer type of prosthesis, in which the head–neck angle and offset could be changed according to the presence of anatomic deformities, became available in 1997 [3].

Until March 2014, only anatomic TSA was available in Japan. In this procedure, the deformed joint (up to the humeral head and glenoid) is replaced. This procedure was not suitable for the treatment of glenohumeral arthritis patients with severe cuff function deficiency.

Stanmore TSA has been performed in patients with destructive shoulder and a lack of cuff function as a constrained-type prosthesis [4]. This procedure is no longer in use because of its association with mechanical failure. In the 1970s, reverse shoulder arthroplasty (RSA) was developed as a prosthesis that could be used to replace a destroyed shoulder joint without rotator cuff function [5, 6]. The prosthesis initially had a biomechanical failure, which was caused by the loosening of the glenoid component; however, outcomes are currently satisfactory, and good results have been reported in 89 % of cases since the improvement of the prosthesis [7].

The reverse prosthesis has been allowed in neighboring countries, including South Korea (since 2006), China (since 2008), and Hong Kong (since 2011); thus, its suitability for smaller Asian patients has been proven. RSA has become a standard procedure in shoulder surgery throughout the world. This type of prosthesis has been used in developing countries as well as in advanced countries, with the previous exception of Japan. RSA is indicated for shoulder disabilities in which the patient does not have normal cuff function; however, postoperative complications have been reported to frequently occur in cases in which surgeons fail to properly adhere to the indications and surgical techniques.

RSA was permitted by the Health, Labor, and Welfare Ministry of Japan from April 2014, after the guidelines for the use of RSA were established by the ad hoc committee of the Japan Orthopaedic Association. The guideline describes several points about the use of RSA, including (1) the indications for RSA; (2) complications during and after operations, (3) points to consider for RSA; (3) operating rooms that are suitable for RSA; (4) surgeons who can perform RSA; (5) lecture classes for RSA; and (6) a registration system for RSA. In 2014, 500 RSA procedures were performed in 9 months in Japan. Anatomic TSA is thought to have been performed in fewer than 400 cases during the same period. RSA is currently more popular than anatomic TSA in Japan. This chapter discusses RSA, including the Japanese guideline for its use.

16.2 Development and Characteristics of Reverse Shoulder Arthroplasty

The most remarkable feature of the glenohumeral joint is its ability to precisely stabilize the humeral head in the center of the glenoid while also allowing a wide range of motion. This balance of stability and mobility is achieved by a combination of mechanisms particular to this articulation [8].

A massive cuff tear is required for a diagnosis of cuff tear arthropathy (CTA), but not everyone with a massive cuff tear develops CTA. The exact etiology of CTA is likely multifactorial and can be associated with inflammatory and crystal-induced arthritis [9, 10]. Neer [9] first described the theoretical process that mechanical and nutritional factors might function in the development of CTA. Treatments for CTA have ranged from nonoperative management and glenohumeral arthrodesis to resection arthroplasty and artificial joint replacement. Anatomic shoulder arthroplasty used to be a standard surgical option in the treatment of patients with CTA [1]. Neer determined that the outcomes of unconstrained shoulder arthroplasty were poorer in the case of cuff deficiency.

The anatomic prosthetic replacement has been abandoned because of cuff deficiency, resulting in superior displacement of the humeral component and glenoid loosening [11, 12]. Hemiarthroplasty was observed to provide similar results with respect to pain relief, functional improvement, and patient satisfaction. Shoulders that have undergone hemiarthroplasty gained significantly more active elevation after surgery. Cuff repair was easier when a humeral head prosthesis alone was used because less lateralization of the humerus occurred [12]. However, it has been difficult to predict the outcomes in these patients in terms of mobility and pain relief [13].

Reverse total shoulder arthroplasty (RSA) has become very popular because of its ability to treat patients experiencing severe rotator cuff dysfunction with or without glenohumeral arthritis [14]. An extensive understanding of the shoulder and artificial joint biomechanics makes it possible to accurately design shoulder prostheses.

To address the drawbacks of conventional shoulder prostheses, early models for RSA were developed. However, numerous reverse prosthesis designs of the 1970s resulted in implant breakage and glenoid component loosening because of an underlying design flaw [15, 16].

In 1985, Paul Grammont designed a reverse prosthesis for arthritic shoulders with severe destruction of the cuff, in which standard anatomic prostheses could not be used to restore joint stability and mobility [14, 17]. Boileau et al. [18] explained that the Grammont reverse prosthesis, differing from any previous reverse ball-and-socket design, has introduced two major innovations:

1. In contrast to all previous reverse ball-and-socket prostheses, the Grammont glenoid component is a third of a sphere with a large diameter of 36 or 42 mm and no neck. The back of the glenosphere is in direct contact with the prepared

glenoid surface. This design has the advantage of placing the center of rotation of the joint in contact with the center of the humeral head and provides a fixed center of rotation. Furthermore, the large diameter allows greater range of movement before impingement of the components occurs and provides more stability.

2. The humeral component has a small cup, oriented with a nonanatomic inclination of 155°, that covers less than half of the glenosphere; this has the advantage of lowering the humerus, resulting in overtensioning the deltoid. It allows a greater range of movement to occur before component–bone impingement.

Recently, Berliner et al. [19] reviewed the biomechanics of RSA. Grammont changed the system's center of rotation directly to the bone–implant interface. This design medialized the joint's center of rotation and stabilized the bone–implant interface by converting the shear forces that challenge glenoid fixation into compressive forces [20].

Further, inferior overhang of the glenosphere provides a space between the glenosphere and the scapular neck that may decrease notching. It also creates additional clearance between the greater tuberosity and coracoacromial arch, allowing greater impingement-free range of motion during abduction. The system is designed both to retension and to reposition the deltoid in relation to the joint's center of rotation. A medialized center of rotation increases the deltoid's moment arm by 20–42 % and recruits additional fibers of the anterior and posterior deltoid to serve as abductors (Fig. 16.1) [18, 20, 21] (figure explanation by Kapandji [22] is cited). Compared with native anatomy, the deltoid abduction moment arm in a reverse shoulder has much greater fluctuation peaking at 90° of abduction, the position at which the weight of the arm creates its largest adducting moment [20]. The enhanced torque-producing capacity of the deltoid, particularly in early abduction, may compensate for impairment in the initiation of torque resulting from supraspinatus deficiency. A distalized center of rotation restores tension to a shortened deltoid in the setting of cuff tear arthropathy, effectively improving the muscle's efficacy by approximately 30 % [21]. In addition, distalization of the center of rotation is necessary to provide space for the proximal humerus, allowing less restricted range of motion. Anatomic TSA has a large prosthetic head with a small shallow glenoid. In general, the radius of curvature of the glenoid is at least 5.5 mm longer than that of the humeral component. Grammont's reverse prosthesis, designed with equal radii of curvature, is able to tolerate a joint-reaction force vector of up to 45° [23] whereas the net humeral joint-reaction force vector in conventional total shoulder arthroplasty must be directed within 30° of the glenoid centerline to avoid dislocation [24]. Increased constraint secondary to the deeper and the more conforming concavity of the humeral articular surface prevents glenohumeral translation while providing sufficient stability for functional range of motion. This high degree of intrinsic stability frees the reverse total shoulder prosthesis from dependence on active stabilization by concentric compression and provides a stable fulcrum for the remaining musculature [23]. Total shoulder arthroplasty has a ratio of approximately 1.0 [25, 26], whereas RSA has a stability

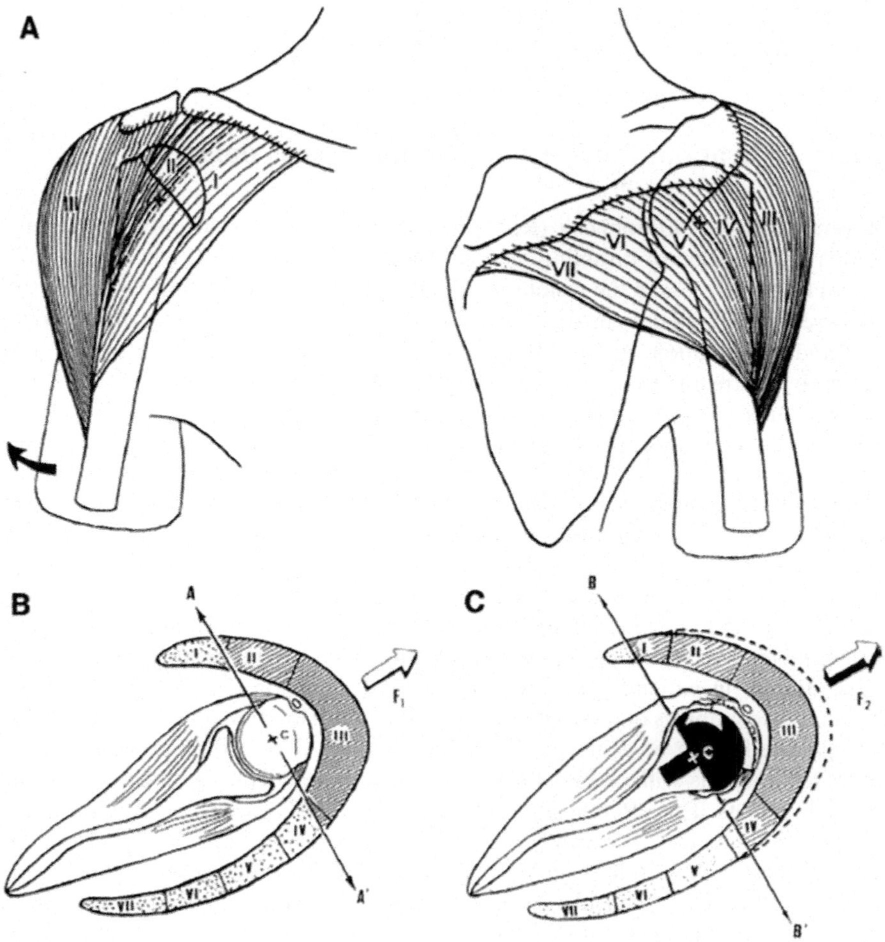

Fig. 16.1 The seven segments of the deltoid, according to Kapandji [22]. (**a**) In a normal shoulder, only the middle deltoid (segment III) and part of the anterior deltoid segment (segment II) can participate to active elevation (**b**). (**c**) After a reverse prosthesis, the medialization of the center of rotation recruits more of the deltoid fibers (segments I and IV) for active elevation. (With permission of Elsevier)

ratio greater than 2.0. With the glenohumeral joint in 90° of abduction, the reverse total shoulder is approximately four to five times more stable than a normal joint and two to three times more stable than an anatomic total shoulder prosthesis [27]. In addition, the net compressive force acting on the glenohumeral articulation is the most important factor of stability [28]. In a reverse shoulder, joint compressive forces are largely produced from deltoid tensioning. Stability also depends on glenoid component positioning.

Although new prostheses have been developed to improve on Grammont's original design, they continue to follow Grammont's core principles [19].

16.3 Indications for Reverse Shoulder Arthroplasty

Reverse shoulder arthroplasty (RSA) was initially recommend only for patients with a combination of disabling glenohumeral arthritis and cuff deficiency. However, clinical success in the restoration of stability, balance, and function has given rise to expanded indications such as a cuff-deficient shoulder without arthritis. With the gradual evolution of the indications, RSA has become an important surgical option in the treatment of a variety of conditions [29].

The Japanese guidelines for RSA list five basic concepts as indications for reverse shoulder arthroplasty (Table 16.1). RSA may be considered when the following conditions are fulfilled. (1) The patient complains of shoulder symptoms caused by irreparable rotator cuff tear associated with pseudo-paresis of anterior elevation and/or abduction in spite of conservative therapy for a certain period of time. Patients with a reparable cuff tear should undergo arthroscopic or open rotator cuff surgery. (2) Degenerative diseases of the shoulder joint, such as cuff tear arthropathy and rheumatoid arthritis, are good conditions for RSA. However, anatomic total shoulder arthroplasty is recommended for the treatment of degenerative disease in patients with intact rotator cuff function (such as patients with primary osteoarthritis of the glenohumeral joint). (3) The strengthening of elevation and pain relief can be achieved, but a full recovery of elevation power is not be expected. Patients with reverse prostheses have reduced strength in comparison to normal patients. This effect is most apparent in external rotation and might explain the clinical outcomes in which a moderately strong relationship is observed. It has been suggested that limited strength is a major factor in reduced range of motion (ROM) [30]. (4) In consideration of the previously reported outcomes, RSA basically should be performed in patients who are older than 70 years. (5) RSA is a final procedure, not a preventive procedure.

Despite demonstrating the early improvement of function and pain, there is limited information regarding the durability and longer-term outcomes of RSA. Survivorship free of revision surgery was 89 % at 10 years with a marked break occurring at 2 and 9 years. Survivorship with a Constant-Murley score less than

Table 16.1 Basic principles for reverse shoulder arthroplasty (RSA) according to the Japanese guidelines for RSA

1. Patients with pseudo-paralysis of the shoulder
2. Degenerative changes in the roentgenographic findings with rotator cuff deficiency
3. The strengthening of elevation and pain relief can be achieved, but the surgeons do not expect a full recovery of elevation power
4. Essentially limited to patients older than 70 years of age
5. A final procedure, not a preventive procedure

30 was 72 % at 10 years with a marked break observed at 8 years [7]. Although the need for revision of reverse shoulder arthroplasty was relatively low at 10 years, the Constant-Murley score and radiographic changes showed deterioration over time. These findings regarding the potential longevity of reverse shoulder arthroplasty are concerning, and caution must therefore be exercised in performing the procedure, especially in younger patients. In consideration of this fact, reverse shoulder arthroplasty has primarily been indicated for patients older than 70 years with symptomatic rotator cuff deficiency, poor function, and pain. The average life expectancy of Japanese individuals in 2014 is approximately 86.83 years in women and more than 80.5 years in males. Japanese individuals have one of the longest lifespans in the world. According to the guidelines, rotator cuff function deficiency and shoulder pain are good indications of RSA when patients are older than 70 years. However, there might be some other indications, including (but not limited to) the salvage of failed total shoulder arthroplasty or the presence of a tumor around the shoulder area.

16.3.1 Absolute Indication

16.3.1.1 Cuff Tear Arthropathy (Hamada Classification [31]: Grade 4, 5)

Cuff tear arthropathy (CTA), a term which was coined by Neer [9] in 1983, describes a state of severe disorganization of the glenohumeral joint following a massive cuff tear. CTA patients are typically elderly and present with a history of long-standing shoulder pain, weakness, decreased active motion, and limited function [32, 33]. CTA occurs in women more frequently than men, and the dominant side is more commonly affected than the nondominant side. Such patients frequently receive multiple injections of corticosteroids and may have undergone one or more surgical interventions. In 1990, Hamada et al. [34] radiographically classified massive rotator cuff tears into five grades. Walch et al. [35] subsequently subdivided grade 4 to reflect the presence or absence of subacromial arthritis and to emphasize glenohumeral arthritis as a characteristic of grade 4.

Hamada et al. [31] examined whether patient characteristics and magnetic resonance imaging (MRI) findings differed between the grades at the initial examination and found that patients with grade 3, 4, or 5 tears had a higher incidence of fatty muscle degeneration of the subscapularis muscle than patients with grade 1 or 2 tears. Currently, the most common indication for a RSA is pain and altered function resulting from glenohumeral arthritis with the compromise of the rotator cuff. When pain or loss of motion is resistant to conservative treatment, alternative treatments should be considered. Arthroscopic debridement or biceps tenotomy may improve pain; however, the results have not been consistent. Glenohumeral arthrodesis may be considered for patients with a nonfunctional deltoid muscle [36]. RSA has become the most common surgical treatment option for patients with

CTA: the ideal candidate for RSA is a CTA patient with severe pain and pseudoparesis [14, 29, 37–39]. The survival rates with the replacement of the prosthesis and glenoid loosening as the end points were 91 % and 84 %, respectively, at 120 months, with a significantly better result demonstrated in shoulders that had arthropathy with a massive rotator cuff tear in comparison to disorders of other etiologies [40].

The presence of a preoperative acromial stress fracture is not considered to be a contraindication to RSA [41]. Boileau et al. [37] suggested that a history of previous infection and a nonfunctional deltoid muscle are two major contraindications to a reverse prosthesis. Gerber also stated that complete axillary nerve palsy is considered a contraindication because of the very high probability of recurrent instability and the minimal potential gain in function [42]. In addition, infection, neuroarthropathy, and substantial glenoid bone erosion or defects are contraindications to RSA.

16.3.1.2 Irreparable, Massive Cuff Tear (Hamada Classification [31]: Grade 2, 3)

Many authors currently define a tear as massive if there is a detachment of at least two complete tendons. The management of patients with irreparable, massive rotator cuff tears in the absence of glenohumeral arthritis remains a challenge for orthopedic surgeons. A variety of arthroscopic treatment options have been proposed for patients with irreparable rotator cuff tears without the presence of arthritis of the glenohumeral joint: these include subacromial decompression [43], simple debridement with a biceps tenotomy [44], partial rotator cuff repair [45], tuberoplasty [46], graft interposition of the rotator cuff [47], superior capsule reconstruction [48], and insertion of a biodegradable spacer [49] to depress the humeral head. In cases of irreparable massive cuff tear with or without glenohumeral pathology, several studies have shown that RSA can predictably restore functions including overhead elevation, improve pain, and increase external rotation, particularly if the patient has a functioning teres minor [38, 40]. Mulieri et al. [50] evaluated the indications for and outcomes of RSA in patients with massive rotator cuff tears but without glenohumeral arthritis. Their indications for RSA include persistent shoulder pain and dysfunction despite the provision of nonoperative treatment for a minimum of 6 months, the presence of at least a two-tendon tear, and Hamada stage 1, 2, or 3 changes in a patient for whom a non-arthroplasty option does not exist. The authors concluded that when non-arthroplasty options have either failed or have a low likelihood of success, RSA provides reliable pain relief and a return of shoulder function in patients with massive rotator cuff tears without arthritis at the time of short- to intermediate-term follow-up examinations.

16.3.2 Relative Indications

16.3.2.1 Complex Three- and Four-Part Proximal Humerus Fractures in Elderly Patients

The use of reverse shoulder arthroplasty is becoming increasingly popular in the treatment of complex three- and four-part proximal humerus fractures in elderly patients [51].

Proximal humerus fractures account for nearly 5 % of all fractures and are increasing in frequency in aging populations. Although three- and four-part fractures and fracture dislocations account for 5 % of all proximal humerus fractures, elderly patients are more prone to sustaining complex fracture patterns in comparison to younger patients [52–54]. Fragility fractures of the proximal humerus are often highly comminuted and displaced and involve poor bone quality, which makes them difficult to treat with open reduction and internal fixation or hemiarthroplasty. Concerns regarding plate osteosynthesis include humeral head osteonecrosis, loss of fixation, and screw penetration through the humeral head. Hemiarthroplasty offers a good solution for irreparable fractures and provides good pain relief; however, the functional outcomes are not always predictable [55]. Hemiarthroplasty outcomes are often bimodal and are divided between excellent and poor outcomes, with the main determinant being the healing of the tuberosities [56]. Consequently, RSA has been advocated for the treatment of complex fractures because the results are often more consistent and predictable [55].

16.3.2.2 Fracture Sequelae of the Proximal Humerus, Including Malunion and Nonunion

Late complications in the proximal humerus, such as malunion, avascular necrosis, and nonunion are frequent and often lead to articular incongruence [57]. Patients can be severely handicapped and may experience considerable pain, stiffness, and important functional impairment. Stiff shoulders with a distorted proximal humerus, soft tissue damage, a scarred deltoid, and rotator cuff tears make shoulder arthroplasty a challenging procedure. The sequelae of a proximal humeral fracture can cause shoulder pain and functional impairment. Hemiarthroplasty or total shoulder arthroplasty are considered after failure of nonoperative treatment [1], although the results have often been poor and unpredictable [58–60]. The procedure is associated with a high risk of complications [57]. The overall results of patients with old trauma are inferior to those that are currently obtained in patients with primary osteoarthritis or with recent four-part fractures who are initially treated with humeral head replacement. In elderly patients in whom there is significant distortion of the proximal humerus, poor bone quality, rotator cuff lesions, or muscle atrophy, reverse shoulder arthroplasty can be proposed instead of non-constrained arthroplasty. Fracture sequelae of the proximal part of the humerus are challenging conditions, and various treatment options have been described. The nonunion of the proximal humerus can be treated with reverse shoulder arthroplasty. The clinical outcomes of RSA have shown significant improvement [57, 61]. Martinez et al. [62] reported on a case series of 44 patients who underwent RSA for proximal humeral sequelae. The Constant score of the patients improved from 28 to 58 points, the anterior elevation improved from 40° to 100°, and range of external rotation improved from 15° to 35°. The most common complication was prosthesis instability. Zafra et al. [63] reviewed the results of 35 patients who underwent RSA for the treatment of nonunion of a fracture of the proximal humerus. The patients reported a significant decrease in pain, and significant improvements were observed in their flexion, abduction, external rotation, and Constant scores. A total of nine complications were recorded in seven patients including dislocation ($n = 6$). Reverse shoulder replacement may lead to a significant reduction in pain, improvement in function, and a higher degree of satisfaction. However, the rate of complications, particularly dislocation, is high.

16.3.2.3 Rheumatoid Shoulder with Cuff-Function Deficiency

Rheumatoid arthritis represents the majority of inflammatory arthritis cases and affects 1 % of the world's population [64–67]. Furthermore, shoulder symptoms are reported in up to 91 % of patients with long-standing rheumatoid arthritis. A system popularized by Laine et al. [68] categorized rheumatoid arthritis into three stages of disease. Stage II is characterized by a marked limitation in the range of motion and radiographic changes in all cases, with limitations that vary from slight to severe. Stage III disease includes patients in whom the disease has "burned out" and is characterized by severe limitations of movement and radiographic changes, including bone erosion and joint space narrowing. Stage II or III patients in whom the disease shows progression and who have disabling pain should be considered for arthroplasty [69]. The attenuated soft tissue of the rheumatoid shoulder, including the increased frequency of rotator cuff tears, must be considered when planning shoulder arthroplasty. RSA is attractive in patients with end-stage rheumatoid arthritis associated with a massive, irreparable rotator cuff tear (Barlow shoulder arthroplasty [67].

One systemic review showed that the mean increases in Constant score and ASES score after RSA surgery were 42.4 and 54 points, respectively [70]. The mean postoperative forward elevation was 120.6°, with the average increase in elevation being 51°. The mean increase in abduction was 58.5°. Revision surgery was performed for eight prostheses (because of infection in four cases). The authors concluded that RSA appeared to achieve similar results in RA patients to those obtained in patients with massive cuff tears with or without arthropathy.

16.3.2.4 Revision Surgery for Failed TSA

Total shoulder arthroplasty is one of the most effective procedures for relieving pain and improving function. The implant survival of total shoulder prostheses was previously reported to be inferior to that of hemiprostheses [71]. According to the Norwegian Arthroplasty Register, the 5-year survival rates for hemiprostheses and anatomic total prostheses and reverse total prostheses inserted from 2006 to 2012 were 95 % (compared to 94 % in 1994–1999), 95 % (75 % in 1994–1999), and 93 % (91 % in 1994–1999), respectively [72]. The findings indicated that the survival of anatomic total shoulder prostheses has improved. Risk factors for revision include young age, male gender, and shoulder arthroplasty for trauma-related sequelae [73, 74]. Singh et al. [75] examined the factors that were predictive of revision in 2207 patients who underwent total shoulder arthroplasty (TSA) and found that male gender and rotator cuff disease were independent risk factors for revision after TSA. If it is uncertain whether the revision of failed anatomic hemiarthroplasty or total shoulder arthroplasty will preserve or restore satisfactory rotator cuff function, conversion to reverse total shoulder arthroplasty has become the preferred treatment, at least for elderly patients. Wall et al. [76] reported that the postoperative Constant scores of revision arthroplasty patients were significantly worse than those of three other groups of patients (cuff tear arthropathy, massive cuff tear, and primary osteoarthritis). Patients in the revision arthroplasty group also had significantly worse postoperative ranges of elevation in comparison to the other three groups. In addition, the percentage of patients who stated that they were very satisfied or satisfied with the outcome was lower in the revision arthroplasty group than in the other three groups; however, this difference did not achieve statistical significance. A humeral fracture occurred during removal of the primary prosthesis or cement mantle during 13 of the 54 (24.1 %) revision procedures.

16.3.2.5 Primary Osteoarthritis of the Glenohumeral Joint with Glenoid Deformity

Neer et al. [1] observed the existence of posterior glenoid erosion and humeral head subluxation in some cases of primary glenohumeral arthritis and advised that erosion of the eccentric glenoid be corrected at the time of implantation of a polyethylene glenoid. The results of shoulder arthroplasty in the presence of a biconcave glenoid have been analyzed as part of a larger series of shoulders with and without this specific pathology [77, 78]. Humeral head replacement is associated with poor functional results. Levine et al. [79] found that only 63 % of results were satisfactory in patients with posterior glenoid wear. Iannotti and Norris [80] analyzed the influence of humeral head subluxation and posterior glenoid erosion in patients with primary osteoarthritis and found that shoulders with posterior subluxation of the humeral head (as quantified by preoperative axillary radiographs) had lower functional results and more pain regardless of whether the patient underwent hemiarthroplasty or total shoulder arthroplasty (TSA). Walch et al. [81] reported on 92 TSAs that were performed for B2 glenoids which were reviewed at a mean of 77 months after surgery. Revision surgery was required in 16 % of the cases and glenoid loosening was observed in 21 % of the cases. Mizuno et al. [82] reported the results of 27 RSAs in patients with primary glenohumeral arthritis with a B2 glenoid at a mean of 54 months after surgery. The mean Constant score increased from 31 to 76, and no recurrence of posterior instability was observed.

The B2 glenoid presents a difficult reconstructive problem with high failure rates caused by early glenoid loosening or recurrent posterior instability with the use of anatomic arthroplasty. In particular, unacceptably high rates of complications have been observed in cases where posterior humeral head subluxation is more than 80 % or neoglenoid retroversion is greater than 27° [82]. When posterior erosion cannot be adequately corrected with eccentric reaming, particularly in older patients, primary reverse shoulder arthroplasty may be a more predictable means of addressing bone deficiency and restoring stability.

16.3.2.6 Proximal Humerus Tumors Requiring the Resection of Rotator Cuff Insertions

The proximal humerus is the third most common site for primary bone tumors and soft tissue tumors [7]. Even in cases for which oncological treatment is essential, the preservation of shoulder function is important after a wide resection of the proximal humerus and the rotator cuff tendons. The salvage of limb and shoulder function after proximal humeral resection for tumors still presents a challenge. Several techniques of shoulder reconstruction have been reported, including arthrodesis [83], allograft [84], and massive shoulder arthroplasty [85]. Limb-sparing surgery for tumors of the proximal humerus yield good oncological results, but regardless of the technique that is used, the patients are left with functional impairment of the shoulder, which almost always precludes activities above shoulder level.

Wilde et al. [7] retrospectively reviewed 14 patients who underwent reverse total shoulder arthroplasty for tumors of the proximal humerus; 4 of the patients died, leaving 9 for review. The minimum follow-up period was 0.6 years (mean, 7.7 years; range, 0.6–12 years). At the most recent follow-up examination, the mean active abduction was 157° and the mean functional Constant-Murley score was 76 %. One patient had a deep infection and 1 developed a loose prosthesis; both were treated with single-stage exchange. Their study, with a medium-term follow-up period, suggests that reverse total shoulder arthroplasty is a reasonable option for tumors of the proximal humerus. However, a prerequisite for this therapeutic option is the preservation of the axillary nerve and the deltoid muscle [37].

16.4 Surgical Technique

Preoperative planning is performed using X-ray templates of known magnification in the frontal and sagittal views to determine the implant size and positioning. The use of a computer tomography (CT) scanner is recommended to determine the orientation of the glenoid and bone stock quality. The X-ray templates allow the surgeon to assess the size and the optimal length of the glenohumeral implants and the diameters of the metaphysis, the polyinsert, and the glenoid sphere.

The patient is placed in a beach-chair position with the shoulder positioned sufficiently lateral to allow full arm extension. In every case, general anesthesia with a scalene block or an indwelling scalene catheter is used, and perioperative antibiotics are administered.

Either the deltopectoral or anterosuperior approach can be used. Most surgeons are more familiar with the deltopectoral approach for arthroplasty. The anterosuperior approach is also used for reverse shoulder arthroplasty, which is an intermediate between the transacromial approach originally proposed by Paul Grammont [14] and the anterosuperior approach described by D.B. Mackenzie [86] for shoulder arthroplasty [87]. As an alternative to the deltopectoral approach, the anterosuperior approach has the advantages of simplicity and postoperative stability in cases with massive cuff tears (Fig. 16.2). A deltopectoral approach was found to be much better than an anterosuperior approach in terms of better orientation of the glenoid component, glenoid loosening, inferior scapular notching, and access to the humeral shaft in prosthetic revisions. The transacromial approach is complicated by failure of acromial synthesis [88]. Surgeons must select the approach according to their experience and patient-specific factors. I prefer the deltopectoral approach.

During the procedure, an incision is made from the tip of the coracoid along the deltopectoral groove, slightly lateral to the axillary fold. The pectoralis major is identified. The deltoid and cephalic veins are retracted laterally to open the deltopectoral groove. The coracoid process is identified, and a Hohmann retractor is positioned behind the coracoid. Care should be taken to preserve the origin and insertion of the deltoid. The clavipectoral fascia is incised at the external border of the coracobrachialis. The biceps tendon sheath is opened and extended proximally to the rotator interval. The long head of the biceps is released from the superior attachment to the glenoid and tenodesed to the pectoralis major tendon. The axillary nerve is then identified by digital palpation before opening the subscapularis. When it is intact, the subscapularis is tenotomized close to the musculotendinous junction to repair it in an original position at the end of the procedure. Some previous studies have found that subscapularis repair decreases the rate of instability by creating anterior soft tissue [89], but others did not observe this finding [76, 90].

With the arm externally rotated, an anterior and inferior capsule may be released from the surgical neck of the humerus to the glenoid. With adequate releases, the humeral head can be dislocated into the deltopectoral interval by abduction of the arm and progressive external rotation and extension. In cases of severely restricted

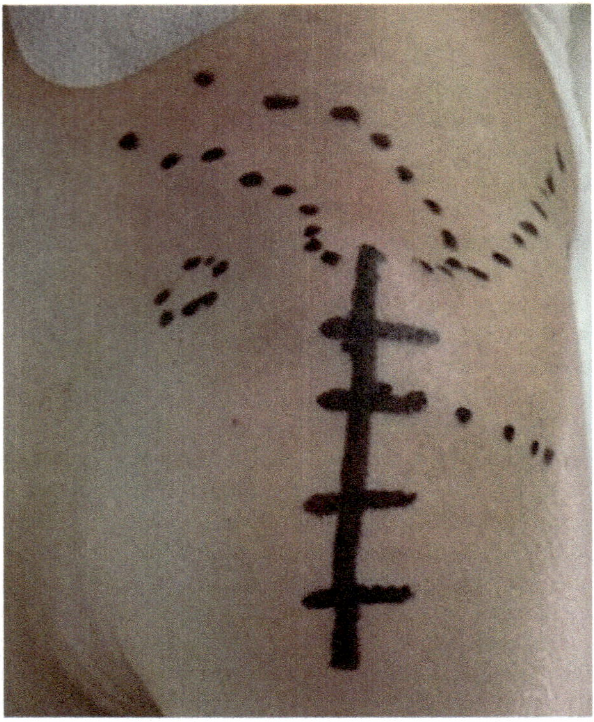

Fig. 16.2 Anterosuperior approach

external rotation, the upper 1 cm of the pectoralis major tendon is released. The joint capsule is split in line with the bicipital groove and extended into the rotator cuff interval. The humeral head is generally deformed, and anatomic reference points may be missing or distorted. Once the retroversion between 0° and 20° has been determined, the head is then resected with an oscillating saw, respecting the greater and lesser tuberosities. After head resection, aggressive removal of osteophytes around the humerus should be performed to improve the range of motion and allow for easier exposure during the remainder of the surgery [91]. Residual posterior osteophytes commonly prevent adequate posterior retraction of the humerus during glenoid preparation.

After retracting the humerus posteriorly, a partial capsulotomy and resection of the remaining glenoid labrum are performed to expose the glenoid. The capsule is released circumferentially. In cases with significant preoperative stiffness, it may be difficult to regain postoperative mobility. Removal of soft tissue adhesions may be required in conjunction with a capsulotomy. A retractor is positioned at the inferior border of the glenoid. The two-pronged retractor is seated at the posterior aspect of the glenoid. Additional retractors are positioned superior and inferior. Glenoid osteophytes are removed to further reveal the anatomic shape. The exact positioning and orientation of the guidewire for the reamer are important (Fig. 16.3). Preoperative planning must ascertain that reaming can be performed without

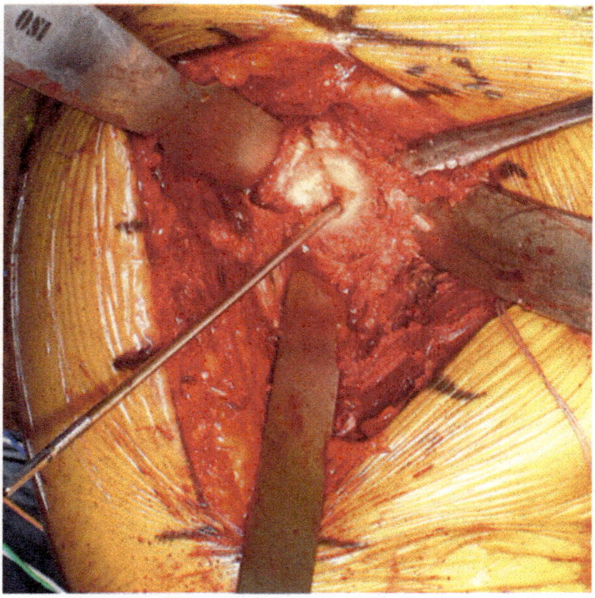

Fig. 16.3 Exposure of glenoid. A guidewire is tilted superiorly

creating glenoid anteversion or retroversion, or a superior glenoid tilt (Fig. 16.4). Compression and locking screws are used to provide stability of the baseplate. To secure fixation, they are anchored in the lateral pillar of the scapula and in the base of the coracoid. An appropriately sized glenosphere is then placed on the baseplate.

Reaming is then performed using a metaphyseal reamer for the metaphysis of the humerus. During this maneuver, the tuberosities may disappear in small patients, as is commonly seen in Japanese females. The diameter of the metaphysis may be too small. The diaphysis of the humerus is manually reamed using cylindrical reamers that progressively increase in diameter. Reaming is complete when the reamer contacts diaphyseal cortical bone. Additional reaming should be avoided to prevent humeral fracture. The last reamer used determines the final implant diameter and length. The assembly of the diaphyseal and metaphyseal components is inserted into the reamed medullary canal. An appropriately thick trial spacer is placed on the metaphyseal component, reduction is performed, and the tension of the deltoid is checked.

The chosen trial insert of the desired thickness is inserted into the trial metaphysis for trial reduction. The humeral trial component is then reduced into the joint to check the deltoid tension, stability, and range of motion. In cases with severe bone defects or inadequate deltoid tension, the final implant is inserted into the canal with appropriate retroversion and a polyinsert with an appropriate thickness. The prosthesis is then reduced using the reducer and the stability is checked. The arm is pulled away from the body after reduction to ensure that there is no pistoning effect. A complete separation of the humeral insert from the glenoid sphere indicates inadequate tensioning of the deltoid. Reverse shoulder arthroplasty

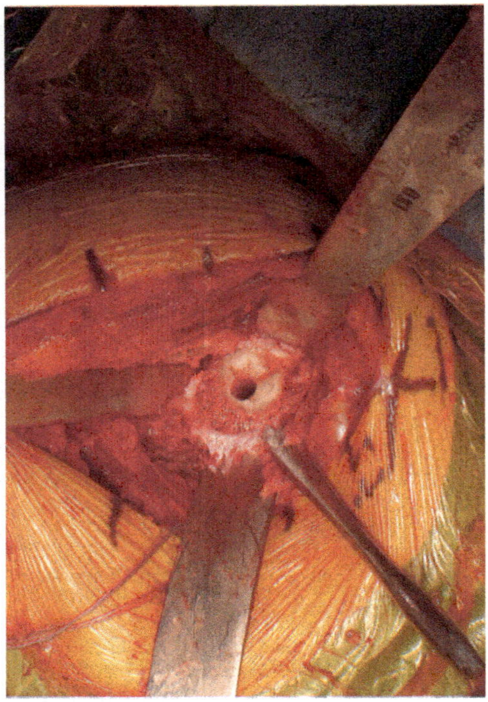

Fig. 16.4 Smile sign. After reaming of glenoid, smile sign should be seen

requires a retensioning of the deltoid to obtain active elevation and stability of the implant.

In patients with a rotator cuff-deficient shoulder, a combined loss of active elevation and external rotation (CLEER) can occur when both the infraspinatus and teres minor muscles are absent. A modified L'Episcopo procedure [latissimus dorsi (LD) and teres major (TM) transfer] is recommended in such cases, because it restores active elevation and external rotation [92].

Abduction of the arm is performed to check that there is no impingement and that the anterior elevation and abduction have been restored. External rotation with the elbow at the side checks for mobility and the risk of subluxation. Internal rotation is performed with the elbow at the side and in abduction. The arm is adducted to check that there is no impingement between the pillar of the scapula and the humeral implant. After reduction, the conjoined tendon should show sufficient muscular tension, which is similar to the deltoid. However, there is no objective and reliable technique that has been described for the preoperative planning of reverse shoulder prosthesis or for the postoperative evaluation of deltoid tension and arm lengthening.

Lädermann et al. [93] described a technique to preoperatively plan adequate deltoid tensioning using radiographs of the contralateral arm, and showed that the arm was lengthened 23 ± 12 mm after reverse shoulder arthroplasty. In cases of postoperative instability, both the humeral and overall arm lengthening were significantly less. He suggested that subjective intraoperative criteria to evaluate deltoid tension should be replaced by objective measures to prevent insufficient or excessive deltoid tension.

Next, the subscapularis is reattached to the lesser tuberosity. Gerber [42] did not initially repair it, because after RSA it becomes an adductor rather than an abductor, but they found that leaving the subscapularis unrepaired consistently led to an inability of the patient to reach behind their back. Thus, they readapted the subscapularis at the end of the procedure. Edwards et al. [89] found that a subscapularis tendon that cannot be repaired using a deltopectoral approach results in a statistically significant risk for postoperative dislocation, and they suggested that repairing the subscapularis can decrease the likelihood of postoperative dislocation after reverse shoulder arthroplasty.

Finally, the wound is closed over two drains, and the patient is placed in a commercially available shoulder immobilizer. The arm is placed in a brace with the elbow close to the body in neutral or internal rotation postoperatively. A single anteroposterior radiograph of the glenohumeral joint should be taken in the recovery room to assess the immediate postoperative stability and component position and to identify any intraoperative fractures that may have occurred. Passive range of motion (ROM) of the elbow and active and passive ROM of the wrist and hand are permitted the next day. The drains are left in place for 24–48 h. Rehabilitation is performed with passive pendulum exercises five times per day at 5 min per session.

16.5 Activities of Daily Life and Sports After RSA

The main goals of reverse shoulder arthroplasty (RSA) are to obtain relief of pain, regain function, and enhance the quality of life in a patient with cuff function deficiency. Wall et al. [76] reported the clinical outcomes of Grammont-type RSA in 240 cases, and found that patients with primary rotator cuff tear arthropathy, primary osteoarthritis with a rotator cuff tear, and a massive rotator cuff tear without arthritis had the best final outcomes. These three groups did not differ significantly from one another with respect to the postoperative Constant scores, range of motion, or the subjective rating of the outcome. In contrast, the patients in the posttraumatic arthritis and revision arthroplasty groups had significantly worse postoperative Constant scores in comparison with the other three groups. The patients in the posttraumatic arthritis and revision arthroplasty groups also had significantly worse postoperative ranges of elevation in comparison with the other three groups. In addition, the percentage of patients who stated that they were very satisfied or satisfied with the outcome was lower in the posttraumatic arthritis and revision arthroplasty groups (89 %) than in the other three groups (96 %), although this difference did not achieve significance ($p = 0.083$). The postoperative Constant scores were significantly related to the patients' subjective ratings. The postoperative Constant scores were also significantly related to the postoperative active range of elevation in all the etiology groups. Other reports have shown similar results [37].

In contrast to these reports, Schwartz et al. [94] found that the intraoperative forward flexion was the strongest predictor of the final postoperative ROM, followed by gender and the preoperative ROM. Because intraoperative forward flexion was the most powerful predictor of postoperative motion, the importance of trying to attain additional soft tissue release in the operating room cannot be overstated. It has been suggested that a limited active ROM of reverse shoulder prostheses is related to a lack of strength.

Alta et al. [30] identified correlations between the clinical outcome scores (Constant-Murley, DASH, and Simple Shoulder Test score) and the abduction and external rotation torque values, which supports that impaired shoulder strength is likely one of the causes of active ROM limitations. The functional outcome is probably not determined by simple ROM ranges alone, but also by the actual capacity for material handling in elevated and axially rotated arm positions.

In our experience, some patients treated with RSA recovered more rapidly than our expectation in terms of the pain and active range of motion (Fig. 16.5). We have never experienced such rapid patient recovery after rotator cuff surgery or artificial joint surgery. Although the patient expectations after anatomic TSA and RSA relate to sustained improvements in pain, function, and motion, the time necessary to reach these goals is unclear. Levy et al. [95] evaluated the time needed to achieve a plateau in maximal improvement after both TSA and RSA, and found that those treated with TSA can anticipate a more consistent and effective recovery of pain, function, and shoulder rotation. Patients receiving RSA can expect a variable length of recovery, with greater improvements in forward elevation and abduction.

Although patients can raise their arms over their heads after this procedure, significant concerns exist regarding the limitations that a RSA prosthesis places on internal rotation (IR), and the concomitant difficulty with activities of daily living, specifically perineal care [96]. Surgical treatment for bilateral, symptomatic CTA with an RSA prosthesis was thought to result in unsatisfactory outcomes and dysfunction in activities in daily living because of patient difficulty with internal rotation [96]. Patients require internal rotation of the shoulder in abduction to reach their back pocket, perform perineal hygiene, wash their back, and so on. Stevens et al. [96] found that perineal care is not a problem for most patients after bilateral RSA; all patients were able to perform perineal hygiene, and their patients experienced a median improvement in the IR of three vertebral levels on each side at final follow-up, although this was not significant. In many patients with a massive rotator cuff tear, the external rotation is restricted by a torn infraspinatus tendon preoperatively. Although Werner et al. [38] found that external rotation decreased from 17° to 12° after RSA, Wall et al. [76] and Rhee et al. [97] reported that the external rotation remained unchanged after RSA. Further, Rhee et al. [97] compared outcomes after a humeral component retroversion of 20° with 0° during RSA for cuff tear arthropathy, and no significant difference was seen in the ROM. However, they observed a better result for back washing and fastening a bra in the back when the retroversion was 0°.

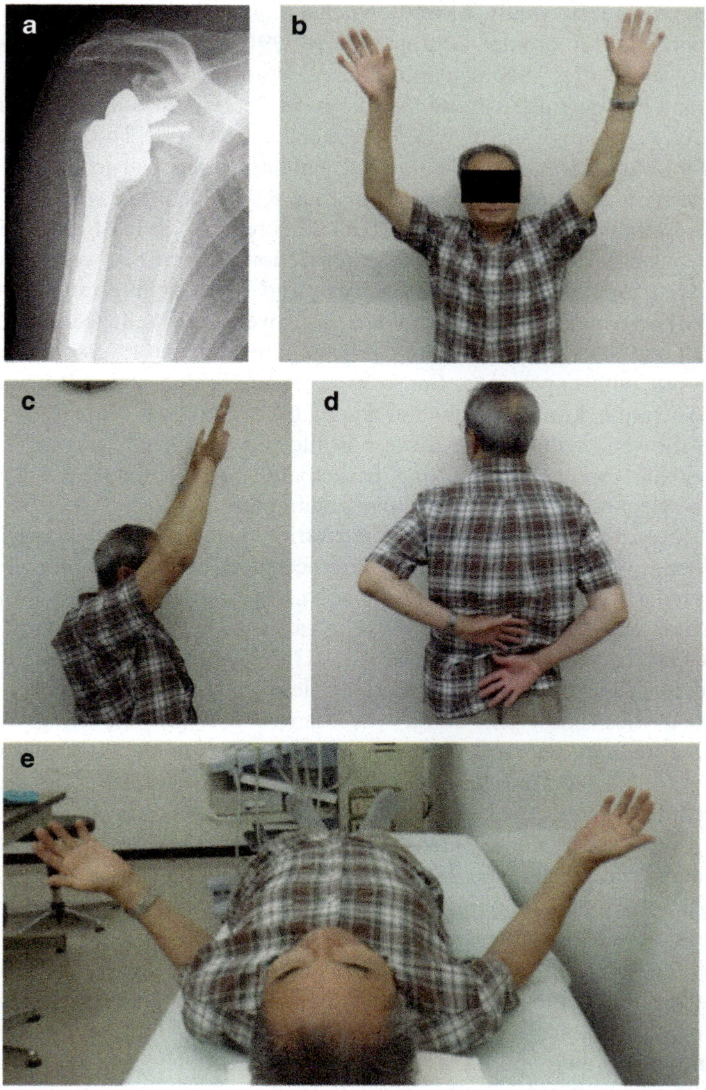

Fig. 16.5 Images obtained after reverse shoulder arthroplasty for cuff tear arthropathy. (**a**) Anteroposterior (AP) radiograph shows humeral and glenoid implants in place. Clinical photographs show postoperative active range of motion in abduction (**b**), forward elevation (**c**), internal rotation (**d**), and external rotation (**e**)

A major component of an improved quality of life after RSA is the ability to resume activities that were not possible or accomplished with difficulty before shoulder replacement surgery. Advances in RSA, creating early positive outcomes, have heightened the patients' expectations for a return to their previous levels of activity. Several recent studies have shown that most patients maintain their athletic participation after hip or knee arthroplasty [98, 99], but much less is known about the activity level after shoulder arthroplasty. With the support of the American Shoulder and Elbow Surgeons and the European Society for Surgery of the Shoulder and Elbow, an online survey was performed in 2010 [100]. The survey indicated that 56 % of shoulder surgeons permitted patients to proceed to their maximum allowed activity level after 5–7 months after RSA, 22 % allowed this level of activity 2–4 months after, and an additional 20 % required at least 8 months before this level of activity was allowed. The restrictions after RSA were much more conservative than those after hemiarthroplasty and TSA. Jogging/running, walking, stationary bicycling, and ballroom dancing were allowed. Numerous other low-impact activities, such as hiking, golf, table tennis, and cross-country skiing, were allowed with experience. Surgeons were undecided about doubles tennis, bowling, downhill skiing, and rowing, among other activities. Numerous activities were not allowed, including all those not allowed with TSA, as well as singles tennis, football (soccer), weightlifting, basketball, and track and field. Surgeons are advised to select older patients with lower demands.

The surgeon recommendations on the restrictions after RSA are largely anecdotal; generally, low-demand activities are accepted, but it is recommended that high-demand activities be avoided for concerns over implant loosening or failure. Seventy-eight patients (average age, 73 years) after RSA were assessed to define the patient-reported activities following RSA [101]. A significant proportion of patients continued to perform medium- (gardening, leaf raking, lawn mowing) or high-demand activities (snow shoveling, wheelbarrow use, dirt shoveling) following RSA. These findings are similar to those for other types of shoulder arthroplasties. Barns et al. [102] reported that 18 of 78 patients with RSA (23.1 %) returned to 24 different high-intensity activities, such as hunting, golf, and skiing; 38 patients (48.7 %) returned to moderate-intensity activities, such as swimming, bowling, and raking leaves; and 22 patients (28.2 %) returned to low-intensity activities, such as riding a stationary bike, playing a musical instrument, and walking. Four patients played golf before and after RTSA, but neither of the two patients who played tennis before RTSA were able to do so after the surgery. Simovitch et al. [103] reported that 95 % of their 40 patients with RSA were able to return to sports at the same level as before surgery or at a higher level, and only 13 % reported increased pain from playing their sport after undergoing an RSA. They therefore concluded that RSA in senior athletes can be safely performed with good clinical results, and that no prominent mode of mechanical or clinical failure has been identified based on a short-term follow-up.

16.6 Complications of Reverse Shoulder Arthroplasty

Accumulated experience with RSA has led to expanded surgical indications, including rotator cuff arthropathy [14, 18, 29, 38, 39], massive rotator cuff tears [38, 40, 50], fracture sequelae [57, 61], rheumatoid arthritis (RA) [70], acute fractures [51], tumors, or as a revision procedure for failed anatomic or reverse prostheses [104]. Although the complication rates vary widely because of the differences in what is considered to be a complication, the number has increased with the increasing indications, with reported rates ranging from 10.8 % to 68 % [29, 76, 88].

Kemptom et al. [105] reviewed an initial series of 200 reverse total shoulder arthroplasties performed by a single surgeon to characterize the early complication-based learning curve for RTSA to determine the types and severity of complications most affected by surgeon experience; they found that the early complication-based learning curve for reverse total shoulder arthroplasty is approximately 40 cases. There was a trend toward more complications in revision versus primary reverse total shoulder arthroplasty and more neuropathies in revisions. Walch et al. [29] compared two consecutive series of 240 RSA procedures to evaluate if the increase in surgeon experience modified the rate of complications. The postoperative complication rate decreased with increased experience (from 19 % to 10.8 %), with dislocation cases showing a reduction from 7 % to 3.2 % and infection cases showing a reduction from 4 to 0.9 %. However, the number of nerve palsies increased. The rate of glenoid notching remained stable, but the severity of notching decreased. The problem and complication rates differed among the different etiologies, and were both twice as common in the revision patients as in the combined primary arthroplasty group [106]. Surgeons must be aware that these patients may have neurological injury, infection, inferior scapular notching, instability, and so on.

16.6.1 Hematoma

The design of the RSA provides a large, empty subacromial space; in an early series, hematoma formation was the most frequently reported complication [38]. Sonography is most commonly used postoperatively to demonstrate the presence of a hematoma. Previous studies have indicated that a hematoma occurs in 1–20 % of patients following RSA [37, 38, 107], whereas a postoperative hematoma occurs in 0.3 % following anatomic TSA [108]. The placement of the glenosphere more inferiorly increases the acromiohumeral distance and increases the subacromial space. Hematoma was higher in failed rotator cuff repair, revision of anatomic prosthesis, and revision of reverse prosthesis [109].

To treat postoperative hematoma, Gerber [42] made the following recommendations: (1) draining should be allowed for 24–48 h, (2) a sling should be used postoperatively, (3) the arm may be used for activities such as brushing the teeth or eating, and (4) sling use should be discontinued after 4–6 weeks.

16.6.2 Neurological Injury

Neurological injury after shoulder arthroplasty has been reported and is transient in most cases [29, 42, 110, 111]. Clinical and subclinical neurological injury after reverse shoulder arthroplasty (RSA) may jeopardize the functional outcomes because of the risk of irreversible damage to the axillary nerve. It may be attributed to intraoperative traction, manipulation of the arm, retractor placement, or relative lengthening of the arm [111]. Lynch and Cofield et al. [112] observed that the presumed mechanism of injury was traction on the plexus occurring during the operation in most cases. The prognosis for neurological recovery was usually good [29, 42, 111]. In addition, neurological injury after total shoulder arthroplasty did not interfere with the long-term outcome of the arthroplasty itself [112]. During exposure of the glenoid, the humerus is posteriorly retracted, externally rotated, and abducted, which may accentuate the traction across the brachial plexus; this places excessive traction on the axillary nerve, in particular.

Walch et al. [29] reported that neurological complications increased from three (1.5 %) in the first cohort to eight (3.6 %) in the second, five of which persisted at follow-up. Of the three cases with transient nerve palsies, one involved the axillary nerve with sensory and motor deficits confirmed by EMG, which resolved in 5 months without sequelae; one had paresthesia in the ulnar nerve distribution, which resolved in a few weeks; and one involved partial sensory and motor dysfunction of the median, ulnar, and radial nerves, which also disappeared in a few weeks without sequelae. Of the five cases with persistent neurological deficits, three had dysesthesia of the fourth and fifth fingers, and one had recurrent median nerve paraesthesia corresponding to carpal tunnel syndrome.

Subclinical neurological lesions after reverse shoulder arthroplasty are common, mainly those involving the axillary nerve. One of the major reported risk factors is postoperative lengthening of the arm. Lädermann [110] observed subclinical postoperative electromyographic changes in 9 of 19 shoulders, with most involving the axillary nerve; 8 resolved in less than 6 months. In the anatomic shoulder arthroplasty group, a brachial plexus lesion was evident in 1 of 23 shoulders. The prevalence of acute postoperative nerve injury was significantly higher in the reverse shoulder arthroplasty group. The mean lengthening of the arm after reverse shoulder arthroplasty was 2.7 ± 1.8 cm compared with the normal, contralateral side. Arm lengthening with a reverse shoulder arthroplasty may be responsible for these nerve injuries.

Marion et al. [113] undertook a simple anatomic study using fresh human cadavers to assess the macroscopic effects on the axillary nerve when lowering the humerus was performed during RSA implantation, and measured the effects of a lateralization of the humerus on the axillary nerve. When the humerus was lowered, clear macroscopic changes appeared below the middle of the glenoid. With regard to the lateralization of the humerus, a macroscopic study and measurements confirmed the absence of stretching of the nerve in those positions. Lowering of the humerus below the equator of the glenoid changes the course and tension of the axillary nerve and may lead to stretching and irreversible damage, compromising the function of the deltoid.

16.6.3 Infection

Postoperative infection is a devastating complication that can follow a total joint arthroplasty. Infection is a relatively common complication associated with RSA, with a reported incidence of approximately 1–10 % [76, 107, 111, 114, 115]. Patients undergoing primary RSA had a six times greater risk of infection compared with patients undergoing primary TSA [115]. However, Florschütz et al. [116] reported that of 814 primary TSA performed, deep periprosthetic infections were confirmed in 16 shoulders. Infections occurred in 6 TSAs and 10 RSAs, with no significant difference among the prosthesis types. Morris reported that the greatest risk factors for infection after RSA were a history of a prior failed arthroplasty and age younger than 65 years [117]. RSA-related infection is generally the result of the formation of a hematoma caused by to the presence of a large amount of dead space and the revision setting after multiple prior surgeries. In a retrospective multicenter study, Jacuot et al. [118] reported that infections were largely caused by coagulase-negative staphylococci and *Propionibacterium acnes* in 32 cases. Implant revision (one- or two-stage) led to better functional results than implant removal, with similar healing rates. Revision of the implant preserves the shoulder function, with no higher rate of residual infection compared with implant removal.

Preventative measures are absolutely necessary to decrease the overall rate of periprosthetic joint infection following RSA procedures [119] (Table 16.2). These strategies are best understood and employed when the risk factors are divided and tackled on three fronts: host, operating room environment, and surgical variables. Similar to other joint arthroplasty procedures, the intraoperative strategies for preventing infection include perioperative administration of intravenous antibiotics; adequate skin preparation; appropriate use of gowns, gloves, and antibiotic cement; limiting OR traffic; and selection of the optimal method of wound closure. Preoperative antibiotic administration decreases the rate of infection following surgical procedures.

Appropriate preoperative antibiotics are administered within 1 h of the incision, and they are mandatory for prophylaxis. Antibiotic prophylaxis can be delivered through antibiotic-impregnated bone cement. In the Finnish Arthroplasty Register, Jämsen et al. [120] found that the combined use of systemic antibiotic prophylaxis and antibiotic-impregnated bone cement lowered the rate of infection (0.68 % of

Table 16.2 Indications for RSA according to the Japanese guidelines for RSA

A. Absolute indications
1. Cuff tear arthropathy (Hamada classification, grade 4, 5)
2. Irreparable, massive cuff tear (Hamada classification, Grade 2, 3)
B. Relative indications
1. Complex three- and four-part proximal humerus fractures in elderly patients
2. Fracture sequelae of the proximal humerus, including malunion and nonunion
3. Rheumatoid shoulder with cuff function deficiency
4. Revision surgery for failed TSA
5. Primary osteoarthritis of the glenohumeral joint with glenoid deformity
6. Proximal humerus tumors requiring the resection of rotator cuff insertions

32,918 knees) more than the use of systemic antibiotics alone (1.05 % of 6,550 knees).

Propionibacterium acnes infection is a significant problem after shoulder surgery [118, 121]. Residual *P. acnes* is found on the skin up to 29 % of the time immediately after surgical skin preparation, and in 70 % of dermal biopsy specimens [122]. These residual bacteria may be one source of infection. Recently, Sabetta et al. [122] reported that the application of topical benzoyl peroxide with chlorhexidine for skin preparation is an effective way to reduce *P. acnes* on the skin at the beginning, and importantly, at the end, of a surgical procedure.

As with other types of joint arthroplasty, infection is diagnosed based on a combination of symptoms, laboratory tests, and findings on physical examination, such as a draining sinus, radiologic evidence of loosening of the prosthesis, radioisotope scanning, and analyses of intraoperative specimens [123]. The management of deep sepsis in RSA involves increased concerns about bone loss compared to traditional TSA [124]. Acute infection can be managed with irrigation, debridement, and polyethylene exchange. Chronic infection is best managed with two-stage revision. Stage one consists of hardware removal, irrigation and debridement and the placement of an antibiotic spacer, followed by a minimum 6-week course of parenteral antibiotics. During stage two, prosthesis reimplantation is performed, but should be deferred until all cultures and blood test results are negative. There is some evidence to suggest that chronic infections can be managed with a one-stage exchange involving irrigation and debridement, reimplantation, and parenteral antibiotics [111, 123, 125]. Beckman et al. [125] retrospectively reviewed 11 consecutive patients with an infected reverse shoulder prosthesis treated by a one-stage revision. All but one patient was considered to be free of infection after one-stage revision after a median follow-up of 24 months, and without antibiotic treatment for a minimum of 6 months. They concluded that a one-stage revision arthroplasty reduces the cost and duration of treatment.

16.6.4 Scapular Notching

The most common problem observed in the radiologic findings was scapular notching, which was noted in approximately 49.8–96 % of patients with a Grammont-type prosthesis [38, 76, 88, 126]. Scapular notching, which is a defect of the bone in the inferior part of the glenoid component, is caused by direct mechanical collision of the superomedial part of the humeral implant against the pillar of the scapula. Particulate polyethylene debris may aggravate inferior notching and lead to osteolysis. Impingement-free range of motion in all planes is essential [111]. In one study, 34 of 77 shoulders had inferior scapular notching, 23 had posterior notching, and 6 had anterior notching. The angle between the glenosphere and the scapular neck, as well as the craniocaudal position of the glenosphere, were highly correlated with inferior notching [127]. Inferior placement of the baseplate on the glenoid plate has been shown to prevent the occurrence of notching and also improve the range of motion [128].

In patients with a Grammont-style prosthesis in which the center of rotation of the glenosphere is on the face of the glenoid, the overall incidence of notching is high [18, 38, 76, 111, 127]. Several authors have recommended inferior placement of the Grammont-style glenosphere relative to the glenoid face to reduce the risk of notching [18, 38, 76, 111, 127].

Impingement may contribute to prosthetic instability, unexplained pain, and long-term loosening. The current prosthetic designs attempt to alleviate this conflict. Some authors lateralize the center of rotation [39, 42], which increases the tilting forces at the interface but also increases the impingement-free ROM. In patients with laterally offset glenospheres, the incidence of scapular notching has been reported to be between zero and 13 % [39, 106, 107, 111]. Zumstein et al. [106] reported that notching is a problem associated with RSA, but not a complication. They defined a problem as an intraoperative or postoperative event that was not likely to affect the patient's final outcome, including radiographic scapular notching, hematomas, heterotopic ossification, algodystrophy, phlebitis, intraoperative dislocations, intraoperative cement extravasation, or radiographic lucent lines of the glenoid.

16.6.5 Periprosthetic Fracture

Intraoperative periprosthetic fractures are common in patients who undergo RSA and can be challenging to manage [111]. Meticulous attention should be paid to prevent intraoperative glenoid fractures, especially when handling the glenoid baseplate reamer and when reaming the osteoporotic glenoid surface. An uncemented glenoid baseplate is used in all RSA systems. The baseplate is attached using a variably sized central screw or post. Wierks et al. [129] recommended reaming the glenoid with a reamer of an appropriate size for the baseplate by hand, because they experienced nondisplaced fractures of the glenoid when using a pneumatic power drill because of its high torque. When a glenoid fracture occurs, the surgeon should consider the company-dependent strategy to achieve rigid fixation again. Frequently, the proximal humerus is osteopenic and easy to break. Careful attention should therefore be paid when preparing the humerus. Wierks et al. [129] initially prepared the proximal humerus before inserting the glenoid baseplate and experienced a high number of rim fractures in the proximal humerus with this sequence. They subsequently recommended that the glenoid component be inserted first, followed by preparation of the proximal humerus and insertions of the humeral component.

16.6.6 Dislocation

One of the most common complications limiting the outcomes of RSA is postoperative instability. In the literature, the reported rates of instability range from 2.4 % to 31 % [130]. The direction of instability is usually anterior, occurring following extension, adduction and internal rotation. The stability in RSA is dependent on adequate soft tissue tensioning. Surgical factors related to the prosthesis design, such as the glenosphere offset and size, humeral neck–shaft angle, and polyethylene thickness and constraint, have been shown to affect the tensioning and stability. There are also surgical techniques that have been shown to alter the stability by increasing the length of the arm and consequently the deltoid muscle tension, such as the level of humeral osteotomy, offset placement of the humeral socket and the baseplate position on the glenoid.

Compared with the deltopectoral approach, the anterosuperior approach has the advantages of providing better postoperative stability in cases with massive cuff tears [87]. In the deltopectoral approach, Edwards et al. [89] quantified the risk of postoperative dislocation after reverse total shoulder arthroplasty in patients with a subscapularis tendon that was irreparable at the time of surgery. Seven postoperative dislocations occurred; all dislocations were in patients whose subscapularis was irreparable. Dislocations were more likely to occur in patients with complex diagnoses, including proximal humeral nonunion, fixed glenohumeral dislocation, and failed prior arthroplasty. They concluded that an irreparable subscapularis tendon at the time of RSA using a deltopectoral approach results in a statistically significant risk for postoperative dislocation. Chalmers et al. [131] reported that atraumatic instability occurred in 11 patients (incidence, 2.9 %) treated with RSA before 3 months post surgery. The most commonly associated factors were a body mass index (BMI) greater than 30 kg/m^2, male gender, subscapularis deficiency , and previous surgery; in these patients, they use an abduction orthosis. Closed reduction alone was successful in 44 % of cases. Five of the 11 RSAs required polyethylene exchange. Teusink et al. [94] experienced 21 patients with dislocation after RSA, and the average time from surgery until the first dislocation event was 200 days. All dislocations were anterosuperior dislocations. Of these, 62 %

occurred within the first 90 days postoperatively. After an average follow-up of 28 months, 62 % of these shoulders remained stable, 29 % had required revision surgery, and 9 % remained unstable.

16.6.7 Scapula Fractures

Fractures around the acromion are a known complication of reverse total shoulder arthroplasty, and have occurrence rates between 0.9 % and 7.2 % based on the literature [37, 132–135]. A fulcrum in RSA is provided by an appropriately tensioned deltoid, which actively elevates the upper arm and stabilizes the prosthesis. The acromial origin of the deltoid is important in deltoid tensioning and in the ultimate performance of the implant. Fractures of the acromion commonly occur as a result of a preexisting acromial lesion, overtensioning of the deltoid, or osseous fatigue from the loading of an osteopenic acromion [23]. Acromion wear of the shoulder, as seen in cuff tear arthropathy, may have a deleterious effect on the acromion, such as thinning, fatigue failure or fragmentation. Osteoporosis is a significant risk factor for scapular fractures after RSA [135]. Fractures that disrupt the appropriate tension of the deltoid may lead to deleterious consequences for the function of the implant. Teusink et al. [136] found that the incidence of scapular fractures after RSA was 3.1 %. Postoperative scapular fractures may occur at any point postoperatively; an increasing incidence is likely as longer follow-up becomes available. This complication leads to inferior clinical results compared with controls. However, patients show improvement compared with their preoperative measurements, even after longer-term follow-up. Scapular fractures after RSA can be treated either surgically or nonsurgically.

In most cases, the fractures can be treated without surgical intervention. After conservative management, most patients who had an acromial fracture returned to a functional level that was comparable to that achieved before fracture [137]. Crosby et al. [132] proposed a classification system based on the relationship of the fracture to the acromioclavicular joint. They showed three discrete patterns of scapula fractures: avulsion fractures of the anterior acromion (type I), fractures of the acromion posterior to the acromioclavicular joint (type II) and fractures of the scapular spine (type III), and they suggested that type I fractures have a high likelihood of symptom relief. For type II fractures, they recommend acromioclavicular joint resection if the joint is stable, but open reduction internal fixation if it is unstable. They believe type III fractures are best treated with open reduction internal fixation.

Otto et al. [135] advocated a different classification system for postoperative acromial fractures. Type I included fractures through the midpart of the acromion, involving a portion of the anterior and middle deltoid origin. Type II were defined as fractures involving at least the entire middle deltoid origin with a portion, but not all of, the posterior deltoid origin. Type III fractures involved the entire middle and posterior deltoid origin, similar to the acromial base fracture. Once an acromial fracture was identified clinically, patients were managed with a shoulder immobilizer for 6 weeks and were instructed to limit activity to pendulum shoulder exercises. After this nonsurgical regimen, significant improvements in the range of motion were seen for all measured movements for the type II group, for there were no improvements in the movements for the type I group, and there were only improvements for external rotation for the type III group. No good or excellent results were observed for type III fractures.

Although postoperative fracture of the acromial spine has a significant effect on the patient outcome [132, 135]. Walch et al. [138] reported that patients with *os acromiale* had a statistically superior mean Constant score when compared to normal subjects after RSA. A significant difference was also found for the activity and mobility portions of the Constant score, but there were no differences in the pain, strength, active elevation or subjective satisfaction. They concluded that acquired and congenital preoperative lesions of the acromion, such as os acromiale, are not a contraindication for RSA.

References

1. Neer CS 2nd, Watson KC, Stanton FJ (1982) Recent experience in total shoulder replacement. J Bone Joint Surg Am 64(3):319–337
2. Fenlin JM Jr, Vaccaro A, Andreychik D, Lin S (1990) Modular total shoulder: early experience and impressions. Semin Arthroplasty 1(2):102–111
3. Boileau P, Walch G (1997) The three-dimensional geometry of the proximal humerus. Implications for surgical technique and prosthetic design. J Bone Joint Surg Br 79 (5):857–865
4. Coughlin MJ, Morris JM, West WF (1979) The semiconstrained total shoulder arthroplasty. J Bone Joint Surg Am 61(4):574–581
5. Buechel FF, Pappas MJ, DePalma AF (1978) "Floating-socket" total shoulder replacement: anatomical, biomechanical, and surgical rationale. J Biomed Mater Res 12(1):89–114. doi:10.1002/jbm.820120109
6. Fenlin JM Jr (1975) Total glenohumeral joint replacement. Orthop Clin North Am 6 (2):565–583
7. Favard L, Levigne C, Nerot C, Gerber C, De Wilde L, Mole D (2011) Reverse prostheses in arthropathies with cuff tear: are survivorship and function maintained over time? Clin Orthop Relat Res 469(9):2469–2475. doi:10.1007/s11999-011-1833-y
8. Skolowsky LJ, Flatow EL, Bigliani LU, Mow VC (1993) Stabilization of the glenohumeral joint by articular contact and by contact in the subacromial space. In: Matsen FA III, Fu FH, Hawkins RJ (eds) The shoulder: a balance of mobility and stability. American Academy of Orthopaedic Surgeons, Rosemont, pp 107–124
9. Neer CS 2nd, Craig EV, Fukuda H (1983) Cuff-tear arthropathy. J Bone Joint Surg Am 65 (9):1232–1244
10. Halverson PB, Cheung HS, McCarty DJ, Garancis J, Mandel N (1981) "Milwaukee shoulder" – association of microspheroids containing hydroxyapatite crystals, active collagenase, and neutral protease with rotator cuff defects. II. Synovial fluid studies. Arthritis Rheum 24 (3):474–483
11. Franklin JL, Barrett WP, Jackins SE, Matsen FA 3rd (1988) Glenoid loosening in total shoulder arthroplasty. Association with rotator cuff deficiency. J Arthroplasty 3(1):39–46

12. Pollock RG, Deliz ED, McIlveen SJ, Flatow EL, Bigliani LU (1992) Prosthetic replacement in rotator cuff-deficient shoulders. J Shoulder Elbow Surg 1(4):173–186. doi:10.1016/1058-2746(92)90011-q
13. Sanchez-Sotelo J, Cofield RH, Rowland CM (2001) Shoulder hemiarthroplasty for glenohumeral arthritis associated with severe rotator cuff deficiency. J Bone Joint Surg Am 83-a(12):1814–1822
14. Grammont PM, Baulot E (1993) Delta shoulder prosthesis for rotator cuff rupture. Orthopedics 16(1):65–68
15. Neer CS 2nd (1990) Cuff tear arthropathy. Shoulder reconstruction. Saunders, Philadelphia
16. Flatow EL, Harrison AK (2011) A history of reverse total shoulder arthroplasty. Clin Orthop Relat Res 469(9):2432–2439. doi:10.1007/s11999-010-1733-6
17. Grammont PM, Trouilloud P, Laffay JP, Deries X (1987) Etude et realization d'une novelle prothese d'epaule. Rhumatologie 39:17–22
18. Boileau P, Watkinson DJ, Hatzidakis AM, Balg F (2005) Grammont reverse prosthesis: design, rationale, and biomechanics. J Shoulder Elbow Surg 14(1 suppl S):147S–161S. doi:10.1016/j.jse.2004.10.006
19. Berliner JL, Regalado-Magdos A, Ma CB, Feeley BT (2015) Biomechanics of reverse total shoulder arthroplasty. J Shoulder Elbow Surg 24(1):150–160. doi:10.1016/j.jse.2014.08.003
20. Kontaxis A, Johnson GR (2009) The biomechanics of reverse anatomy shoulder replacement: a modelling study. Clin Biomech 24(3):254–260
21. Terrier A, Reist A, Merlini F, Farron A (2008) Simulated joint and muscle forces in reversed and anatomic shoulder prostheses. J Bone Joint Surg Br 90(6):751–756. doi:10.1302/0301-620x.90b6.19708
22. Kapandji IA (1970) The physiology of joints, vol 1. Williams & Wilkins, Baltimore
23. Matsen FA 3rd, Boileau P, Walch G, Gerber C, Bicknell RT (2007) The reverse total shoulder arthroplasty. J Bone Joint Surg Am 89(3):660–667
24. Oosterom R, Herder JL, van der Helm FC, Swieszkowski W, Bersee HE (2003) Translational stiffness of the replaced shoulder joint. J Biomech 36(12):1897–1907
25. Halder AM, Kuhl SG, Zobitz ME, Larson D, An KN (2001) Effects of the glenoid labrum and glenohumeral abduction on stability of the shoulder joint through concavity-compression: an in vitro study. J Bone Joint Surg Am 83-A(7):1062–1069
26. Karduna AR, Williams GR, Williams JL, Iannotti JP (1997) Joint stability after total shoulder arthroplasty in a cadaver model. J Shoulder Elbow Surg 6(6):506–511
27. Favre P, Sussmann PS, Gerber C (2010) The effect of component positioning on intrinsic stability of the reverse shoulder arthroplasty. J Shoulder Elbow Surg 19(4):550–556. doi:10.1016/j.jse.2009.11.044
28. Gutierrez S, Keller TS, Levy JC, Lee WE 3rd, Luo ZP (2008) Hierarchy of stability factors in reverse shoulder arthroplasty. Clin Orthop Relat Res 466(3):670–676. doi:10.1007/s11999-007-0096-0
29. Walch G, Bacle G, Ladermann A, Nove-Josserand L, Smithers CJ (2012) Do the indications, results, and complications of reverse shoulder arthroplasty change with surgeon's experience? J Shoulder Elbow Surg 21(11):1470–1477. doi:10.1016/j.jse.2011.11.010
30. Alta TD, Veeger HE, Janssen TW, Willems WJ (2012) Are shoulders with a reverse shoulder prosthesis strong enough? A pilot study. Clin Orthop Relat Res 470(8):2185–2192. doi:10.1007/s11999-012-2277-8
31. Hamada K, Yamanaka K, Uchiyama Y, Mikasa T, Mikasa M (2011) A radiographic classification of massive rotator cuff tear arthritis. Clin Orthop Relat Res 469(9):2452–2460. doi:10.1007/s11999-011-1896-9
32. Ecklund KJ, Lee TQ, Tibone J, Gupta R (2007) Rotator cuff tear arthropathy. J Am Acad Orthop Surg 15(6):340–349
33. Feeley BT, Gallo RA, Craig EV (2009) Cuff tear arthropathy: current trends in diagnosis and surgical management. J Shoulder Elbow Surg 18(3):484–494. doi:10.1016/j.jse.2008.11.003

34. Hamada K, Fukuda H, Mikasa M, Kobayashi Y (1990) Roentgenographic findings in massive rotator cuff tears. A long-term observation. Clin Orthop Relat Res (254):92–96
35. Walch G, Edwards TB, Boulahia A, Nove-Josserand L, Neyton L, Szabo I (2005) Arthroscopic tenotomy of the long head of the biceps in the treatment of rotator cuff tears: clinical and radiographic results of 307 cases. J Shoulder Elbow Surg 14(3):238–246. doi:10.1016/j.jse.2004.07.008
36. Zeman CA, Arcand MA, Cantrell JS, Skedros JG, Burkhead WZ Jr (1998) The rotator cuff-deficient arthritic shoulder: diagnosis and surgical management. J Am Acad Orthop Surg 6 (6):337–348
37. Boileau P, Watkinson D, Hatzidakis AM, Hovorka I (2006) Neer Award 2005: the Grammont reverse shoulder prosthesis: results in cuff tear arthritis, fracture sequelae, and revision arthroplasty. J Shoulder Elbow Surg 15(5):527–540. doi:10.1016/j.jse.2006.01.003
38. Werner CM, Steinmann PA, Gilbart M, Gerber C (2005) Treatment of painful pseudoparesis due to irreparable rotator cuff dysfunction with the Delta III reverse-ball-and-socket total shoulder prosthesis. J Bone Joint Surg Am 87(7):1476–1486. doi:10.2106/jbjs.d.02342
39. Frankle M, Siegal S, Pupello D, Saleem A, Mighell M, Vasey M (2005) The reverse shoulder prosthesis for glenohumeral arthritis associated with severe rotator cuff deficiency. A minimum two-year follow-up study of sixty patients. J Bone Joint Surg Am 87(8):1697–1705. doi:10.2106/jbjs.d.02813
40. Guery J, Favard L, Sirveaux F, Oudet D, Mole D, Walch G (2006) Reverse total shoulder arthroplasty. Survivorship analysis of eighty replacements followed for five to ten years. J Bone Joint Surg Am 88(8):1742–1747. doi:10.2106/jbjs.e.00851
41. Mottier F, Wall B, Nove-Josserand L, Galoisy Guibal L, Walch G (2007) Reverse prosthesis and os acromiale or acromion stress fracture. Rev Chir Orthop Reparatrice Appar Mot 93 (2):133–141
42. Gerber C, Pennington SD, Nyffeler RW (2009) Reverse total shoulder arthroplasty. J Am Acad Orthop Surg 17(5):284–295
43. Ellman H, Kay SP, Wirth M (1993) Arthroscopic treatment of full-thickness rotator cuff tears: 2- to 7-year follow-up study. Arthroscopy 9(2):195–200
44. Liem D, Lengers N, Dedy N, Poetzl W, Steinbeck J, Marquardt B (2008) Arthroscopic debridement of massive irreparable rotator cuff tears. Arthroscopy 24(7):743–748. doi:10.1016/j.arthro.2008.03.007
45. Burkhart SS (1996) Shoulder arthroscopy. New concepts. Clin Sports Med 15(4):635–653
46. Scheibel M, Lichtenberg S, Habermeyer P (2004) Reversed arthroscopic subacromial decompression for massive rotator cuff tears. J Shoulder Elbow Surg 13(3):272–278. doi:10.1016/s1058274604000242
47. Rhee YG, Cho NS, Lim CT, Yi JW, Vishvanathan T (2008) Bridging the gap in immobile massive rotator cuff tears: augmentation using the tenotomized biceps. Am J Sports Med 36 (8):1511–1518. doi:10.1177/0363546508316020
48. Mihata T, Lee TQ, Watanabe C, Fukunishi K, Ohue M, Tsujimura T, Kinoshita M (2013) Clinical results of arthroscopic superior capsule reconstruction for irreparable rotator cuff tears. Arthroscopy 29(3):459–470. doi:10.1016/j.arthro.2012.10.022
49. Savarese E, Romeo R (2012) New solution for massive, irreparable rotator cuff tears: the subacromial "biodegradable spacer". Arthrosc Tech 1(1):e69–e74. doi:10.1016/j.eats.2012.02.002
50. Mulieri P, Dunning P, Klein S, Pupello D, Frankle M (2010) Reverse shoulder arthroplasty for the treatment of irreparable rotator cuff tear without glenohumeral arthritis. J Bone Joint Surg Am 92(15):2544–2556. doi:10.2106/jbjs.i.00912
51. Jobin CM, Galdi B, Anakwenze OA, Ahmad CS, Levine WN (2015) Reverse shoulder arthroplasty for the management of proximal humerus fractures. J Am Acad Orthop Surg 23(3):190–201. doi:10.5435/jaaos-d-13-00190
52. Court-Brown CM, Garg A, McQueen MM (2001) The epidemiology of proximal humeral fractures. Acta Orthop Scand 72(4):365–371. doi:10.1080/000164701753542023

53. Gaebler C, McQueen MM, Court-Brown CM (2003) Minimally displaced proximal humeral fractures: epidemiology and outcome in 507 cases. Acta Orthop Scand 74(5):580–585. doi:10.1080/00016470310017992
54. Bhandari M, Matthys G, McKee MD (2004) Four part fractures of the proximal humerus. J Orthop Trauma 18(2):126–127
55. Gallinet D, Clappaz P, Garbuio P, Tropet Y, Obert L (2009) Three or four parts complex proximal humerus fractures: hemiarthroplasty versus reverse prosthesis: a comparative study of 40 cases. Orthop Traumatol Surg Res 95(1):48–55. doi:10.1016/j.otsr.2008.09.002
56. Sirveaux F, Roche O, Mole D (2010) Shoulder arthroplasty for acute proximal humerus fracture. Orthop Traumatol Surg Res 96(6):683–694. doi:10.1016/j.otsr.2010.07.001
57. Mansat P, Bonnevialle N (2015) Treatment of fracture sequelae of the proximal humerus: anatomical vs reverse shoulder prosthesis. Int Orthop 39(2):349–354. doi:10.1007/s00264-014-2651-0
58. Antuna SA, Sperling JW, Sanchez-Sotelo J, Cofield RH (2002) Shoulder arthroplasty for proximal humeral malunions: long-term results. J Shoulder Elbow Surg 11(2):122–129
59. Beredjiklian PK, Iannotti JP, Norris TR, Williams GR (1998) Operative treatment of malunion of a fracture of the proximal aspect of the humerus. J Bone Joint Surg Am 80 (10):1484–1497
60. Dines DM, Warren RF, Altchek DW, Moeckel B (1993) Posttraumatic changes of the proximal humerus: malunion, nonunion, and osteonecrosis. Treatment with modular hemiarthroplasty or total shoulder arthroplasty. J Shoulder Elbow Surg 2(1):11–21. doi:10.1016/s1058-2746(09)80132-8
61. Raiss P, Edwards TB, da Silva MR, Bruckner T, Loew M, Walch G (2014) Reverse shoulder arthroplasty for the treatment of nonunions of the surgical neck of the proximal part of the humerus (type-3 fracture sequelae). J Bone Joint Surg Am 96(24):2070–2076. doi:10.2106/JBJS.N.00405
62. Martinez AA, Calvo A, Bejarano C, Carbonel I, Herrera A (2012) The use of the Lima reverse shoulder arthroplasty for the treatment of fracture sequelae of the proximal humerus. J Orthop Sci 17(2):141–147. doi:10.1007/s00776-011-0185-5
63. Zafra M, Uceda P, Flores M, Carpintero P (2014) Reverse total shoulder replacement for nonunion of a fracture of the proximal humerus. Bone Joint J 96-b(9):1239–1243. doi:10.1302/0301-620x.96b9.33157
64. Cuomo F, Greller MJ, Zuckerman JD (1998) The rheumatoid shoulder. Rheum Dis Clin N Am 24(1):67–82
65. Petersson CJ (1986) Painful shoulders in patients with rheumatoid arthritis. Prevalence, clinical and radiological features. Scand J Rheumatol 15(3):275–279
66. Chen AL, Joseph TN, Zuckerman JD (2003) Rheumatoid arthritis of the shoulder. J Am Acad Orthop Surg 11(1):12–24
67. Barlow JD, Steinmann SP (2012) Shoulder arthroplasty in inflammatory arthritis. In: Sanchez-Sotelo J (ed) Shoulder arthroplasty, vol 47, Monograph series. AAOS, Rosemont
68. Laine VA, Vainio KJ, Pekanmaki K (1954) Shoulder affections in rheumatoid arthritis. Ann Rheum Dis 13(2):157–160
69. Sperling JW, Cofield RH, Schleck CD, Harmsen WS (2007) Total shoulder arthroplasty versus hemiarthroplasty for rheumatoid arthritis of the shoulder: results of 303 consecutive cases. J Shoulder Elbow Surg 16(6):683–690. doi:10.1016/j.jse.2007.02.135
70. Postacchini R, Carbone S, Canero G, Ripani M, Postacchini F (2015) Reverse shoulder prosthesis in patients with rheumatoid arthritis: a systematic review. Int Orthop. doi:10.1007/s00264-015-2916-2
71. Rasmussen JV, Olsen BS, Fevang BT, Furnes O, Skytta ET, Rahme H, Salomonsson B, Mohammed KD, Page RS, Carr AJ (2012) A review of national shoulder and elbow joint replacement registries. J Shoulder Elbow Surg 21(10):1328–1335. doi:10.1016/j.jse.2012.03.004

72. Fevang BT, Nystad TW, Skredderstuen A, Furnes ON, Havelin LI (2015) Improved survival for anatomic total shoulder prostheses. Acta Orthop 86(1):63–70. doi:10.3109/17453674.2014.984113
73. Fox TJ, Cil A, Sperling JW, Sanchez-Sotelo J, Schleck CD, Cofield RH (2009) Survival of the glenoid component in shoulder arthroplasty. J Shoulder Elbow Surg 18(6):859–863. doi:10.1016/j.jse.2008.11.020
74. Fevang BT, Lie SA, Havelin LI, Skredderstuen A, Furnes O (2009) Risk factors for revision after shoulder arthroplasty: 1,825 shoulder arthroplasties from the Norwegian Arthroplasty Register. Acta Orthop 80(1):83–91
75. Singh JA, Sperling JW, Cofield RH (2011) Revision surgery following total shoulder arthroplasty: analysis of 2588 shoulders over three decades (1976 to 2008). J Bone Joint Surg Br 93(11):1513–1517. doi:10.1302/0301-620x.93b11.26938
76. Wall B, Nove-Josserand L, O'Connor DP, Edwards TB, Walch G (2007) Reverse total shoulder arthroplasty: a review of results according to etiology. J Bone Joint Surg Am 89 (7):1476–1485. doi:10.2106/JBJS.F.00666
77. Boileau P, Avidor C, Krishnan SG, Walch G, Kempf JF, Mole D (2002) Cemented polyethylene versus uncemented metal-backed glenoid components in total shoulder arthroplasty: a prospective, double-blind, randomized study. J Shoulder Elbow Surg 11(4):351–359. doi:10.1067/mse.2002.125807
78. Gerber C, Costouros JG, Sukthankar A, Fucentese SF (2009) Static posterior humeral head subluxation and total shoulder arthroplasty. J Shoulder Elbow Surg 18(4):505–510. doi:10.1016/j.jse.2009.03.003
79. Levine WN, Djurasovic M, Glasson JM, Pollock RG, Flatow EL, Bigliani LU (1997) Hemiarthroplasty for glenohumeral osteoarthritis: results correlated to degree of glenoid wear. J Shoulder Elbow Surg 6(5):449–454
80. Iannotti JP, Norris TR (2003) Influence of preoperative factors on outcome of shoulder arthroplasty for glenohumeral osteoarthritis. J Bone Joint Surg Am 85-A(2):251–258
81. Walch G, Moraga C, Young A, Castellanos-Rosas J (2012) Results of anatomic nonconstrained prosthesis in primary osteoarthritis with biconcave glenoid. J Shoulder Elbow Surg 21(11):1526–1533. doi:10.1016/j.jse.2011.11.030
82. Mizuno N, Denard PJ, Raiss P, Walch G (2013) Reverse total shoulder arthroplasty for primary glenohumeral osteoarthritis in patients with a biconcave glenoid. J Bone Joint Surg Am 95(14):1297–1304. doi:10.2106/jbjs.l.00820
83. Mimata Y, Nishida J, Sato K, Suzuki Y, Doita M (2015) Glenohumeral arthrodesis for malignant tumor of the shoulder girdle. J Shoulder Elbow Surg 24(2):174–178. doi:10.1016/j.jse.2014.05.023
84. Yang Q, Li J, Yang Z, Li X, Li Z (2010) Limb sparing surgery for bone tumours of the shoulder girdle: the oncological and functional results. Int Orthop 34(6):869–875. doi:10.1007/s00264-009-0857-3
85. Moran M, Stalley PD (2009) Reconstruction of the proximal humerus with a composite of extracorporeally irradiated bone and endoprosthesis following excision of high grade primary bone sarcomas. Arch Orthop Trauma Surg 129(10):1339–1345. doi:10.1007/s00402-008-0752-1
86. Mackenzie DB (1993) The antero-superior exposure for total shoulder replacement. Orthop Traumatol 2(2):71–77
87. Mole D, Wein F, Dezaly C, Valenti P, Sirveaux F (2011) Surgical technique: the anterosuperior approach for reverse shoulder arthroplasty. Clin Orthop Relat Res 469 (9):2461–2468. doi:10.1007/s11999-011-1861-7
88. Rittmeister M, Kerschbaumer F (2001) Grammont reverse total shoulder arthroplasty in patients with rheumatoid arthritis and nonreconstructible rotator cuff lesions. J Shoulder Elbow Surg 10(1):17–22. doi:10.1067/mse.2001.110515

89. Edwards TB, Williams MD, Labriola JE, Elkousy HA, Gartsman GM, O'Connor DP (2009) Subscapularis insufficiency and the risk of shoulder dislocation after reverse shoulder arthroplasty. J Shoulder Elbow Surg 18(6):892–896. doi:10.1016/j.jse.2008.12.013
90. Boulahia A, Edwards TB, Walch G, Baratta RV (2002) Early results of a reverse design prosthesis in the treatment of arthritis of the shoulder in elderly patients with a large rotator cuff tear. Orthopedics 25(2):129–133
91. Willis MP, Walker MH, Frankle M (2012) Reverse shoulder arthroplasty. In: Sanchez-Sotelo J (ed) Shoulder arthroplasty, vol 47, Monograph series. American Academy of Orthopaedic Surgeons, Rosemont, pp 49–69
92. Boileau P, Rumian AP, Zumstein MA (2010) Reversed shoulder arthroplasty with modified L'Episcopo for combined loss of active elevation and external rotation. J Shoulder Elbow Surg 19(2 suppl):20–30. doi:10.1016/j.jse.2009.12.011
93. Lädermann A, Williams MD, Melis B, Hoffmeyer P, Walch G (2009) Objective evaluation of lengthening in reverse shoulder arthroplasty. J Shoulder Elbow Surg 18(4):588–595. doi:10.1016/j.jse.2009.03.012
94. Schwartz DG, Cottrell BJ, Teusink MJ, Clark RE, Downes KL, Tannenbaum RS, Frankle MA (2014) Factors that predict postoperative motion in patients treated with reverse shoulder arthroplasty. J Shoulder Elbow Surg 23(9):1289–1295. doi:10.1016/j.jse.2013.12.032
95. Levy JC, Everding NG, Gil CC Jr, Stephens S, Giveans MR (2014) Speed of recovery after shoulder arthroplasty: a comparison of reverse and anatomic total shoulder arthroplasty. J Shoulder Elbow Surg 23(12):1872–1881. doi:10.1016/j.jse.2014.04.014
96. Stevens CG, Struk AM, Wright TW (2014) The functional impact of bilateral reverse total shoulder arthroplasty. J Shoulder Elbow Surg 23(9):1341–1348. doi:10.1016/j.jse.2013.12.012
97. Rhee YG, Cho NS, Moon SC (2015) Effects of humeral component retroversion on functional outcomes in reverse total shoulder arthroplasty for cuff tear arthropathy. J Shoulder Elbow Surg. doi:10.1016/j.jse.2015.03.026
98. Bauman S, Williams D, Petruccelli D, Elliott W, de Beer J (2007) Physical activity after total joint replacement: a cross-sectional survey. Clin J Sport Med 17(2):104–108. doi:10.1097/JSM.0b013e3180379b6a
99. Wylde V, Blom A, Dieppe P, Hewlett S, Learmonth I (2008) Return to sport after joint replacement. J Bone Joint Surg Br 90(7):920–923. doi:10.1302/0301-620x.90b7.20614
100. Magnussen RA, Mallon WJ, Willems WJ, Moorman CT 3rd (2011) Long-term activity restrictions after shoulder arthroplasty: an international survey of experienced shoulder surgeons. J Shoulder Elbow Surg 20(2):281–289. doi:10.1016/j.jse.2010.07.021
101. Lawrence TM, Ahmadi S, Sanchez-Sotelo J, Sperling JW, Cofield RH (2012) Patient reported activities after reverse shoulder arthroplasty: part II. J Shoulder Elbow Surg 21(11):1464–1469. doi:10.1016/j.jse.2011.11.012
102. Fink Barnes LA, Grantham WJ, Meadows MC, Bigliani LU, Levine WN, Ahmad CS (2015) Sports activity after reverse total shoulder arthroplasty with minimum 2-year follow-up. Am J Orthop 44(2):68–72
103. Simovitch RW, Gerard BK, Brees JA, Fullick R, Kearse JC (2015) Outcomes of reverse total shoulder arthroplasty in a senior athletic population. J Shoulder Elbow Surg 24(9):1481–1485. doi:10.1016/j.jse.2015.03.011
104. Flury MP, Frey P, Goldhahn J, Schwyzer HK, Simmen BR (2011) Reverse shoulder arthroplasty as a salvage procedure for failed conventional shoulder replacement due to cuff failure: midterm results. Int Orthop 35(1):53–60. doi:10.1007/s00264-010-0990-z
105. Kempton LB, Ankerson E, Wiater JM (2011) A complication-based learning curve from 200 reverse shoulder arthroplasties. Clin Orthop Relat Res 469(9):2496–2504. doi:10.1007/s11999-011-1811-4
106. Zumstein MA, Pinedo M, Old J, Boileau P (2011) Problems, complications, reoperations, and revisions in reverse total shoulder arthroplasty: a systematic review. J Shoulder Elbow Surg 20(1):146–157. doi:10.1016/j.jse.2010.08.001

107. Cuff D, Pupello D, Virani N, Levy J, Frankle M (2008) Reverse shoulder arthroplasty for the treatment of rotator cuff deficiency. J Bone Joint Surg Am 90(6):1244–1251. doi:10.2106/jbjs.g.00775
108. Gonzalez JF, Alami GB, Baque F, Walch G, Boileau P (2011) Complications of unconstrained shoulder prostheses. J Shoulder Elbow Surg 20(4):666–682. doi:10.1016/j.jse.2010.11.017
109. Alentorn-Geli E, Samitier G, Torrens C, Wright TW (2015) Reverse shoulder arthroplasty. Part 2: systematic review of reoperations, revisions, problems, and complications. Int J Shoulder Surg 9(2):60–67. doi:10.4103/0973-6042.154771
110. Ladermann A, Lubbeke A, Melis B, Stern R, Christofilopoulos P, Bacle G, Walch G (2011) Prevalence of neurologic lesions after total shoulder arthroplasty. J Bone Joint Surg Am 93 (14):1288–1293. doi:10.2106/jbjs.j.00369
111. Cheung E, Willis M, Walker M, Clark R, Frankle MA (2011) Complications in reverse total shoulder arthroplasty. J Am Acad Orthop Surg 19(7):439–449
112. Lynch NM, Cofield RH, Silbert PL, Hermann RC (1996) Neurologic complications after total shoulder arthroplasty. J Shoulder Elbow Surg 5(1):53–61
113. Marion B, Leclere FM, Casoli V, Paganini F, Unglaub F, Spies C, Valenti P (2014) Potential axillary nerve stretching during RSA implantation: an anatomical study. Anat Sci Int 89 (4):232–237. doi:10.1007/s12565-014-0229-y
114. Molé D, Favard L (2007) Excentered scapulohumeral osteoarthritis [French]. Rev Chir Orthop Reparatrice Appar Mot 93(6 suppl):37–94
115. Richards J, Inacio MC, Beckett M, Navarro RA, Singh A, Dillon MT, Sodl JF, Yian EH (2014) Patient and procedure-specific risk factors for deep infection after primary shoulder arthroplasty. Clin Orthop Relat Res 472(9):2809–2815. doi:10.1007/s11999-014-3696-5
116. Florschutz AV, Lane PD, Crosby LA (2015) Infection after primary anatomic versus primary reverse total shoulder arthroplasty. J Shoulder Elbow Surg 24(8):1296–1301. doi:10.1016/j.jse.2014.12.036
117. Morris BJ, Waggenspack WN Jr, Laughlin MS, Elkousy HA, Gartsman GM, Edwards TB (2015) Reverse shoulder arthroplasty for management of postinfectious arthropathy with rotator cuff deficiency. Orthopedics 38(8):e701–e707. doi:10.3928/01477447-20150804-58
118. Jacquot A, Sirveaux F, Roche O, Favard L, Clavert P, Mole D (2015) Surgical management of the infected reversed shoulder arthroplasty: a French multicenter study of reoperation in 32 patients. J Shoulder Elbow Surg. doi:10.1016/j.jse.2015.03.007
119. Adeli B, Parvizi J (2012) Strategies for the prevention of periprosthetic joint infection. J Bone Joint Surg Br 94(11 suppl A):42–46. doi:10.1302/0301-620x.94b11.30833
120. Jamsen E, Huhtala H, Puolakka T, Moilanen T (2009) Risk factors for infection after knee arthroplasty. A register-based analysis of 43,149 cases. J Bone Joint Surg Am 91(1):38–47. doi:10.2106/JBJS.G.01686
121. Horneff JG 3rd, Hsu JE, Voleti PB, O'Donnell J, Huffman GR (2015) Propionibacterium acnes infection in shoulder arthroscopy patients with postoperative pain. J Shoulder Elbow Surg 24(6):838–843. doi:10.1016/j.jse.2015.03.008
122. Sabetta JR, Rana VP, Vadasdi KB, Greene RT, Cunningham JG, Miller SR, Sethi PM (2015) Efficacy of topical benzoyl peroxide on the reduction of *Propionibacterium acnes* during shoulder surgery. J Shoulder Elbow Surg 24(7):995–1004. doi:10.1016/j.jse.2015.04.003
123. Cuff DJ, Virani NA, Levy J, Frankle MA, Derasari A, Hines B, Pupello DR, Cancio M, Mighell M (2008) The treatment of deep shoulder infection and glenohumeral instability with debridement, reverse shoulder arthroplasty and postoperative antibiotics. J Bone Joint Surg Br 90(3):336–342. doi:10.1302/0301-620x.90b3.19408
124. Zavala JA, Clark JC, Kissenberth MJ, Tolan SJ, Hawkins RJ (2012) Management of deep infection after reverse total shoulder arthroplasty: a case series. J Shoulder Elbow Surg 21 (10):1310–1315. doi:10.1016/j.jse.2011.08.047
125. Beekman PD, Katusic D, Berghs BM, Karelse A, De Wilde L (2010) One-stage revision for patients with a chronically infected reverse total shoulder replacement. J Bone Joint Surg Br 92(6):817–822. doi:10.1302/0301-620x.92b6.23045

126. Levigne C, Boileau P, Favard L, Garaud P, Mole D, Sirveaux F, Walch G (2008) Scapular notching in reverse shoulder arthroplasty. J Shoulder Elbow Surg 17(6):925–935. doi:10.1016/j.jse.2008.02.010
127. Simovitch RW, Zumstein MA, Lohri E, Helmy N, Gerber C (2007) Predictors of scapular notching in patients managed with the Delta III reverse total shoulder replacement. J Bone Joint Surg Am 89(3):588–600. doi:10.2106/jbjs.f.00226
128. Nyffeler RW, Werner CM, Gerber C (2005) Biomechanical relevance of glenoid component positioning in the reverse Delta III total shoulder prosthesis. J Shoulder Elbow Surg 14 (5):524–528. doi:10.1016/j.jse.2004.09.010
129. Wierks C, Skolasky RL, Ji JH, McFarland EG (2009) Reverse total shoulder replacement: intraoperative and early postoperative complications. Clin Orthop Relat Res 467(1):225–234. doi:10.1007/s11999-008-0406-1
130. Teusink MJ, Pappou IP, Schwartz DG, Cottrell BJ, Frankle MA (2015) Results of closed management of acute dislocation after reverse shoulder arthroplasty. J Shoulder Elbow Surg 24(4):621–627. doi:10.1016/j.jse.2014.07.015
131. Saltzman BM, Chalmers PN, Gupta AK, Romeo AA, Nicholson GP (2014) Complication rates comparing primary with revision reverse total shoulder arthroplasty. J Shoulder Elbow Surg 23(11):1647–1654. doi:10.1016/j.jse.2014.04.015
132. Crosby LA, Hamilton A, Twiss T (2011) Scapula fractures after reverse total shoulder arthroplasty: classification and treatment. Clin Orthop Relat Res 469(9):2544–2549. doi:10.1007/s11999-011-1881-3
133. Hamid N, Connor PM, Fleischli JF, D'Alessandro DF (2011) Acromial fracture after reverse shoulder arthroplasty. Am J Orthop 40(7):E125–E129
134. Hattrup SJ (2010) The influence of postoperative acromial and scapular spine fractures on the results of reverse shoulder arthroplasty. Orthopedics 33(5) doi:10.3928/01477447-20100329-04
135. Otto RJ, Virani NA, Levy JC, Nigro PT, Cuff DJ, Frankle MA (2013) Scapular fractures after reverse shoulder arthroplasty: evaluation of risk factors and the reliability of a proposed classification. J Shoulder Elbow Surg 22(11):1514–1521. doi:10.1016/j.jse.2013.02.007
136. Teusink MJ, Otto RJ, Cottrell BJ, Frankle MA (2014) What is the effect of postoperative scapular fracture on outcomes of reverse shoulder arthroplasty? J Shoulder Elbow Surg 23 (6):782–790. doi:10.1016/j.jse.2013.09.010
137. Dubrow S, Streit JJ, Muh S, Shishani Y, Gobezie R (2014) Acromial stress fractures: correlation with acromioclavicular osteoarthritis and acromiohumeral distance. Orthopedics 37(12):e1074–e1079. doi:10.3928/01477447-20141124-54
138. Walch G, Mottier F, Wall B, Boileau P, Mole D, Favard L (2009) Acromial insufficiency in reverse shoulder arthroplasties. J Shoulder Elbow Surg 18(3):495–502. doi:10.1016/j.jse.2008.12.002

Chapter 17
Physical Therapy: Tips and Pitfalls

Shinichi Chiba, Takashi Tachibana, Mitsukuni Yamaguchi, Takashi Yusa, Satoshi Suzuki, Hitoshi Nishikawa, and Takayuki Muraki

Abstract Postoperative physical therapy is important to obtain smooth recovery of shoulder functions and satisfactory return to daily living after surgery. In addition, physical therapy as a conservative treatment can lead to enhancement of shoulder function and consequent improvement of symptoms, and furthermore, can validate the indication of shoulder surgery even though the conservative treatment is not effective. In conservative physical therapy for rotator cuff tear, improving function of residual cuff tendons as well as coordination between the glenohumeral and scapulothoracic joint are essential. In postoperative physical therapy after rotator cuff repair, prescription of exercise in line with advances in healing of rotator cuff is necessary. For frozen shoulder, physical therapy intervention needs to be provided according to the phase of the disease. In physical therapy for throwing injuries, contributing factors to shoulder injury as well as functional problems induced by the injury need to be managed. For humeral fracture, therapeutic exercise should be performed without shear stress on the fractured part. In postoperative physical therapy after total shoulder arthroplasty (TSA) and reverse shoulder arthroplasty (RSA), loading during exercise needs to increase with attention to postoperative

S. Chiba
Rehabilitation Center, Showa University Hospital, Tokyo, Japan

T. Tachibana
Department of Rehabilitation, Nobuhara Hospital, Tatsuno, Hyogo, Japan

M. Yamaguchi
Thera-Labo Co., Ltd, Kawasaki, Kanagawa, Japan

T. Yusa
Rehabilitation Center, Matsudo Orthopaedic Hospital, Matsudo, Chiba, Japan

S. Suzuki
Department of Sports Rehabilitation, Funabashi Orthopaedic Hospital, Funabashi, Chiba, Japan

H. Nishikawa
Department of Physical Therapy, Konan Women's University, Kobe, Hyogo, Japan

T. Muraki (✉)
Department of Physical Medicine and Rehabilitation, Tohoku University Graduate School of Medicine, 1-1 Seiryo-cho, Aoba-ku, Sendai, Miyagi 980-8574, Japan
e-mail: takayukimurakipt@yahoo.co.jp

K. Tamai et al. (eds.), *Advances in Shoulder Surgery*,
DOI 10.1007/978-4-431-55988-7_17

complications. In physical therapy after hook plate fixation for acromioclavicular joint dislocation, an exercise program should be designed based on the characteristics of the hook plate.

Keywords Physical therapy • Shoulder function • Rehabilitation

17.1 Rotator Cuff Tear

17.1.1 Conservative Treatment of Rotator Cuff Tears

Improvement of symptom in the patients with rotator cuff tears is attributed to subsiding of bursitis, decrease of muscle spasm, and compensation of adjacent cuff tendons for the torn cuff tendon [1].

In the acute phase, symptoms such as resting pain and elevation deficit emerge. Aggressive therapeutic exercise should be avoided in this phase. Instead, the therapist instructs resting position and Codman's stooping exercise to resolve inflammation reaction and to obtain muscle relaxation.

After confirmation of subsiding of the inflammation reaction, aggressive shoulder exercise will start. Inflammation reaction is considered to have subsided when the shoulder pain becomes localized.

17.1.1.1 Improving Function of Residual Rotator Cuff Tendons

Four muscles form the rotator cuff as a functional unit to stabilize the glenohumeral joint. Therefore, residual cuff tendons can play a role of stabilizing the joint by improving their function, even though a part of the rotator cuff is torn. For example, although infraspinatus tendon tear can result in weakness or deficit of active shoulder external rotation, enhancing the function of the teres minor enables the patients to perform external rotation in arm elevation position (Fig. 17.1).

17.1.1.2 Improving Function of the Scapulothoracic Joint

The humeral head is superiorly migrated by contraction of the deltoid muscle during arm elevation when rotator cuff tear progresses to some extent. The superior migration of the humeral head makes passage of the greater tuberosity under the acromion difficult, and arm elevation is thereby restricted. The superior migration of the humeral head can be avoided if the patients are able to contract the deltoid muscle with downward rotation of the scapula, which means that the glenoid faces inferiorly, although this motion is different from the normal scapulohumeral rhythm. After the greater tuberosity passes under the acromion with the deltoid contraction at lower elevation angle where the arm is less affected by gravity, patients need to practice shoulder elevation with compensatory upward rotation of

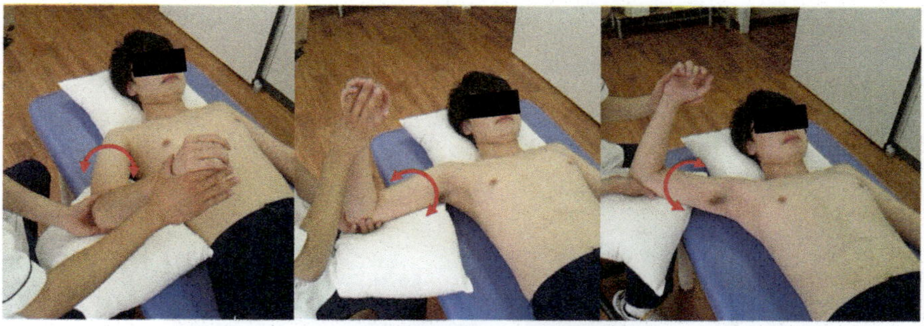

Fig. 17.1 Exercise to improve function of residual rotator cuff muscles. To improve compensatory function of residual cuff muscles, rotation exercises are performed in various shoulder positions. For example, external rotation in arm elevation position can facilitate compensatory function of the teres minor

the scapula. To do so, improving coordination between the glenohumeral and scapulothoracic joint as well as mobility in downward rotation and depression of the scapula is essential (Fig. 17.2).

17.1.2 Postoperative Physical Therapy [2]

After rotator cuff repair, it is important that the therapeutic exercise program proceed in a step-by-step manner according to the healing process of the repaired rotator cuff.

17.1.2.1 Range-of-Motion Exercise

From a couple of days after the surgery, gentle passive range-of-motion exercises for the directions where the repaired rotator cuff is not stretched start to prevent adhesion around the repaired site. For supraspinatus tendon tear, passive elevation in the scapular plane and external rotation starts immediately after the repair, whereas passive range of motion in the direction to adduction, internal rotation, and horizontal adduction, which can add stress to the repaired supraspinatus tendon, start from 5 to 6 weeks after the repair.

17.1.2.2 Muscle-Strengthening Exercise

Active assistive exercises start from 4 weeks after the surgery. Active exercise, followed by resistive exercise, starts with gradual increase of loading from 5 weeks after the surgery.

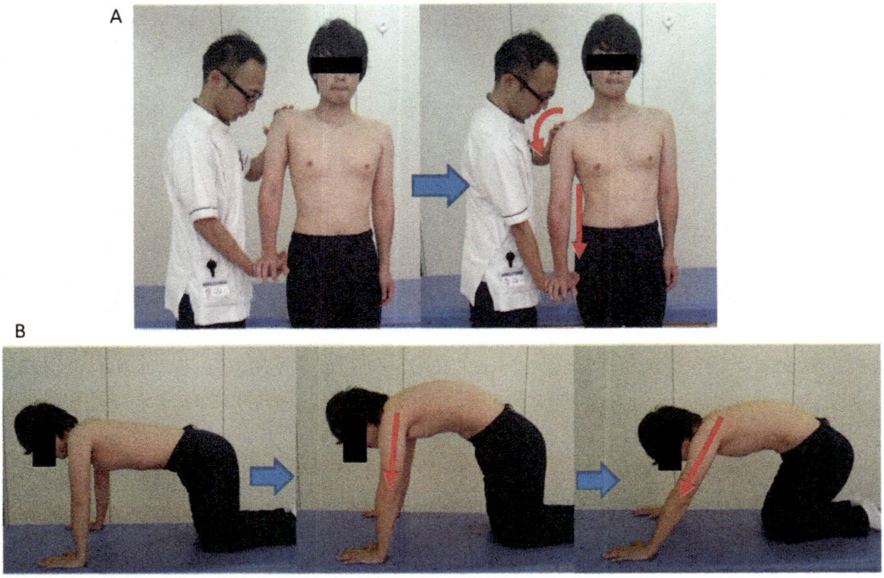

Fig. 17.2 Exercise to improve coordination between the humeral and scapular motions. Patient pushes the therapist's hand down with fully extended elbow. This motion facilitates scapular depression and downward rotation. Consequently, the glenohumeral joint is relatively abducted (**a**). In all-fours position, the patient protracts his scapula by pushing the floor, and then changes the direction of pushing forward so that the patient's trunk moves backward. This exercise can facilitate the scapular motion more dominantly compared to the humeral motion. In addition, this exercise can be performed with less activity of the deltoid muscle causing superior shift of the humeral head because of weight-bearing condition (**b**)

17.1.2.3 Other Tips and Pitfalls

Excessive tension of shoulder girdle muscles is often observed because of pain and immobilization immediately after the surgery. Therapeutic exercise without relaxing the hypertone of shoulder muscles can risk increasing stress to the repaired rotator cuff. Relaxation approaches to the elbow, forearm, and trunk before the exercise for the glenohumeral joint should start immediately after the surgery.

17.2 Frozen Shoulder

17.2.1 Intervention in Each Phase of the Disease

17.2.1.1 Acute Phase After Onset

Although the inflammatory reaction is necessary for the involved tissue to recover from the pathological condition, this reaction should be minimized to prevent a high intensity of scar formation resulting in severe joint contracture. Therefore, keeping the involved shoulder joint at rest is the fundamental intervention strategy in this phase. However, it is a challenge for the patient to do that because the patients never consider the symptoms to be severe and tend to place priority on their daily activities.

17.2.1.2 Peak Inflammation Phase

Unnecessary intervention can disturb a subsiding inflammation reaction and induce broad formation of scar tissue in the joint capsule, although negative effects of prolonged rest are also a problem as is the continuous inflammation. There is no clear way to define exercises that promote recovery while preventing excessive inflammatory reaction. In this phase, the synovium of the joint capsule appears to be red and sore because of active capillary angiogenesis. The shoulder joint should be moved without stimulating the synovium. Pain is the most useful indicator to control the loading to the involved tissues.

17.2.1.3 Late Inflammation Phase

Scar tissues in the capsule are formed in proportion to severity of inflammation reaction. It is anticipated that high-intensity exercises will lead to reactivation of inflammation because of proliferation of capillary vessels in the synovium. Low-intensity exercise such as active assistive or active exercises without pain provocation should be performed to prevent the exacerbation of joint contracture.

17.2.1.4 Frozen Phase

Stretching exercises can be included in the treatment program in this phase when the capillary vessels in the synovium decrease and the process of joint contracture is completed. However, high-intensity stretching to gain immediate and temporal improvement is less meaningful because of scar formation in the joint capsule. Rather, it is more important to provide low-intensity mechanical stress to the scar tissues, to promote circulation around the joint, and thereby to attempt to remodel the connective tissues of the shoulder joint. In that sense, a treatment program including active exercise as well as stretching exercise may be more effective than stretching exercise alone.

17.2.1.5 Thawing Phase

In this phase, the joint contracture, which did not respond stretching exercise, improves naturally. It is common that this “thawing” occurs approximately 1 year after the onset. Stretching exercise is effective in this phase; however, high-intensity stretching exercise ignoring the consideration of pain is not recommended.

17.2.2 Targets and Techniques of Stretching

17.2.2.1 Muscles

Shortening of shoulder muscles also progresses secondary to joint contracture, and then worsen to the degree stretching does not immediately respond to intervention. The main targets of stretching are the rotator cuff muscles, pectoralis major, teres major, etc. Severity of contracture in each muscle is different depending on the patients. Stretching with bone movement, contract–relaxation, press-out stretching, and deep tissue massage are used to regain the flexibility of each muscle.

17.2.2.2 Ligaments

17.2.2.2.1 Coracohumeral Ligament

In the frozen shoulder, serious scar formation tends to occur in the coracohumeral ligament, and the contacted ligament becomes a factor causing severe restriction of shoulder joint motion. In macroscopic finding during open surgery, it appears to be impossible to stretch the contracted coracohumeral ligament. Therefore, physical therapy needs to continue patiently until sufficient improvement in the flexibility of the ligament is obtained. Horizontal abduction, with external rotation at shoulder adduction, or extension stretches this ligament. The stretched ligament can be palpated immediately lateral to the side of the coracoid process.

17.2.2.2.2 Glenohumeral Ligament

As shown in Fig. 17.3, all fibers of the glenohumeral ligament are lengthened at both internal and external rotations in shoulder elevation in the scapular plane compared with that at neutral rotation. External rotation at shoulder elevation or abduction stretches the inferior glenohumeral ligaments. External rotation at shoulder adduction stretches all fibers of the glenohumeral ligament. These motions also stretch the anterior and anteroinferior capsule because the glenohumeral ligament merges with the joint capsule.

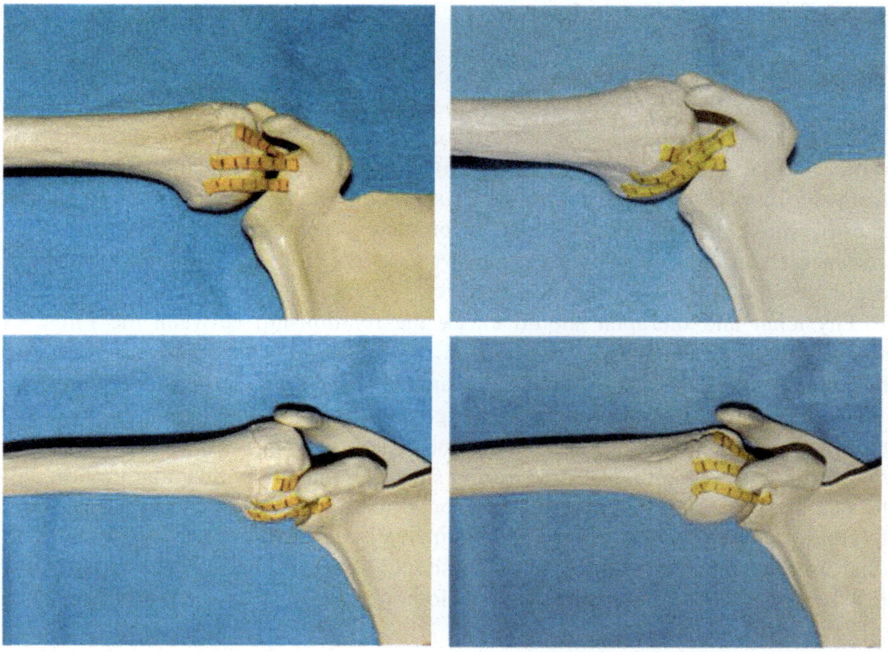

Fig. 17.3 Behavior of the glenohumeral ligament during rotation in shoulder elevation position in the scapular plane. Both internal and external humeral rotation without change of glenohumeral elevation angle lengthens all fibers of the glenohumeral ligament compared to the length at neutral rotation. (**a**) Observation from anterior aspect during internal rotation. (**b**) Observation from anterosuperior aspect during external rotation

17.2.2.3 Capsule

Bone movement (osteokinematic motion), joint distraction, and gliding in closed-pack position are used to stretch the capsule.

17.2.2.4 Flexibility of the Thorax

Patients with kyphosis have poor flexibilities of the thorax as well as of the spine. Adduction of the scapula is restricted by the poor flexibilities of the thorax even though the scapulothoracic joint itself is flexible enough to move because the scapula is positioned more ventrally as the result of kyphosis and poor flexibility of the thorax. In the whole shoulder girdle, the ranges of abduction and horizontal abduction are affected. Passive motion exercises to dorsal, ventral, and caudal directions are performed slowly and carefully to obtain the flexibility of the thorax. Mobilization of the costovertebral joint is also effective. Care should be taken to avoid rib fracture when these techniques are used for elder people.

17.2.2.5 Scapulothoracic Joint

The scapular position is controlled by tethering with the rhomboids and levator scapulae from the spinal side and with the serratus anterior from the anterior side. The trapezius controls scapular upward rotation. It is considered that the pectoralis minor and latissimus dorsi help in stabilizing the scapular so as not to separate it from the thorax. Although the range of scapulothoracic motion is restricted, the cause is most likely hypertonic contraction of scapulothoracic muscles rather than contractures of their muscle tissues. Active assistive exercise to guide directions of optimal scapular motions will be effective.

Physician and therapist should check the relationship between the range of scapular motion and the position of the spine and then judge whether scapular motion is a true problem. For normal scapular motion during shoulder abduction, scapular upward rotation occurs with the glenoid facing forward along the shape of the rib cage around 120° of abduction. Therefore, range of horizontal abduction in the glenohumeral joint is required during shoulder abduction. Scapular motion will be blocked because glenohumeral horizontal abduction is restricted by the lesser flexibility of the anterior capsule and ligaments in the shoulder with contracture. In this case, the anterior connective tissues should be treated because the cause of the restriction is not contracture in the scapulothoracic joint.

17.2.3 Stretching Technique Without Inducing Subacromial Impingement

17.2.3.1 Humeral Neck Axis Rotation (Figs. 17.4 and 17.5)

When the long axis of the anatomic neck of the humerus (humeral neck axis) is placed perpendicular to the glenoid surface, the spinning motion of the humeral head about the long axis can avoid subacromial impingement because the greater and lesser tuberosities do not approach the undersurface of the coracoacromial arch. To place the humeral neck axis perpendicular to the glenoid surface, the glenohumeral joint needs to be manipulated as follows. First, therapists imagine the humeral neck axis as an axis of cone with 90° of apex angle and place it perpendicular to the glenoid surface; then, they need to move the humerus on the slope of the cone (offsetting the neck shaft angle) and to keep the forearm at 30° of external rotation relative to the tangent line wherever the upper arm is located (offsetting the retroversion angle). This maneuver produces a spinning motion of the humeral head in the humeral neck axis. Stretching is performed at the end range of this spinning motion. In healthy people, ranges of external and internal rotations in this motion are approximately 75° and 55°, respectively.

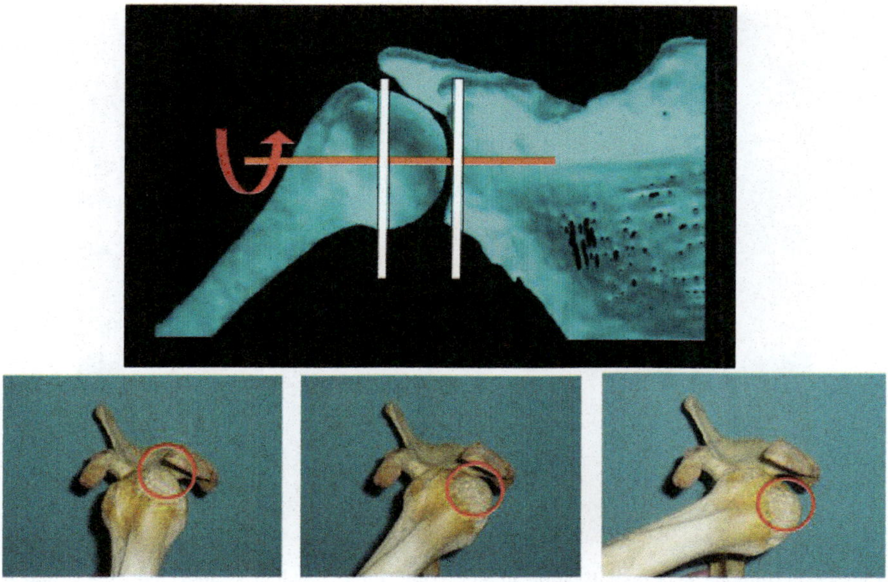

Fig. 17.4 Diagram and photograph of humeral neck axis rotation. The humerus is rotated along the long axis of humeral neck in the glenohumeral position where the plane of the humeral anatomic neck is placed parallel to the plane of the glenoid (**a**). When the humerus is rotated forward on the humeral neck axis, the greater tuberosity moves parallel to the coracoacromial arch (**b**)

17.2.3.2 Press-Out Stretching (Figs. 17.6 and 17.7)

Instead of bone movement, muscle is stretched by pushing it out like a bowstring. This technique can be applied to stretching of the teres major, pectoralis major and minor, triceps brachii, etc., although this technique cannot cover all shoulder muscles because sufficient spaces to push them out are needed.

17.3 Throwing Injuries

17.3.1 Goal of Physical Therapy for Throwing Injuries

The goal of physical therapy for throwing injuries in the shoulder is not only to regain an ability to throw. Regaining the ability to throw is a process to achieve the final goal because it is important not only to improve impairment induced by the injuries but also to manage contributing factors to the injuries, and furthermore to encourage the athletes to change their behavior to prevent the recurrence of injury.

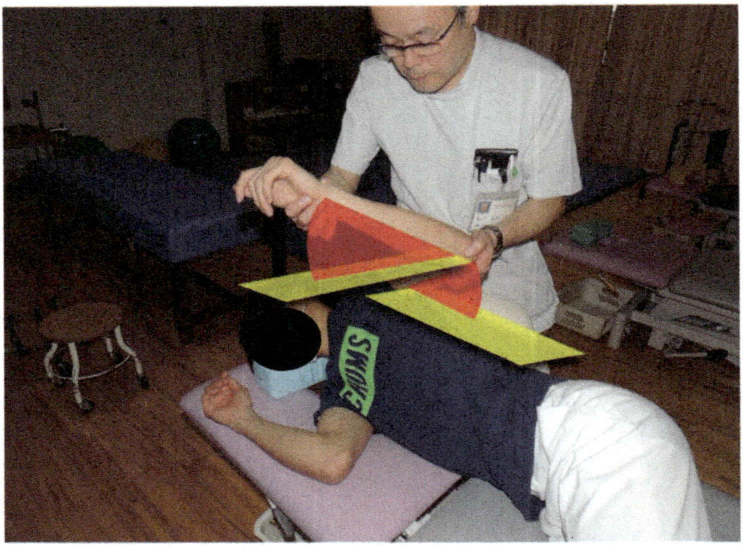

Fig. 17.5 Humeral neck axis rotation in side lying. First, shoulder is abducted by 45° and is rotated externally by 30° in side-lying position. When shoulder is rotated with keeping the elbow and hand position from the ground, the humeral neck axis rotation can be performed in the shoulder joint

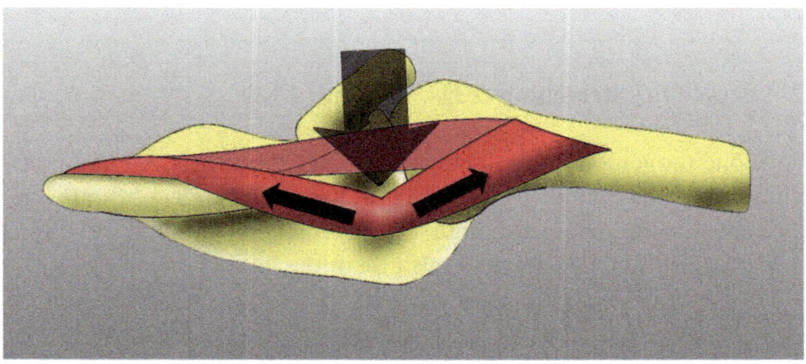

Fig. 17.6 Diagram representing principle of press-out stretch for the teres major. The teres major can be stretched by pressing its muscle belly dorsally

Throwing injuries are injuries induced by repetitive loading to the joint, which come from various causes. Even though athletes regain the ability to throw once, lack of management for contributing factors, which originally led to the throwing shoulder injuries, can cause recurrence of the injuries and, in some cases, may make them more severe. It should be noted that reducing the overload to the shoulder joint and preparing conditions to protect the joint are more important than only regaining the ability to throw.

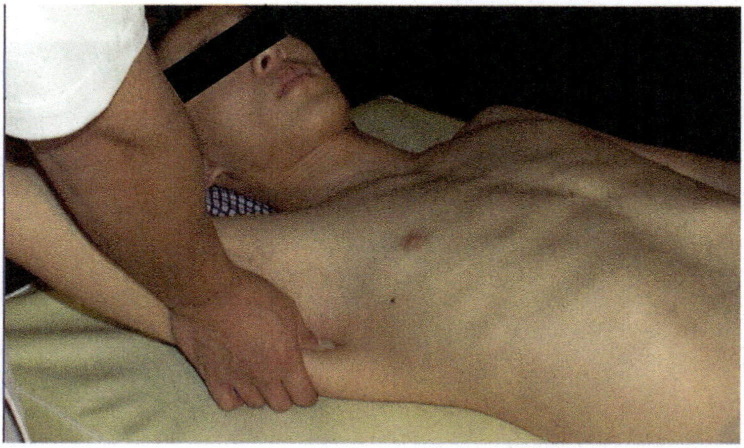

Fig. 17.7 Photograph of press-out stretch

17.3.2 Managements of Local Parts and Whole Body

In throwing shoulder injuries, structural and functional problems around the shoulder exist. Particularly, functional problems induced by damages of the shoulder structure should be managed based on physiological recovery process. This management is an important issue in the physical therapy for the early phase after the throwing injuries. In the process of management, assessment of the local parts related to the injuries needs to be precisely performed while excluding the influences of the other body parts. Management also needs to focus on the local part depending on its purpose.

Functional problems in adjacent joints can cause overload in the shoulder because the shoulder moves on the thorax and is strongly affected by the adjacent joints. In addition, the primary causes of the throwing shoulder injuries, which add overload to the shoulder joint, can be the same as the functional problem of the adjacent joint. Furthermore, subject to throw is required to achieve precisely the aim with speed and trajectory expected by the athletes in throwing, particularly pitching. To do so, each part of the body sequentially and smoothly works together. Therefore, dysfunction of a part of the body makes the stress on other body parts higher. A shoulder problem can be also caused by functional problems of the other body parts [3].

Based on the purpose of the physical therapy for throwing shoulder injuries, management of these contributing factors from various parts other than the shoulder is also another important issue and should be chosen depending on the condition and ability of throwing athletes and the phase of the recovery process. Attitude to select proper management depending on the situation of the cases is essential without premature decision on whether management should be provided to the injured part or contributing factors to the injury.

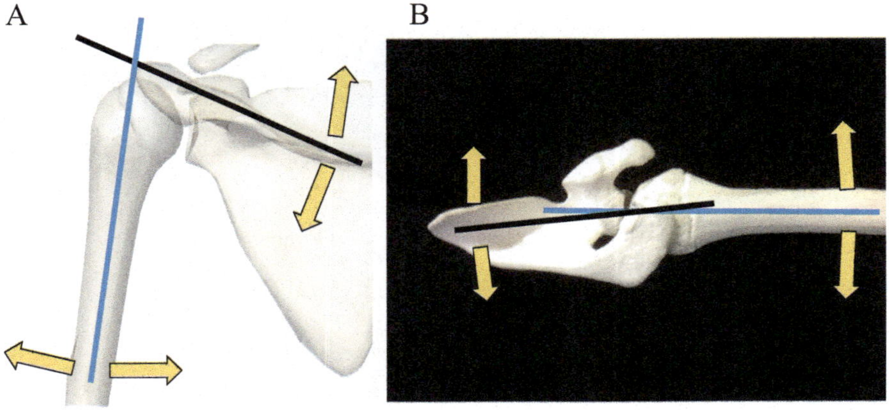

Fig. 17.8 Assessment of relationship between scapula and humerus. (**a**) Changes of spinohumeral angle in scapular plane. (**b**) Changes of scapular plane and humerus in horizontal plane

17.3.3 Functional Assessment

Based on characteristics of shoulder function, the humerus, scapula, and other body parts should work together to keep the appropriate joint position and to thereby protect the joint [4, 5]. Therefore, only assessing either the humerus and scapula in a certain position or condition is insufficient to obtain the information for decision making in physical therapy. From this point of view, not only measuring range of humeral motion relative to the ground, but also assessing the scapular position relative to the ground and the humeral position relative to the scapula are important (Fig. 17.8).

In addition, throwing shoulder injuries are often caused by a combination of various contributing factors rather than a simple cause. Hence, the information from an assessment needs to be considered as the result of the combination of several factors. Interaction of each contributing factor should be examined with information related to other factors.

For example, if manual muscle testing for arm elevation at 45° of elevation in the scapular plane causes scapular downward rotation with pain, this downward rotation may indicate a problem on scapular stabilization. However, there is a possibility of necessary evil, namely compensatory motion to reduce the pain as well, because the scapula and humerus change their positions to each other depending on the situation. To confirm the cause of the scapular downward rotation, the same manual muscle testing should be performed with stabilizing the scapula as well (Fig. 17.9). The pain will decrease in the testing with scapular stabilization if a problem of ability to stabilize the scapular causes scapular downward rotation in the testing without scapular stabilization. On the other hand, the pain will increase in the testing with scapular stabilization if the downward rotation is a compensatory motion to reduce the pain. Moreover, even if there is a problem on scapular

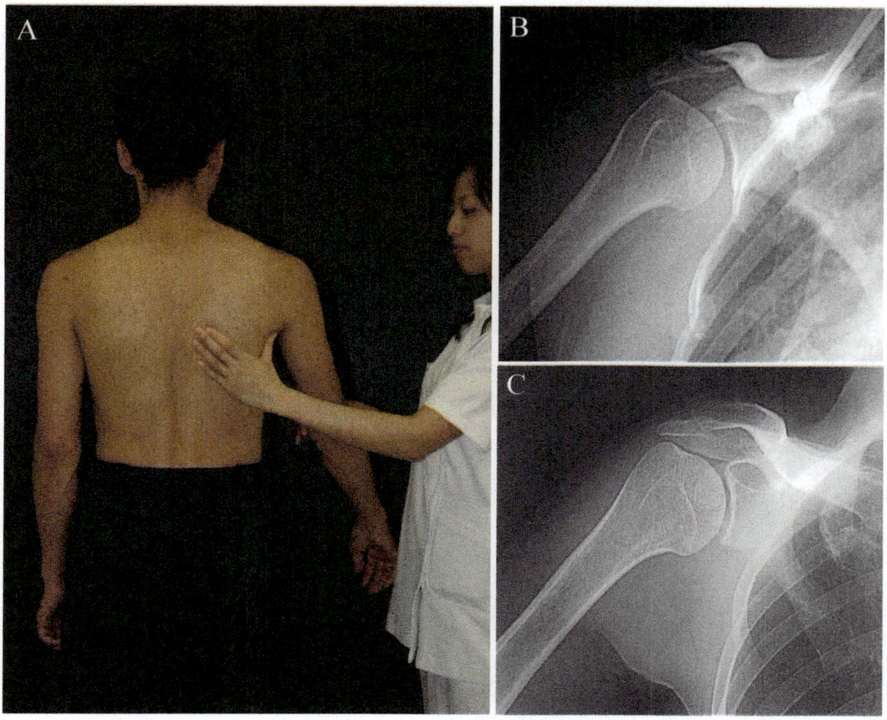

Fig. 17.9 Manual muscle testing for arm elevation at 45° of elevation in the scapular plane. (**a**) Examiner holds the inferior angle of patient's scapula with her thumb and index finger when stabilizing the scapula during the testing. (**b**) X-ray image without examiner's assistance to hold scapula. (**c**) X-ray image with examiner's assist to hold scapula

stabilization during the muscle testing for arm elevation, strengths of all scapular muscles are sometimes normal in the manual muscle testing. In this case, functions of trunk or lower extremity may affect the problem on scapular stabilization.

Figure 17.10 shows muscle strength of the scapular adductors with two different knee positions in healthy subjects and a baseball player who had shoulder pain. The baseball player has injured his medial collateral ligament of the knee and developed shoulder pain when he made a return to play. He showed scapular downward rotation with pain during manual muscle testing for arm elevation at 45° of elevation in the scapular plane, but the pain disappeared with manual stabilization of the scapula. Although dysfunction of the scapular muscles was suspected, strengths of all scapular muscles were normal on the manual muscle testing to evaluate the scapular muscles individually. Because of excessive trunk motion during the scapular muscle testing, the same testing was repeated with trunk stabilization and knee-flexed position, which then revealed the obvious weakness of the scapular adductors. In addition, weakness of the gluteus maximus muscle was also found.

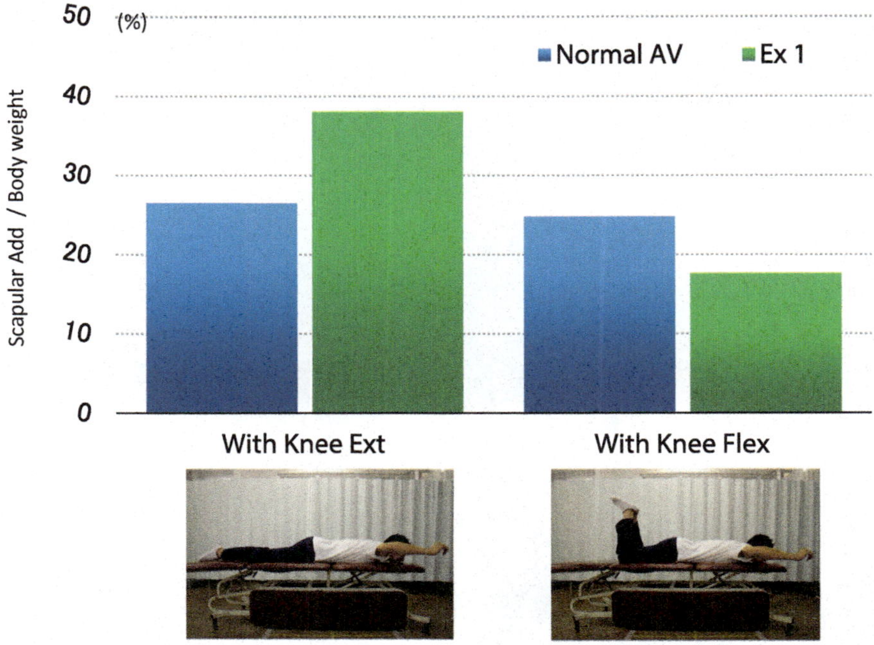

Fig. 17.10 Comparison of strength of scapular adduction between healthy subjects and an example athlete with throwing injury. *Bars* indicate force of scapular adduction normalized by body weight (*Scapular add/Body weight*) during muscle testing in prone position with extended and flexed knee positions. The example athlete (*Ex 1*) shows significant decrease of scapular adduction force in prone with flexed knee position whereas averaged scapular adduction forces in healthy subjects (*Normal AV*) in both knee positions are almost the same

It was speculated that this player did not have enough ability to stabilize the trunk and scapula and to reduce stress on the glenohumeral joint during the stepping phase in a throwing motion because of the weakness of the gluteus maximus muscle, although sufficient recovery of knee muscle strength was obtained. After approaching this problem, this player obtained satisfactory function and ability to throw without pain and could make a return to play.

As mentioned, clinical reasoning needs to be advanced based on the characteristics of the subject, time course, and environmental information as well as evidence obtained from previous studies.

In summary, physical therapy for throwing shoulder injuries is not substantially different from that for other shoulder diseases. However, in addition to management for functional problems induced by the injury, management for contributing factors to shoulder injury such as problems from each part of the body, psychological factors, and environmental factors needs to be emphasized. Because throwing shoulder injuries are affected by various factors, assessment of each factor, including testing condition, environment, and time course, and their interaction, is crucial.

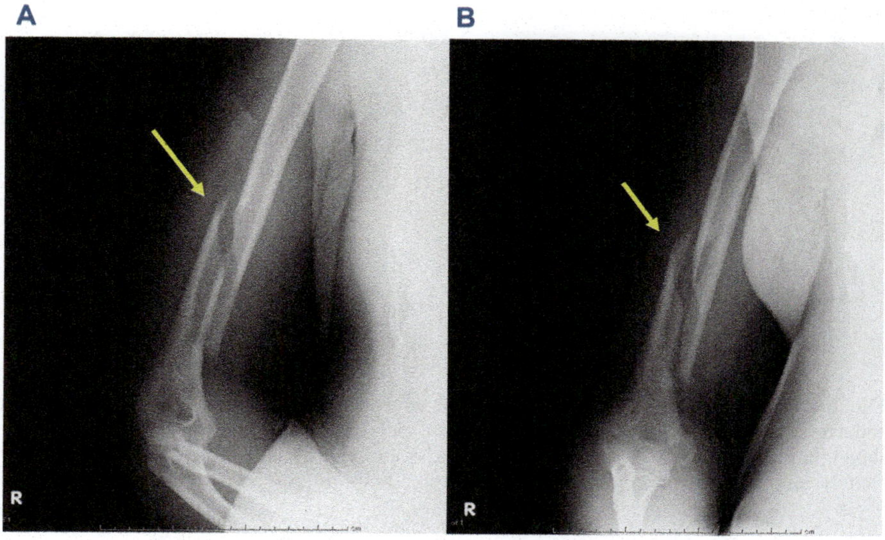

Fig. 17.11 A typical humeral shaft fracture. (**a**) Lateral view. (**b**) Anterior view

17.4 Humeral Shaft Fracture

The purposes of physical therapy for fracture of the humerus are to promote healing of the fracture and to recover shoulder function [6]. The important tips in the physical therapy are presented next with an example of typical fracture (Fig. 17.11).

17.4.1 Improvement of Scapular Motion

It is very important for obtaining shoulder function to improve scapular mobility without loading to the fractured part (Fig. 17.12) [7].

17.4.2 Techniques to Grasp the Fractured Part and to Improve Range of Motion

Excessive rotational and shear stresses to the fractured part can disturb bone healing [6]. When therapists attempt to improve range of shoulder abduction, they grasp the fractured part as shown in Fig. 17.13 and move the shoulder with compression

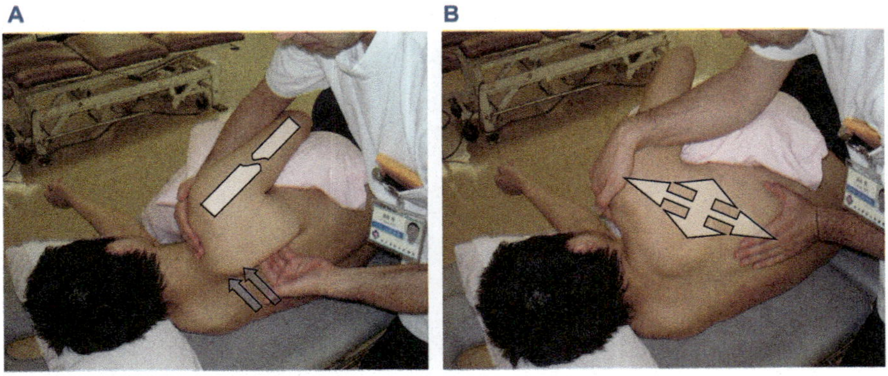

Fig. 17.12 Stretching and exercise to improve scapular mobility. (**a**) Stretching of scapular adductors by lifting the medial border of the scapula to dorsal and lateral directions while supporting the humerus with a pillow. (**b**) Passive exercise of the scapula to diagonal directions, namely, anterosuperior–posteroinferior and anteroinferior–posterosuperior directions

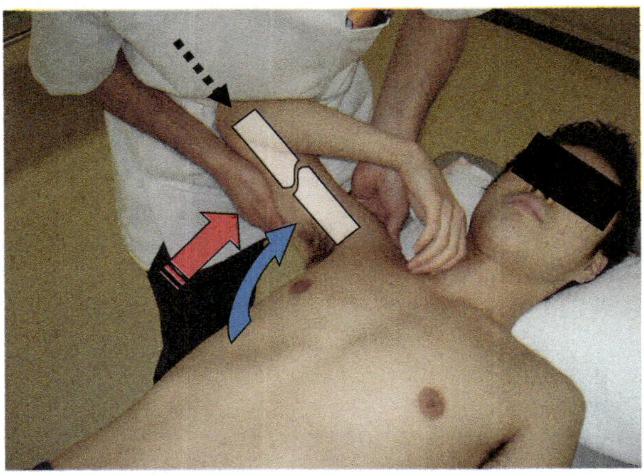

Fig. 17.13 Passive shoulder abduction exercise. The therapist grasps the fractured part with his right hand (*red arrow*) and slightly compresses the humerus along the long axis of the humerus with his abdomen (*dotted black arrow*) to prevent displacement of the distal humerus, and then abducts the patient's shoulder. The therapist simultaneously prevents superior migration of the humeral head with his left hand

along the long axis of the humerus and with depression of the humeral head according to concave-convex rule [8]. When improving range of shoulder rotation, therapists need to control the whole part of the humerus and then move as shown in Fig. 17.14.

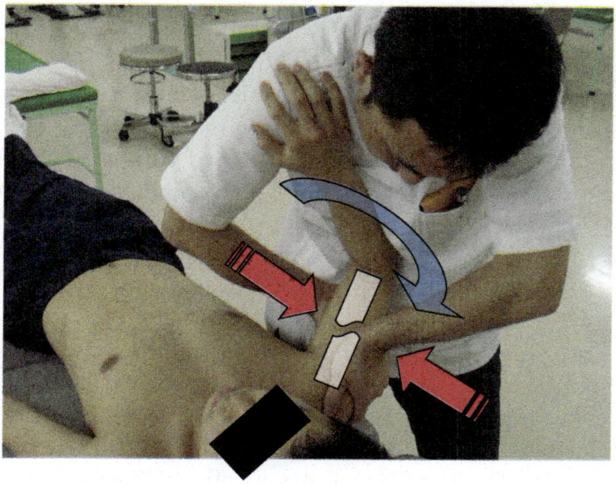

Fig. 17.14 Passive shoulder rotation exercise. The therapist grasps the fractured part with his both hands (*red arrows*). Then, with slight compression along the long axis of the humerus with his abdomen, the therapist rotates the patient's humerus with his whole body movement

17.5 Total Shoulder Arthroplasty

17.5.1 Total Shoulder Arthroplasty (TSA)

TSA is indicated for patients who have severe pain and restriction of shoulder motion resulting from osteoarthritis in the glenohumeral joint and who have resistance to oral medication, intraarticular injection, and physical therapy. In addition, the requirements for TSA are sufficient function of rotator cuff muscles and the glenoid with small bone defect where a glenoid component can be inserted.

17.5.1.1 Tips and Pitfalls in Postoperative Physical Therapy After TSA

Postoperative physical therapy starts under the supervision of physical therapists from the day after surgery. The patients wear a shoulder abduction orthosis for 3 weeks after TSA to protect the affected part in shoulder and to obtain relaxation.

An important point in this phase is to obtain range of shoulder flexion and external rotation proactively while therapists give attention to pain. Passive exercise for range of external rotation should be carefully performed to avoid shoulder anterior dislocation in the early phase after the surgery, because the subscapularis is repaired in the TSA. From 3 weeks after TSA, the patients start active assistive exercises, followed by active exercises in antigravity position, with the supervision of physical therapists. In addition, patients are encouraged to use the involved shoulder actively in daily living. From 6 weeks after TSA, strengthening exercises of shoulder muscles are gradually promoted so that the patients can obtain an ability to do lightly loaded work and, from 12 weeks after the surgery, can completely return to daily activities.

17.5.2 Reverse Shoulder Arthroplasty

RSA is indicated for elderly patients more than 70 years old who show pseudo-paralysis with irreparable massive rotator cuff tear or have cuff tear arthropathy.

In contrast to TSA, which is based on normal shoulder anatomy, a socket and prosthetic ball are placed in the proximal humerus and on the glenoid, respectively.

17.5.2.1 Tips and Pitfalls in Postoperative Physical Therapy After RSA

Postoperative physical therapy starts under the supervision of physical therapists from the day after surgery as done after TSA. The patients wear a shoulder abduction orthosis for 3–4 weeks after RSA to protect the affected part of the shoulder. Because the main purpose of wearing the orthosis is not to immobilize the affected shoulder, the patients are allowed to move their elbow on the affected side and to use their hand during washing the face and eating.

A primary shoulder position of postoperative dislocation is the combined position of shoulder extension, adduction, and internal rotation, so-called "hand behind back." This position is prohibited in the early phase after RSA. In addition, touching the contralateral axilla is prohibited to prevent the dislocation in this phase. With increase of loading from 6 weeks after RSA, risks of fracture, dislocation in shoulder hyperextension, and loosening and breakage of the components and implants need to be taken into consideration. The patients and therapists aim at complete return to daily activities from 12 to 24 weeks after the surgery.

17.6 Acromioclavicular Joint Dislocation

Acromioclavicular (AC) joint dislocation is usually categorized with Rockwood classification [9]. Type III–VI indicates complete dislocation and are generally surgical indications. Of various surgery methods for AC joint dislocation, hook plate fixation is reported as a common surgery for the acute phase of the dislocation [10, 11]. It is necessary to consider the characteristics of the hook plate fixation on the postoperative physical therapy after AC joint reconstruction.

17.6.1 Considerations in Physical Therapy After Surgery Using Hook Plate

Hook plate fixation is a noninvasive to the inside of the AC joint and can hold the AC joint by using the hook portion under the acromion as leverage. As it also allows some degree of AC joint motion, range-of-motion exercise can be conducted in the early phase of postoperative rehabilitation [12]. However, even though the hook plate enables a good fixation of the AC joint, there is a chance of developing complications such as acromion fracture ("cut-out"), expansion of the hook hole [12, 13], erosion in the bottom side of the acromion [14], and subacromial bursitis from impingement if there is concentrated stress on the hook portion of the acromion. Therefore, it is necessary to consider the stress on the hook portion during the range-of-motion exercises in postoperative rehabilitation. In addition, in case of severe damage or detachment of the upper trapezius and anterior deltoid on the clavicle, the repair of these muscles is necessary in the type III–VI. These two muscles are important because the upper trapezius and anterior deltoid pull the clavicle up and down, respectively, and thereby stabilize the AC joint.

17.6.2 Five Tips and Pitfalls in Postoperative Physical Therapy

17.6.2.1 Stress on the Hook Portion

Because the hook portion is placed underneath the acromion, subacromial bursitis may occur because of subacromial impingement. Improvement of range of shoulder motion should carefully proceed with caution to the subacromial impingement sign. There are also possibilities for erosion and cut-out of the hook portion to occur. Ludewig et al. [15] have reported that the scapula posteriorly tilts by 19° and upwardly rotates by 11° relative to the clavicle during shoulder elevation. Immoderate shoulder elevation exercise at early phase of postoperative treatment (postoperative 1–2 weeks) may cause concentrated stress on the hook portion underneath the acromion. It is important to set a limit of the range of elevation to proceed with therapeutic exercise as planned. It is also necessary to pay attention to trick motion of the scapula associated with contracture of the glenohumeral joint because it may produce a load on the hook portion.

17.6.2.2 Setting the Limit of Shoulder Elevation Angle

Inman [16] has reported the rotation of the clavicle on the long axis increase from 90° elevation. Although fixation with the hook plate has excellent stability, the protection of the surgical site is more important than obtaining a larger range of shoulder elevation at the early phase after the surgery. Setting the limit of range of shoulder elevation at 90° is an important first step to progress with postoperative rehabilitation successfully.

17.6.2.3 Recovery of Upper Trapezius and Anterior Deltoid

During the early postoperative stage, before scar tissue forms in the muscle repair process, the repair of the upper trapezius and anterior deltoid should not experience interference. Active or resistive shoulder elevation that induces contraction of both muscles and shoulder extension (hand behind the back) which stretches both muscles should be avoided.

At a month after the surgery, increasing the range of shoulder motion exercise and muscle-strengthening exercise will carefully start with observing the responses of the muscles (e.g., stretching sensation and pain) to active flexion and passive extension.

17.6.2.4 Home Exercise and Activity of Daily Living (ADL) Guidance

Therapists should explain the purpose of the surgery, the advantages and cautions of the surgery method, postoperative course, how to proceed with exercises, and guidance in ADL, and they need to place emphasis on communication to obtain cooperation from the patient. No matter how carefully therapists conduct postoperative physical therapy, it will hinder the recovery of the surgical site and impaired shoulder function if patients fail to comply with guidance in home exercise and ADL.

17.6.2.5 Timing of the Hook Plate Removal

The hook plate is used to hold the AC joint in reduced position and to allow shoulder exercises for postoperative physical therapy without hindering the recovery of the continuity of the damaged ligament. The hook plate needs to be placed for 3 months after the surgery at a minimum [17, 18], as more than 3 months are necessary for healing of the ligaments [19]. After hook plate removal, patients will be permitted to move their shoulder in the full range of motion, and then the treatment will be completed.

References

1. Tabata S, Kida H, Takahara M et al (1986) Follow-up study of non-operative complete tear of the rotator cuff. Shoulder Joint 10:191–194 (in Japanese)
2. Chiba S (2010) Therapeutic exercise of tendon rupture. In: Yoshio M (ed) Standard physical therapy: detailed discussion in therapeutic exercise, 3rd edn. Igaku-Shoin, Tokyo, pp 38–46 (in Japanese)
3. Miyasita K (2013) Therapeutic exercise for shoulder impingement syndrome from perspective of lower extremity and trunk. J Clin Sports Med 30:473–478 (in Japanese)

4. Yanai T (2011) Three-dimensional lashing movement of pelvis, thorax, and scapula during pitching motion. J Health Phys Educ Recreat 61:484–490 (in Japanese)
5. Yamaguchi M, Tsutsui H (2009) The movement of the shoulder girdle on the basis of the humerus position. Shoulder Joint 33:805–808 (in Japanese)
6. Neer CS II (1970) Displaced proximal humeral fractures. Part 1: Classification and evaluation. J Bone Joint Surg Am 52:1077–1089
7. Adler S, Beckers D, Buck M (2000) PNF techniques. In: Adler S (ed) PNF in practice, 2nd edn. Springer, Berlin, pp 19–35
8. Kaltenborn FM (1999) The Kaltenborn method of joint examinations and treatment. In: Vollowitz E (ed) Manual mobilization of the joint, vol 1. Olaf Norlis Bokhandel, Oslo, pp 20–30
9. Rockwood CA Jr, Williams GR, Young DC (2004) Disorders of the acromioclavicular joint. In: Rockwood CA Jr (ed) The shoulder, vol 1, 3rd edn. Saunders, Philadelphia, pp 521–595
10. Kienast B, Thietje R, Queitsch C et al (2011) Mid-term results after operative treatment of Rockwood grade III–V acromioclavicular joint dislocations with an AC-hook-plate. Eur J Med Res 16:52–56
11. Koukakis A, Manouras A, Apostolou CD et al (2008) Results using the AO hook plate for dislocations of the acromioclavicular joint. Expert Rev Med Devices 5:567–572. doi:10.1586/17434440.5.5.567
12. Habernek H, Weinstabl R, Schmid L et al (1993) A crook plate for treatment of acromioclavicular joint separation: indication, technique, and results after one year. J Trauma 35:893–901
13. Muramatsu K, Shigetomi M, Matsunaga T et al (2007) Use of the AO hook-plate for treatment of unstable fractures of the distal clavicle. Arch Orthop Trauma Surg 127:191–194
14. Meda PV, Machani B, Sinopidis C et al (2006) Clavicular hook plate for lateral end fractures: a prospective study. Injury 37:277–283
15. Ludewig PM, Phadke V, Braman JP et al (2009) Motion of the shoulder complex during multiplanar humeral elevation. J Bone Joint Surg Am 91:378–389. doi:10.2106/JBJS.G.01483
16. Inman VT, Saunders JB, Abbott LC (1944) Observations on the function of the shoulder joint. J Bone Joint Surg 26:1–30
17. Gstettner C, Tauber M, Hitzl W et al (2008) Rockwood type III acromioclavicular dislocation: surgical versus conservative treatment. J Shoulder Elbow Surg 17:220–225. doi:10.1016/j.jse.2007.07.017
18. Fraser-Moodie JA, Shortt NL, Robinson CM (2008) Injuries to the acromioclavicular joint. J Bone Joint Surg (Br) 90:697–707. doi:10.1302/0301-620X.90B6.20704
19. Nadarajah R, Mahaluxmivala J, Amin A et al (2005) Clavicular hook-plate: complications of retaining the implant. Injury 36:681–683

Printed by Printforce, the Netherlands